DEVELOPMENTAL TOXICOLOGY: RISK ASSESSMENT AND THE FUTURE

Ronald D. Hood, Ph.D, Editor

Sponsored by

Reproductive and Developmental Toxicology Branch
Human Health Assessment Group
Office of Health and Environmental Assessment
Office of Research and Development
U.S. Environmental Protection Agency
Washington, D.C.

Carole A. Kimmel, Ph.D., Project Manager

Funding for this book was provided by the U.S. Environmental Protection Agency. Although the manuscript has been reviewed in accordance with Agency policy and approved for publication, it does not necessarily reflect the views and policies of the Agency, and no official endorsement should be inferred. The opinions expressed within respective chapters reflect the views of the authors, and mention of trade names or commercial products does not constitute endorsement by the Agency or recommendation for use.

Library of Congress Catalog Card Number: 90-12232
ISBN 0-442-00422-2

Printed in the United States of America

Van Nostrand Reinhold
115 Fifth Avenue
New York, New York 10003

Van Nostrand Reinhold International Company Limited
11 New Fetter Lane
London EC4P 4EE, England

Van Nostrand Reinhold
480 La Trobe Street
Melbourne, Victoria 3000, Australia

Nelson Canada
1120 Birchmount Road
Scarborough, Ontario M1K 5G4, Canada

16 15 14 13 12 11 10 9 8 7 6 5 4 3 2 1

Library of Congress Cataloging-in-Publication Data

Developmental toxicology: Risk assessment and the future.
Ronald D. Hood, editor; sponsored by [the] Reproductive and Developmental Toxicology Branch, Human Health Assessment Group, Office of Health and Environmental Assessment, Office of Research and Development, U.S. Environmental Protection Agency, Washington, D.C.
    p. cm.
    "December 1989."
    Includes bibliographical references.
    ISBN-0-442-00422-2
    1. Developmental toxicology. 2. Health risk assessment. I. Hood, Ronald D. II. United States. Environmental Protection Agency. Office of Health and Environmental Assessment. Human Health Assessment Group. Reproductive and Developmental Toxicology Branch.
    [DNLM: 1. Abnormalities. 2. Data Interpretation, Statistical. 3. Prenatal Exposure Delayed Effects. 4. Risk Factors. 5. Toxicology. QS 675 R432]
RA1224.2.R48 1990
618.3'2--dc20
DNLM/DLC
for Library of Congress

CONTENTS

PREFACE

The Reproductive and Developmental Toxicology Branch of the Human Health Assessment Group within the EPA's Office of Health and Environmental Assessment (OHEA) was responsible for the preparation of this book as an outgrowth of their work on the Guidelines for the Health Assessment of Suspect Developmental Toxicants (U.S. EPA, 1986b). In that document, several general areas of research were identified that were needed to fill data gaps or to reduce uncertainties associated with estimating risks for human developmental effects due to exposure to hazardous substances.

This book focuses on the research needs for risk assessment indicated in the Guidelines, expanding with an update and review of each area. Each chapter focuses on the specific issues within a particular area that hold promise in addressing uncertainties for risk assessment and regulatory decision-making. A comprehensive listing of relevant literature is included.

We gratefully acknowledge the helpful suggestions and guidance of the following individuals who generously gave of their time to review parts or entire drafts of this manuscript: Nigel A. Brown, Ph.D., Gary Burin, Elaine Z. Francis, Ph.D., Bryan D. Hardin, Ph.D., Andrew G. Hendrickx, Ph.D., E. Marshall Johnson, Ph.D., Robert J. Kavlock, Ph.D., Gary L. Kimmel, Ph.D., Heinz Nau, Ph.D, Godfrey P. Oakley, Jr., M.D., James L. Schardein, Bernard A. Schwetz, D.V.M., Ph.D., William J. Scott, Jr., D.V.M., Ph.D., Richard G. Skalko, Ph.D., M. Kate Smith, and John F. Young, Ph.D.

We would like to acknowledge the tremendous editorial support provided by Judy Theisen, without whom this effort would not have been completed. We would also like to thank William D. Theriault, Ph.D., Linda C. Bailey, and Theresa M. Konoza for their efforts in producing this book.

Ronald D. Hood

Carole A. Kimmel

CONTRIBUTORS

Dr. Carole Kimmel of the Reproductive and Developmental Toxicology Branch of the Human Health Assessment Group within EPA's Office of Health and Environmental Assessment provided overall direction and coordination of this effort. Dr. Ronald Hood acted as editor and, in addition to authoring several chapters, identified and recruited expert scientists to prepare other chapters.

Vernon M. Chinchilli, Ph.D., Associate Professor of Biostatistics, Department of Biostatistics, Medical College of Virginia, Virginia Commonwealth University, Richmond, VA

Elaine M. Faustman, Ph.D., Associate Professor, Department of Environmental Health, University of Washington, Seattle, WA

Maureen C. Hatch, Ph.D., Assistant Professor of Public Health, Division of Epidemiology, Columbia University, New York, NY

Ronald D. Hood, Ph.D., Professor, Department of Biology, The University of Alabama, Tuscaloosa, AL, and Principal Associate, R. D. Hood and Associates, Consulting Toxicologists

Donald E. Hutchings, Ph.D., Research Scientist, New York State Psychiatric Institute, New York, NY

Donald R. Mattison, M.D., Associate Professor of Obstetrics, Gynecology and Pharmacology, Department of Obstetrics and Gynecology, University of Arkansas for Medical Sciences, Little Rock, AR

Roman Osman, Ph.D., Associate Professor of Physiology and Pharmacology, Department of Physiology and Biophysics, Mt. Sinai School of Medicine, New York, NY

Paul Ribeiro, Ph.D., Postdoctoral Fellow, Department of Pathology, University of Washington, Seattle, WA

Todd W. Thorslund, Sc.D., Vice President, Clement Associates, Incorporated, Fairfax, VA

Charles V. Vorhees, Ph.D., Associate Professor, Institute for Developmental Research, Children's Hospital Research Foundation, Cincinnati, OH

1.
EXECUTIVE SUMMARY

Investigations that should aid the regulator in making enlightened decisions are summarized here and covered in more detail in Chapter 3. The sections in this summary correspond to those covered in that chapter. It is hoped that these suggestions will aid in prioritization of future research. The projects recommended were selected to provide specific information for use in improving the provision and assessment of data essential for regulation of potential developmental toxicants. It is realized that opinions may differ with regard to the order of priority of topics and of specific projects within topic areas. Due to the inherent subjectivity of prioritization, it is necessarily subject to future modification. Nevertheless, it is hoped that this document will aid in focusing attention on specific areas of inquiry and that it will facilitate planning of a coherent program of research.

MECHANISMS OF DEVELOPMENTAL TOXICITY

Because it is difficult to single out specific areas for targeted support, promising studies proposed by knowledgeable investigators should be funded. As areas of research begin to appear especially promising, they can be emphasized, based on significant findings.

CHEMICAL INTERACTIONS

Superior protocols should be developed to assess interactive effects, followed by testing of combinations of agents in order to investigate mechanisms and interactions with commonly encountered agents. The outcome of exposure to low doses of multiple chemicals might also be explored.

PREIMPLANTATION EFFECTS

The data on preimplantation effects appear to indicate a need for some increased funding for mechanistic studies.

MATERNAL vs. DEVELOPMENTAL TOXICITY

Needs in this area include determining if there are specific developmental toxicity end points for maternally mediated effects and assessing which are the most useful end points for maternal toxicity. Attempts should be made to determine which toxicity-induced changes in the internal environment of the dam can cause developmental toxicity, and their relationship to the type of stress. The relationship between chemically induced behavioral teratogenesis and maternal toxicity and the potential for maternally mediated developmental toxicity in humans are also of interest.

PATERNALLY MEDIATED EFFECTS

Information should be obtained on the generality of developmental toxicity due to paternal chemical exposure, followed by a focus on mechanisms.

EVALUATION OF BEHAVIORAL EFFECTS

The most pressing issue in behavioral teratology is validation, including consideration of criterion validity (ability to reflect changes in a given criterion), predictive validity (ability to extrapolate to another setting), construct validity (ability to assess a specific function), and susceptibility (ability of a test to respond to the damage to the underlying central nervous system [CNS] that it is designed to reflect). Research is also needed on dose-response relationships, particularly to determine if responses are monotonic or nonmonotonic, and on end point relationships (e.g., relationships between maternal toxicity, embryolethality, malformation, ponderal teratogenicity, and behavioral dysfunction). Further considerations should include permanence of effect, developmental stage dependent relationships, use of additional species for evaluation of behavioral teratogenesis, and decision criteria for various behaviors that can be used prospectively for sorting performance.

ISSUES OF EXTRAPOLATION IN BEHAVIORAL TERATOLOGY

Known behavioral teratogens should be tested in laboratory rats using state-of-the-art protocols, and the results systematically compared with findings on the same compounds in man.

NONBEHAVIORAL FUNCTIONAL EFFECTS

This includes refinement, standardization, and validation of tests to assess neonatal renal, cardiac, and lung function, evaluation of the permanence of effects and whether they compromise function and survival, and definition of the "critical periods" of development for production of functional effects. Additional aspects of function, such as immune system, hepatic, and nonreproductive endocrine functions, gut motility, and hematological parameters, could also be assessed.

TRANSPLACENTAL AND PERINATAL CARCINOGENESIS

The critical cellular determinants for transplacental carcinogenesis must be established to allow quantitative risk extrapolation. Investigations of the practicality of short-term in vitro assays for transplacental and perinatal carcinogens are needed, as are investigations of the likely etiological factors involved in childhood cancer and of the potential for increased tumor incidence in their offspring following preconception exposure of one or both parents to carcinogens. It would also be useful to determine the likelihood that human cancers of middle or old age may originate from transplacental or neonatal exposure to carcinogens and to assess the potential of a Solt-Farber (1976) type protocol as a short-term in vivo assay for transplacental carcinogenicity.

PHARMACOKINETIC CONSIDERATIONS IN DEVELOPMENTAL TOXICITY

Pharmacokinetic evaluations are required to define differences in species susceptibility to developmental toxicants, and these pharmacokinetic considerations must be extended to the cellular and molecular level and incorporated into biochemical epidemiology studies. Molecular dosimetry studies may provide the missing link in these cross-comparison studies.

FETAL PHARMACOKINETIC AND PHYSIOLOGICAL MODELS

A range of in vitro, in vivo, and mathematical models should be explored to increase our understanding of normal and pathological development. Qualitative and quantitative models of maternal, fetal, and placental physiological and pharmacokinetic changes across species during pregnancy should be developed, using available data and collecting additional data on maternal, placental, and fetal physiological parameters.

TESTS FOR DEVELOPMENTAL TOXICITY

The issues to be examined include sensitivity of current developmental toxicity tests, the utility of a priori calculation of numbers of test animals per dosage group, and whether either moderately or highly inbred mouse strains or strain crosses are superior animal models. Individual end points and indices made up of their combinations should be evaluated to determine whether some end points could be omitted or grouped. Biochemical end points could also be assessed, especially for maternal toxicity. Data regarding whether chronically dosed pregnant test animals should be given a constant amount per animal or a constant dosage, adjusted for changes in body weight, are needed as well. The most promising currently suggested prescreens should be put through a well-devised validation procedure, and the Chernoff-Kavlock assay should be refined and validated in terms of longer postnatal assessment.

MALFORMATIONS vs. VARIATIONS AND "MINOR DEFECTS"

A categorization of anomalies should be published, with each malformation, minor defect, variation, and manifestation of delayed development adequately described, and even illustrated when necessary.

ANIMAL MODELS OF EFFECTS OF PRENATAL INSULT

The available literature could be examined and appropriate new data developed for comparison of developmental toxicity outcomes in test animals and man on the basis of pharmacokinetic end points to determine if more accurate risk extrapolation would result. The true significance of placental type in choice of animal models or interpretation of experimental outcomes should be further investigated.

USE OF HUMAN DATA

Health workers and patients should be encouraged to report suspected associations, "new" syndromes, and "unexpected" concentrations to a central source, where they could be cross-indexed, merged with existing toxicologic data, and reviewed for testable hypotheses. Techniques such as meta-analysis could be used to identify likely toxins in the existing literature, and these compounds should be studied to confirm hazard in humans, develop dose-response data, and investigate processes. Investigations should include the natural history of end points, use of special diagnostic studies to develop data on the mode of action in humans, and use of biological markers of exposure and subclinical effect for human tests of developmental toxicity. Mechanisms are needed for promoting regular exchange of research questions and findings and collaboration between epidemiologists, clinicians, and toxicologists.

Further studies are needed of the relationship of head circumference to CNS damage. Research opportunities presented by changes in medical practice, such as increased record keeping in obstetric routines, should be exploited. Clinical or epidemiological research on developmental toxicity should give consideration to uses of (1) populations potentially available through the Agency for Toxic Substances and Disease Registry, (2) exposed cohorts enrolled in ongoing medical surveillance programs, (3) infertility patients, and (4) existing national health surveys.

STRUCTURE-ACTIVITY RELATIONSHIPS

Large data sets derived from compounds with diverse structures that share the same biological end point should be used to classify compounds into major classes—active and inactive—and more detailed subclassifications. Sets of descriptors for the data set should be defined or generated and processed, and methods for generation of descriptors based on structure should be improved, emphasizing chemical reactivity.

The definition of a proper steric parameter is needed for structurally related compounds with the classical Hansch quantitative structure-activity relationship (QSAR). Also, the relationship between the parameters (experimentally or computationally derived) and molecular reactivity for both the ADAPT and Hansch methods should be more clearly defined, and attempts to refine the molecular superposition method should continue.

Relationships between the QSAR parameter and specific molecular reactivities should be defined using molecular superposition techniques combined with depiction of properties related to the parameters that correlate structure and activity.

Molecular parameters that reflect reactivities related to causal relationships should be defined by statistically grouping compounds according to elements of similarity correlated with activity, formulating discriminant properties as parameters, and calculating such parameters for other molecules from the data sets obtained above. Attempts should be made to correlate biological activity with these parameters.

STATISTICAL ANALYSIS OF DEVELOPMENTAL TOXICITY DATA

An exhaustive simulation should be employed to clarify the capabilities and limitations of the beta-binomial probability model, and other aspects of that model's development should be addressed, including goodness-of-fit tests and diagnostic criteria. The beta-binomial model should also be extended for situations encountered in developmental toxicity studies, particularly with regard to litter size distributions and inclusion of random litter sizes in analyzing continuous variables. Statistical methods that adjust for random litter sizes should be developed for performing rank tests and analyses of variance on transformed data. An attempt should also be made to develop statistical models that incorporate a threshold effect for analysis and risk assessment with developmental toxicity data. Finally, a general consensus should be obtained among statisticians as to an appropriate statistical model or class of models for development of statistical decision rules for handling dichotomous end points.

MATHEMATICAL MODELING OF TERATOGENIC EFFECTS

New models for developmental toxicity data should incorporate both the biology of development and the mechanisms of action for toxic agents. Feasibility studies, in which delivered doses are related using pharmacokinetic models, should be conducted to look at in vivo and in vitro test systems. Other models examining series of end points suggesting continuous progression of fetal damage should be explored, and teratogenesis at early or late stages should be investigated relative to dose-response curves and the implications on mechanisms of action. New mathematical models might be verified by sorting and evaluating the available information from human and animal dose-response studies. Also, even epidemiological studies with ill-defined exposures, limited number of end points, and small sample sizes could be used to provide information in the form of rate estimates for a given exposure, basing these upper-bound estimates on conservative exposure values and statistical confidence limits on elevated rates. It might be feasible to independently verify the general shape of dose-response curves by using simple test subjects, such as *Hydra attentuata* and artificial "embryos" derived from them, and by using multiple exposure scenarios. Further, if extrapolation to humans is problematic because inbreeding of laboratory animals may cause too homogeneous a response, equal sensitivity between humans and laboratory animals could be assumed with imposition of human variability assumptions on the animal model.

APPLICATION OF EXPERIMENTAL DATA IN RISK ASSESSMENT

No obvious research projects were apparent from the reviewed material.

2.
INTRODUCTION

Research efforts in developmental toxicology have significantly increased during the last 10 years, as more emphasis has been directed toward protecting the overall health of workers and the general population. Even though much research has been done and a large information base compiled, there are still numerous barriers to our ability to evaluate and predict developmental toxicology end points. Past research has shown that a proper evaluation of the developmental toxicity potential of an agent requires an interdisciplinary approach. This approach should be an assessment of information from several related scientific fields, such as developmental toxicology, reproductive toxicology, genetic toxicology, and pharmacokinetics. The complex nature of this area of toxicology mandates a significantly expanded funding and research effort if significant progress is to be made.

Even though past research experience has increased our knowledge of the various types of agents that may cause adverse effects in developing mammals, it has also opened many new and diverse areas that require attention. Since there has been no recent in-depth review of the current state of developmental toxicology for the purpose of identifying research needs (with one partial exception: Dixon et al., 1986), a concerted effort is urgently needed to address the gaps in our knowledge base. It is hoped that the current undertaking will encourage the proper focus of research funds and promote an increase in the level of research activities needed to close the information gaps that this project has exposed. These new data should enhance current efforts to make valid risk assessments in developmental toxicology.

To ensure that this document would be comprehensive in its coverage of areas of direct importance, additional experts were secured as authors to provide sections of the document in the following areas:

- pharmacokinetics
- behavior
- epidemiology
- structure-activity relationships
- quantitative risk assessment
- statistical analysis

Once prepared, the original draft of the document was reviewed by additional experts, to ensure its timeliness and accuracy, and was appropriately revised by the authors.

The Executive Summary (Chapter 1) and Summary of Research Needs (Chapter 3) are arranged in subsections in the same order as the following detailed supporting review chapters. The order in which they are presented was originally based on two considerations: the presumed relative significance of the desired information, and the apparent likelihood that useful results could be obtained under reasonable time and funding constraints. Because of the diversity of opinion regarding any conceivable order of priority, as pointed out by numerous reviewers of previous drafts, the order in which topics are presented has been changed to a logical sequence and should no longer be considered a prioritization. Suggested specific research projects or areas of concentration are discussed within each subsection and are categorized as of high, medium, or low priority on a document wide basis.

Any attempt at prioritization of areas or specific projects for research funding is relatively subjective and likely to be subject to future modifications. Nevertheless, this document will serve as a source of information needed to allow funding to be allocated on a logical basis and with greater efficiency. It received its impetus from questions raised in the Guidelines for the Health Assessment of Suspect Developmental Toxicants (U.S. EPA, 1986b) and is a logical follow-up to that document. In particular, it must be kept in mind that this document was prepared to assist in the identification of research gaps to be addressed because of their perceived relevance to risk assessment in developmental toxicity. Thus, it is not a review of overall basic research needs in the field and should not be used or evaluated as such. Further, since no review can be entirely comprehensive and all-inclusive, it is recognized that specific research projects and even entire areas of need have likely been omitted from the current document.

3.

SUMMARY OF RESEARCH NEEDS

A number of unresolved issues in developmental toxicology have been raised by the authors in this book. Those that appear to have the greatest potential for providing information that would allow the regulator to make enlightened decisions are included in this chapter. Within each topic area, levels of priority for research are assigned, based on their importance and potential for addressing uncertainties in risk assessment. Although it is realized that neither this nor any other list could include every needed study, it is hoped that these suggestions will provide useful information to aid in prioritization of future research in the area of developmental toxicology. Supporting documentation is included in the following chapters, which appear in the same order as the sections in this chapter. Also, please note that explanatory supporting material is particularly extensive in the section on validity of behavioral effects evaluation. This area has been widely discussed in terms of behavioral effects, but may be unfamiliar to readers concerned with other areas.

MECHANISMS OF DEVELOPMENTAL TOXICITY

It is widely recognized that the lack of knowledge regarding mechanisms is a major impediment to our ability to identify and control developmental toxicants (Skalko, 1981; Wolkowski-Tyl, 1981; Johnson, 1983a; Environmental Health Criteria 30, 1984). Nevertheless, relatively few recommendations have been put forth in the literature regarding specific approaches to the problem.

Certain areas involving direct effects on the conceptus, such as interaction of teratogens with specific receptors in target tissues of the embryo, have been particularly fruitful topics for research and appear to deserve continued support. We know relatively little about the role of the placenta in this regard, and studies of the role of placental structure and function, including effects of chemicals on placental endocrine function (Goodman et al., 1982), are also likely candidates for pursuit. Maternally mediated effects are also of interest and are addressed in the section on maternal vs. developmental toxicity.

Because it is difficult to single out specific areas for targeted research support, it is essential that as many as possible of the promising studies proposed by knowledgeable investigators be funded. As areas of research begin to appear especially promising, they can be emphasized, but this emphasis must be based on significant findings rather than a priori assumptions. *High priority.*

CHEMICAL INTERACTIONS

This area appears to be critical in terms of needed information. Although there is a considerable amount of evidence that interactions are common, little has been established in terms of the mechanisms for such interactions. It is important that we achieve a better understanding of why and how interactions occur, because pregnant women and immature individuals are often concurrently exposed to a number of pharmacologically active agents.

1. If superior protocols for assaying for interactive effects could be developed and validated, their use could save time and expense in future testing. Thus, protocol design and assessment is an important need. *High priority.*

2. Combinations of agents must be tested from the point of view of elucidating mechanisms of interactive effects. Thus, tests will require planning in terms of both the agents studied and the temporal relationships of exposure. The possibility of interactions of a variety of compounds with common licit (and illicit) drugs, pollutants, pesticides, and the like should be further explored. This should be done to determine if, for example, maternal alcohol consumption or cigarette smoking might result in increased (or decreased) hazard from other known or potential developmental toxicants. If adverse effects were enhanced, this could affect the relative margin of safety for the offspring. *Medium priority.*

3. Further, some effort might be expended in attempts to better understand the likely outcome of concurrent exposure to low doses of multiple chemicals, as this more closely approximates a realistic situation. Until we know more about the mechanisms involved in determining the outcome of chemical interactions, however, the expense and complexity of such systems probably warrant only exploratory studies intended to assess the likely relative importance of such exposures. *Low priority.*

PREIMPLANTATION EFFECTS

According to the currently available data, in many cases preimplantation exposure to toxic insult results in the predicted "all-or-none" phenomenon of early death or repair and recovery. In some cases, however, death occurs significantly later in development, and increases in malformed fetuses have been seen in several studies.

Recent data on preimplantation effects (e.g., Generoso et al., 1987, 1988b; Katoh et al., 1988; Pillans et al., 1988) are of some concern and indicate a need for research. Studies should be aimed at determining whether the primary mechanism resulting in delayed manifestation of developmental toxicity is the indication of mutations, as has been suggested (e.g., Iannaccone et al., 1987), or if other effects may be involved. If potent mutagens are the most likely agents capable of causing irreparable damage to the preimplantation conceptus, this would aid in a priori identification of early acting developmental toxicants. Conversely, if nongenotoxic chemicals are found to have similar effects, this would be of considerable concern, as current testing regimens might miss agents that cause delayed effects. It seems likely, however, that most such agents would also have noticeable effects following exposure of postimplantation embryos and would be detected by Segment II or III type tests. *Medium priority*.

MATERNAL vs. DEVELOPMENTAL TOXICITY

1. In order to deal with this issue, it is essential to determine if there are developmental toxicity end points that are at least relatively specific for maternally mediated effects. For example, Kavlock et al. (1985) and Beyer and Chernoff (1986) found an apparent association of fetal supernumerary ribs with maternal toxicity in mice, but not in rats. Khera (1984b, 1985), on the other hand, suggested that a number of different end points were primarily associated with maternal effects and that they varied somewhat by species. Thus, it is also important to explore the issue of possible species or strain specificity.

Such questions could be addressed in various ways. The work of Kavlock et al. (1985) and Beyer and Chernoff (1986), which looks at fetal outcome following induction of maternal toxicity, could be continued with additional compounds in various mouse and rat strains and in the rabbit. Developmental toxicity data from such efforts may be compared with data obtained from tests that largely eliminate the effects of maternal toxicity, such as the use of intra-amniotic test chemical administration (Dostal and Jelinek, 1979).

Experimental studies might be supplemented with a review of reports submitted in support of pesticide registration by contract laboratories (U.S. EPA, 1986a). Such reports contain relevant systematically collected data on both developmental and maternal toxicity and could give useful guidance regarding expected findings in safety evaluation studies. Such information should be superior to that obtainable from the open literature, especially in terms of maternal toxicity end points. The data would generally be much more uniform and complete and not biased toward positive effects on the conceptus. *High priority*.

2. It would be useful to know what toxicity-induced changes in the maternal physiology or biochemistry act upon the conceptus to bring about developmental toxicity. If a variety of toxic effects on the dam are translated into a relatively low number of developmentally toxic alterations, perhaps we should be testing for these changes in the mother's internal environment, rather than surrogate toxicity end points. We already have reason to suspect that increases in maternal glucocorticoid and/or catecholamine secretion could lead to secondary effects on the offspring. Additional changes in the internal milieu could be assayed for and attempts made to correlate them with effects on the conceptus. At the same time, attempts should be made to determine if different types of stress elicit different maternal responses (and perhaps different developmental effects as well) and whether dams or animal strains that were more sensitive to stress had more affected offspring. *High priority.*

3. It is important to know what the most sensitive, reliable end points are for maternal toxicity. Further information is needed, such as whether end points differ among species, and at what times during gestation, with what frequency, and in what detail they should be monitored.

Such information might be obtained by testing compounds covering a range of toxicity mechanisms. Starting with obviously toxic doses, a variety of end points could be monitored throughout the period of dosing. Then, using large numbers of dams and a series of lower doses, the end points identified at the high dose could be followed until they were no longer distinguishable from background "noise." It could then be determined which end points were the most sensitive and consistent and at what times and how frequently they would have to be measured to achieve the best balance between expense and test sensitivity. A similar protocol could be evaluated in the rat and rabbit and any other test species of interest. *High priority.*

4. Some maternally mediated effects have been said to result in behavioral effects on the offspring. This seems well established in the case of feminization of male rats due to failure of sufficient enzymatic production of testosterone at the critical period for sexual imprinting; we know less about other behavioral effects. It would be useful to know whether chemically induced behavioral teratogenesis is often secondary to maternal toxicity, and the types of possible mechanisms involved. *Medium priority.*

5. Knowledge of the potential for maternally mediated developmental toxicity in man would be useful to further our understanding of the relative significance of such effects. Screening for such effects would be difficult. Records of birth outcomes in times of stress (e.g., famine, war) might offer some insight, although stress would be confounded with other factors, such as lack of key nutrients. *Low priority.*

PATERNALLY MEDIATED EFFECTS

The occurrence of adverse developmental outcomes in the offspring of toxicant-exposed sires has been reported by a number of researchers. Its validity appears to be established, but our knowledge of this aspect of developmental toxicology is extremely limited at present.

1. Initially, we need more information on how general the phenomenon is. Thus, tests of various classes of toxicants could allow some perspective on how significant the hazard from paternally mediated effects may be, and what kinds of agents are likely to cause such effects. *High priority.*

2. Once more is known regarding the scope of the problem, research can focus on possible mechanisms. Although logically one would expect genotoxic agents to be the major candidates for causing male-mediated effects, apparently nongenotoxic agents (e.g., ethanol) are among the compounds implicated by previous research. A thorough understanding of the mechanistic basis of such effects should allow regulation of potentially hazardous chemicals on a more logical basis. Until much more is known about the types of agents that can or cannot cause paternal effects, however, defining mechanisms involved will be more difficult. *High priority.*

EVALUATION OF BEHAVIORAL EFFECTS

The occurrence of functional impairment in laboratory species and in man as a consequence of pre- or neonatal toxic insult is now well established, but this issue has been inadequately addressed in terms of safety evaluation. In part, this has occurred because the study of functional end points is a relatively recent development. Further, the time and expense associated with current testing requirements is great. Without a major impetus, addition of many further required tests is unlikely, as they are not seen as cost-effective. Nevertheless, further study of the issue is warranted. Refinement of possible functional tests will facilitate their use in cases where functional effects are suspected, and they would be available if any event comparable to the thalidomide disaster compelled their extensive use.

1. Validity

An important issue in behavioral teratology is validation. As discussed elsewhere (Vorhees, 1985a) there are at least three types of validity to be addressed, and perhaps four, depending on how one conceptualizes the area. The three types of validity studies needed are those dealing with criterion, predictive, and construct validity, and the fourth area is what might be termed experimental susceptibility.

a. Criterion Validity[1]

New research is needed using positive control agents. These studies should be conducted using standardized behavioral teratology protocols. Preferably, they should be done as an experimental series of positive control trials with standardized methods under rigorous protocols. This would allow the maximum acquisition of criterion validity data, as well as providing as a by-product a wealth of information on susceptibility and test sensitivity. Positive control agents worthy of consideration are trans-retinoic acid, methylmercury, phenytoin, methimazole, ethanol, trimethadione, x-irradiation, 5-azacytidine, 2-ethoxyethanol, methylazoxy-methanol, and lead. Chlordecone, polychlorinated biphenyls (PCBs), aspirin, valproic acid, and carbon monoxide might also be considered as "putative," but not proven, behavioral teratogens. Any good criterion validation experimental trial would include negative control test agents, such as d-amphetamine at doses below 2.0 mg/kg or acetazolamide at doses below 500 mg/kg. It is important that dose and duration be carefully limited in any negative control test agent studies to those previously found to be negative. Deviations from this approach or the testing of any hypothesized negative control agents could easily lead to problems which would destroy the intent of the experiment. *High priority.*

b. Predictive Validity[2]

New research is needed on the comparability of animal findings to outcomes discovered in humans with known behavioral teratogens. Such data are important for establishing that animal experimental methods are predictive of adverse human outcomes. Predictive validity is a cornerstone of all good preclinical toxicological methods, but in practice is seldom investigated systematically. The cross-species validity of most methods in toxicology is based on face validity or retrospective review of lists of test agents investigated in both animals and humans. The technique of awaiting the accumulation of large quantities of data cannot be entirely short-circuited. There is no substitute for "weight of evidence," but a proactive approach to this issue might save time. Enough human behavioral teratogens exist now to allow us to begin to compare the human and animal data.

---

1. Criterion validity refers to whether a test accurately reflects changes in an established criterion. In this context, the criterion would be established evidence of developmental neurotoxicity, using neuropathological evidence as the criterion. In other words, this is the use of positive control test agents.
2. Predictive validity refers to the characteristic in which a test result provides an accurate estimate of an effect in another setting. In this context, it is the extent to which test results in animals predict findings obtained in humans with the same agents.

The optimal approach appears to be the development of a new animal experimental data base using a standardized set of test methods, similar to the approach used to validate tests such as the Chernoff-Kavlock (1982) assay and various in vitro assays. A select group of test agents would be used. Agents to be considered are ethanol, methylmercury, 13-cis-retinoic acid and/or trans-retinoic acid (probably both should be used in a single experimental protocol for maximum advantage), PCBs, anticonvulsants, lead, and marijuana (or delta-9-tetrahydrocannabinol). Note that this set of agents is, with one exception, a subset of those listed above under criterion validity studies needed, in which known animal behavioral teratogens are used. This overlap suggests that some experimental efficiencies may be realized from careful planning of research aimed at meeting the needs of both criterion and predictive validity. *High priority.*

c. Construct Validity[3]

Discussions arising from the Collaborative Study (Kimmel et al., 1985) and elsewhere (e.g., Vorhees, 1985a) have pointed out the necessity of developing testing strategies that take into account our knowledge of central nervous system (CNS) function. As an obvious example, one could not conceive of an academic test of abilities for humans that did not assess expressive and receptive language capacities. It is similarly incomprehensible that a behavioral teratology test system could be developed blindly, without regard for categories of behavior (functional domains) and their CNS substrates. Some have questioned the value of such considerations in methods development research (Geyer and Reiter, 1985), but it is difficult to proceed rationally without consideration of constructs, whether implicitly or explicitly defined.

The central research question is how to approach construct validity experimentally. A common method is the development of an extensive test system involving multiple dependent measures and analysis of the findings obtained by factor analysis. Factor analysis yields groups or factors that are statistically, and therefore presumably biologically, related. These factors may be viewed as one approach to defining CNS functional domains.

Another approach would be to use accumulated knowledge about CNS functional domains. Thus, in reviewing the psychological and neuroscience literature, one finds concepts such as activity, reactivity, learning, memory, reproductive behavior, parental behavior, social behavior, sensory acuity, motoric competence, etc., as areas previously identified as functional domains. The task then becomes one of trying to identify tests that assess

---

3. Construct validity refers to test development in which selected constructs or hypothesized functions are intended to be measured.

each of these domains. Comparisons of tasks are then needed to address the question of which tests are optimal and/or sufficient to provide coverage of each domain. This is the issue raised in question "e," as originally put forth by the Collaborative Study planners.

Research to address this is complex, but crucial. At present, the functional domains identified as requiring coverage in behavioral teratology screening are based primarily on the end points that researchers have most experience in measuring and on what can be measured well, rather than on theoretical considerations of what might be measured to reflect full functional integrity. Research in this area may benefit from a more theoretical approach.

A fresh analysis of this area should draw upon the best of what has been already developed, but might also delve into areas not touched previously. Once assembled, this new test battery must undergo evaluation with the positive controls identified above. This would be a more straightforward task than development of the older test batteries. The list of positive controls is more soundly based and is more extensive than it was 10-15 years ago, when the first of the present batteries began being developed. *Medium priority.*

d. Susceptibility

In the present context, susceptibility refers to the test's capacity to reflect damage to underlying CNS functions. It is well known that rats with hippocampal damage show impairments on tests of activity, passive avoidance, radial arm maze, Morris maze, spontaneous alternation, etc. It is reasonable to ask, "Which test best reflects hippocampal damage?" Surprisingly, there is virtually no answer to this question that can be extracted from the vast literature on hippocampal lesions, because no one working on hippocampal lesions has been interested in toxicity screening, but from the applied perspective of behavioral teratology screening, this is precisely the way the point needs to be addressed.

If a simple test (such as activity monitoring) could detect hippocampal damage as readily as complex tests (such as radial maze testing), then radial maze testing might not be appropriate for screening potential behavioral teratogens. Research is needed using both lesion studies and known behavioral teratogens to specifically compare methods that might respond to a particular type of CNS damage and determine the degree of damage each test requires to detect a significant difference. *Medium priority.*

2. Dose Response

There is need in behavioral teratology for more research on dose-response relationships. Some have suggested that monotonic dose-response relationships might not exist in this field (Nelson, 1981). Others have argued that this problem is more apparent than real, reflecting artifactual rather than biological circumstances (Vorhees and Butcher, 1982). It has also been suggested that nonmonotonic dose-response relationships may be more probable in this field than monotonic ones (Mactutus and Tilson, 1986), yet new evidence shows that linear dose-response patterns can be demonstrated in behavioral teratology (Vorhees, 1987).

Which is the more common state of affairs? Research on positive control agents must be dose-response studies, and should include three, not merely two, exposed groups plus a vehicle control group. These studies must also use multiple, standardized, behavioral tests conducted according to a strict protocol, in order to fully resolve these issues. *Medium priority.*

3. Relationships among End Points

The relationship between maternal toxicity, embryolethality, malformation, growth differences, and behavioral dysfunction continues to be a major unresolved issue. Some have suggested that behavior represents a potentially more sensitive index of embryotoxicity than does malformation. Others restrict this point of view only to those instances where the agent in question is able to produce both types of effects, implying that this relationship is not universal. It has been suggested by Brent (1983) that behavioral and physical defects are inextricably linked, and knowing one provides knowledge of the other. Still others maintain that any possible ordered relationship among these end points may occur, with no consistent pattern emerging. Using a series of both known behavioral and structural teratogens, dose-response studies that measure all four possible manifestations of developmental disorder should be compared, along with evidence of maternal toxicity. This research could resolve the proper use of behavioral analysis in developmental toxicology.

Finally, it has been proposed that the dose-response curve describing body weight effects usually lies in between those for malformations and behavioral dysfunction (Vorhees, 1986). Research on the relationship among these end points will go a long way toward verifying or refuting this recent hypothesis. *High priority.*

4. Permanence of Effect

Another issue of debate has been the extent to which early behavioral changes, primarily developmental delays, are indicative of permanent injury. Few investigations exist that have sought to determine the predictive value of early tests (preweaning) as markers for later (postweaning) dysfunction. This problem has long plagued researchers of human infant behavior, but there is no reason to believe that a definitive resolution cannot be obtained in animals.

Now that a list of positive control agents exists, studies of these agents can simultaneously track individual offspring through all tests; i.e., all offspring receive all tests with no split-litter or crossover designs, these having been obviated by the Collaborative Study findings. Using such data, correlations can be computed to determine the predictive value of each early test on later performance. This research may also provide crucial information toward another goal of applied research, namely that of streamlining behavioral teratology test batteries. *Medium priority.*

5. Stage-Dependent Relationships

The empirical principle of critical periods of susceptibility to injury is deeply rooted in teratology. There are sufficient data available showing that administering agents at different stages of ontogeny produces different behavioral dysfunctions. What is missing is more precise information about CNS vulnerability as it accompanies each phase of brain development.

Research is needed to systematically describe what the vulnerability is during different stages of pre- and postnatal development. Using a series of positive control agents and a set of standardized behavioral tests, this research should compare various stages of developmental exposure: early, middle, and late organogenesis, fetogenesis, and early postnatal development, using a constant dose of the test agent. Comparisons between prenatal and postnatal drug dosage may be difficult and should probably rely upon fetal and newborn blood levels as the criteria of comparison. Agents for which maternal and embryonic/fetal concentrations are identical can be found, thus simplifying sampling problems. Such research should ultimately determine the period or periods of maximum vulnerability of the CNS.

Stage sensitivity is not a trivial matter from either a practical or theoretical standpoint. Practically, evidence resolving this matter will provide needed guidance in determining where behavioral teratology testing fits best in the overall picture of developmental toxicity evaluation. Theoretically, evidence on this matter will help resolve a long-standing debate: Does vulnerability of the conceptus tend to decline with maturation, or are there organ-by-organ windows of vulnerability that open and close at different stages of ontogeny, each with its own unique timetable that does not fit into any overall rule? *Medium priority.*

6. Multispecies Research

Testing for teratogenesis in at least two species has been a fundamental tenet since the post-thalidomide revisions in government reproductive regulations. This approach grew logically out of thalidomide's well-known effect of producing species-specific teratogenesis. Is this same safeguard needed for behavioral teratogenesis? How can an informed decision concerning this point be reached until a series of positive control agents is tested in at least two species? In turn, how can the latter be done until an adequate second species test system for behavioral dysfunction is developed?

The first step that must be carried out in this area is the development of a behavioral test system using a second species. The system should then be evaluated for reliability, sensitivity, and all types of validity and compared to the best methods used in rats.

From the perspective of current regulatory practice, an ideal second species is the rabbit. Is the rabbit a good candidate for behavioral testing? It is clear that some kind of feasibility study should be conducted on rabbits prior to undertaking a full-fledged behavioral test battery development program. It could be that rabbits are suitable for structural, but not behavioral, teratogenesis testing because of species-specific behavioral response characteristics that make behavioral assessment unduly complex. However, new data suggest that the rabbit may be suitable for behavioral teratology research (Hudson and Distal, 1986). *Medium priority.*

7. Decision Criteria

For malformations, it is clear that there are affected and unaffected members of each litter. No such dichotomy has been revealed in analyses of body weight effects; instead, a continuous distribution of effects prevails. What is found in the case of behavioral dysfunction? Past research has only dealt with group means, and no attempt has been made to set "affected vs. unaffected" decision criteria for behavioral effects and then use these prospectively. (Such dichotomizations are used in research retrospectively, but in these cases, the dividing points are pragmatically chosen and apply only on a study-by-study basis.)

Using a small number of positive control agents and a few behavioral measures, research should be undertaken to determine the feasibility of setting "normal vs. abnormal" criteria for various behaviors that can be used prospectively for sorting performance. To be optimally effective, such research must carefully map the distribution of responses, initially on test-by-test and litter-by-litter bases, and search for highly reliable boundaries between subgroupings. Statistically based dichotomizations, empirically derived by examining an already collected data set, are not satisfactory if they merely divide groups at the 50th percentile or some other mathematically determined point; to be useful, the criteria of abnormality must be found to be distinctive. If the data within litters are found to be continuously distributed, then dichotomization approaches will be rejected for measures of behavioral dysfunction. *Low priority.*

ISSUES OF EXTRAPOLATION IN BEHAVIORAL TERATOLOGY

The combined animal and human data lead to the unequivocal conclusion that a variety of compounds can produce subtle to severe damage in the developing CNS, with functional effects ranging from minor impairments of attention, impulse control, and activity to mental retardation. As with birth defects, these deficits may be of genetic origin or arise spontaneously. Therefore, in the clinical situation, one must take care to distinguish the primary toxic effects of a compound from the secondary (environmental interactive) effects and, in addition, consider that a genetic disorder might also contribute to the long-term clinical outcome.

For example, there is no question that the opioids produce a neonatal abstinence syndrome characterized by CNS arousal. Clinical observations suggest that this altered state results in a less alert and less attentive newborn, with the result that the mother-infant interaction is compromised. This, in turn, may lead to secondary impairments of both cognitive and emotional development that emerge during the first year of life. (For a detailed discussion of possible effects on mother-infant interaction, see Hutchings and Fifer, 1986.) Additionally, if a genetically transmitted behavior disorder of minimal brain dysfunction is associated with or contributed to the mother's becoming a drug abuser in the first place, the clinical picture in her offspring may be even more complex. This could include a mixture of neonatal abstinence effects, the postnatal sequel as described above, and a genetically transmitted behavior disorder of attention deficit and impulse disorder, giving rise to school failure in middle childhood and emerging drug abuse in adolescence.

It is these sorts of complex multifactorial or multietiological effects that we must appreciate and that animal studies might help sort out. What must first occur is the development of more precise animal research techniques; several laboratories will have to study the same compounds from a basic research perspective in order to generate a reliable data base and consensus of effects. Most important, the animal findings, when possible, must be compared with the clinical observations. This mutual trade-off cross-validates both the human and animal findings in a way that is impossible when the same observations are made independently and in isolation. The result could be a powerful and meaningful set of comparative observations that test systems.

As a first step in carrying out such comparative studies, it is recommended that the following compounds, using state-of-the-art behavioral assessment techniques, be studied in the laboratory rat and the findings compared with existing and developing findings from human clinical studies:

Isotretinoin is a retinoic acid analogue of vitamin A that is teratogenic in laboratory animals and humans. During the past 12 years, many reports have appeared on the behavioral teratogenicity of vitamin A and retinoic acid (for review, see Hutchings, 1983). Moreover, a recent report in the New England Journal of Medicine (Lammer et al., 1984) indicates that behavioral/clinical studies of human infants prenatally exposed to isotretinoin are currently in progress. Thus, comparative data for this compound should be forthcoming.

Diphenylhydantoin is a widely prescribed anticonvulsant medication that has been demonstrated to be teratogenic in humans and produce behavioral effects in rats following prenatal exposure. Groups of exposed children are currently being studied for behavioral effects in San Diego and at Massachusetts General Hospital in Boston.

Delta-9-tetrahydrocannabinol (THC) is the major psychoactive ingredient in marijuana and does not appear to be teratogenic in humans or rats. It does, however, produce behavioral effects in both species. There are currently several behavioral studies of infants and children whose mothers smoked marijuana during pregnancy, and there is a large animal literature. These would afford comparison between laboratory animals and man. THC is particularly interesting in that it appears to target fetal neuroendocrine systems and not produce the sort of CNS damage associated with classical teratogens. *High priority.*

NONBEHAVIORAL FUNCTIONAL EFFECTS

1. An important need is the refinement, standardization, and validation of tests that have been developed to assess neonatal renal (Kavlock et al., 1986), cardiac (Grabowski and Payne, 1983a,b), and lung function (Daston, 1983; Newman and Johnson, 1983). Evaluation of the degree to which observed effects are permanent and truly compromise function and survival would be a valuable addition. It would also be useful to further define the "critical periods" of development, both pre- and postnatal, when the affected systems are especially vulnerable to toxic effects. Some of these effects are likely causes of the "spontaneous neonatal deaths" sometimes seen in postnatal evaluations. *Medium priority.*

2. Development of standard protocols for assessment of functional deficits of the immune system is another worthwhile goal. Problems arise in that the immune system is highly complex, and many functions can be tested.

Nevertheless, an effort must be made to sort out which functional aspects among the many possible candidates are the best indicators of biologically significant damage. *Medium priority*.

3. Assessment of additional aspects of function should be addressed. Hepatic and nonreproductive endocrine functions are examples of areas in which little if any work has been published. Gut motility and hematological parameters are further examples—they have been shown to be affected during in utero development (Christian, 1983), but little is known about the prevalence or significance of such effects, or whether they are transient or permanent. *Medium priority*.

TRANSPLACENTAL AND PERINATAL CARCINOGENESIS

There is increasing evidence that transplacental carcinogenesis may be a significant health hazard for humans, but relatively little is definitely known regarding a number of aspects of this area of interface between developmental toxicology and chemical carcinogenicity. Nevertheless, this is one area in which it appears that research may readily answer a significant proportion of the remaining important questions.

1. According to Anderson et al. (1985), we can currently make apparently reasonable inferences in terms of qualitative risk assessment for potential transplacental carcinogens, based on animal data. What we lack is the ability to quantify this risk. Before quantitative risk extrapolation can be done, it is important to establish which are the critical cellular determinants for this end point. Thus, more definitive experimental evidence must be obtained regarding such aspects as: (a) the numbers of target cells and the proportions of dividing cells in target tissues during critical periods for initiation of transplacental carcinogenesis; (b) the relative abilities of embryonic, fetal, and neonatal tissues to activate or inactivate carcinogens; and (c) the abilities of such tissues to repair carcinogen-induced damage to the DNA. Such information is needed for both the usual test species (e.g., rat, mouse) and for primates. At least in the case of fetal metabolism, some human data may be obtained by culture of fetal lymphocytes (from cord blood) and maternal lymphocytes (cf., Pelkonen et al., 1981). Follow-up by epidemiology could greatly increase the value of such information. *High priority*.

2. Another particularly useful endeavor would be the establishment of a practical, relatively rapid, valid assay for transplacental and perinatal carcinogens. A particularly promising test system that is a candidate for validation studies is the in vivo-in vitro mutagenesis assay of Dean (Dean and Senner, 1977; Dean and Hodson-Walker, 1979) as modified by Anderson et

al. (1985). This test system has the added potential benefit of being a possible rapid test system for adult carcinogens as well. *High priority.*

3. It would also be very helpful to know what etiological factors are involved in childhood cancer. The relative roles of transplacental, perinatal, and perhaps parental exposure to carcinogens, anticarcinogens, promotors, and the like must be better understood and placed in the proper perspective with other influential factors, such as developmental stage during time of exposure. This is obviously not an easy task, but it may be approached initially by epidemiological studies. Further testing of hypotheses thus generated could be done by means of animal experimentation or further, more narrowly targeted epidemiological approaches. The influence of developmental stage on carcinogenesis could be further explored by use of primate models. *Medium priority.*

4. Evidence has accumulated from animal studies to the effect that preconception exposure of one or both parents may result in increased tumor incidence in their offspring. If this is a real effect, it is likely due to germ-cell mutation, and it has serious implications for regulation of known and potential carcinogens. The potential for such effects should be evaluated systematically. This can be done by use of known carcinogens, including agents with different potencies, as suggested by Anderson et al. (1985). A worthwhile goal could be the establishment of a practical test system, if preconception effects are confirmed and found to occur frequently enough to be of likely biological significance. *Medium priority.*

5. It may be worthwhile to investigate the potential of a Solt-Farber (1976) type protocol as a short-term in vivo assay for transplacental carcinogenicity. This would be especially true if the in vivo-in vitro test proposed in 2 above proves unreliable. *Medium priority.*

6. Another question of significance asks whether human cancers of middle or old age may originate from transplacental or neonatal exposure to carcinogens. If at least some types of adult tumors in humans are commonly induced early in life, this too would have regulatory implications in terms of the relative risk from early vs. late carcinogen exposures. According to data from experimental animals, late-occurring tumors can be initiated by transplacental carcinogen exposure. There is also suggestive human data as well, but more clear-cut data are needed. Such data can only be obtained by epidemiological studies, but it is often difficult to differentiate accurately between effects of early and later exposures and in particular to pin down causation to specific events. The main approach to date has been studies of changing patterns of tumorigenesis in emigrants vs. the populations of their old and new homes. Even in such studies, it has been impossible to distinguish between effects due to early carcinogen exposure and possible modification by postemigration changes in life-style (Anderson et al., 1985).

Thus, although this is an important question, it is likely to be difficult to answer. *Low priority.*

PHARMACOKINETIC CONSIDERATIONS IN DEVELOPMENTAL TOXICITY

1. Molecular dosimetry studies identifying target organ doses (biologically effective doses) versus administered doses. Among the greatest needs in pharmacokinetic analysis of developmental toxicity are molecular dosimetry studies determining target doses or biologically effective doses rather than just citing administered dose information or even serum level concentrations. Available markers of human biologically effective doses that have been used in dosimetry studies of other toxicities include protein and DNA adducts, cytogenetic effects (e.g., sister chromatid exchanges, chromosomal aberrations, micronuclei), DNA damage and repair, and somatic cell mutations (Pedersen, 1987). In developmental toxicity, where nonmutagenic but reactive agents can be positive teratogens, critical focus on biologically effective doses could be conducted by identifying reactions with protein, such as hemoglobin adducts. Such biological markers could form the link for more exact species-species comparisons and allow for comparisons to humans as well as to laboratory animals. It is the lack of suitable comparisons across species that pharmacokinetic analysis first set out to conquer. Now these approaches need to be applied to extend such analyses to the cellular and molecular levels. *High priority.*

2. Definition of a series of pharmacokinetic parameters in a consistent manner for the most commonly used laboratory animals and, whenever possible, define comparable parameters in humans and primates. Although the proliferation of recent reports on pharmacokinetic studies in developmental toxicity attests to the extensive research efforts in this area, there are still major gaps in pharmacokinetic parameters and information on the most commonly used laboratory animals. It appears that many of these studies focus on one or two parameters in making cross-species comparisons, and the next study may choose two different parameters to investigate. This rather disconnected approach to defining the importance of pharmacokinetics in developmental toxicity will eventually lead to comprehensive information; however, there appears to be a need for well-organized and well-funded cross-laboratory projects. Perhaps the most successful attempts in this approach have been by Nau and his collaborators, whose efforts have shown that it is important that the same pharmacokinetic parameters (metabolism, repair, timing, pregnancy-related changes in physiology) be investigated across species (rat, mouse, rabbit, primate, and, whenever possible, human) for a specified series of compounds of interest (Nau, 1986a; Nau

and Scott, 1987). The 10 or so most likely candidate compounds, of course, would be those with the most dramatic species-related differences in teratogenicity (e.g., glucocorticoids, thalidomide, warfarin, valproic acid, etc.). *High priority.*

3. Characterization of the potential of ecogenetic differences in explaining human differences in response to developmental toxicants. In addition to characterizing the cross-species differences that are observed with developmental toxicants, the role of ecogenetic differences in explaining intraspecies differences in developmental toxicity should be defined. The important observations by Spielberg of potential differences in susceptible and nonsusceptible diphenylhydantoin-exposed offspring indicate the significance of looking for genetic polymorphs that would define susceptibility to developmental toxicity (Spielberg, 1987). Such polymorphisms, which have been extensively investigated for other toxicities, have rarely been examined in the context of defining susceptibility to birth defects, yet their identification would be of critical importance in defining human risk. Identification of these polymorphisms should be conducted through biochemical epidemiology studies, as well as through the development of animal models that reflect these differences. Many genetic differences in animal species exist that would be useful in answering such questions. *High priority.*

4. Improve correspondence of in vitro models to the in vivo situation by incorporation of pharmacokinetic considerations. The utilization of molecular dosimetry studies would also enhance our ability to make comparisons and predictions from in vitro studies. Examples of such initial efforts in this area are discussed in the in vitro section of Chapter 13. The incorporation of other pharmacokinetic considerations into in vitro studies is also of critical importance if any potential for extrapolation to in vivo results exists. These pharmacokinetic considerations would include characterization of metabolism (both activation and detoxification pathways), repair processes, and dose/timing exposure considerations. *Medium priority.*

FETAL PHARMACOKINETIC AND PHYSIOLOGICAL MODELS

This is an exciting era for research in reproductive and developmental toxicology. A range of in vitro, in vivo, and mathematical models are being explored that offer promise for understanding normal and pathological development. These models also offer toxicologists the opportunity to define common links between species for the formulation of defined risk assessments with well-characterized uncertainty.

The availability of risk assessments across species will, however, not come without research funding and research efforts in several areas. The areas that are ripe for initiation of funding fall into three categories: model development, data collection, and model validation (Table 3-1). It is apparent that it is necessary to develop qualitative and quantitative models of maternal, fetal, and placental physiological and pharmacokinetic changes across species during pregnancy. Because of past research interests, a considerable amount of data is available on maternal, placental, and fetal physiological parameters for both humans and sheep. These data should be collected into a computerized data base and made freely available to any interested investigator. Finally, it will be necessary to support the development of in vivo and in vitro models to validate the physiological-pharmacokinetic models and collect additional data for a parameter data base. *High priority.*

TESTS FOR DEVELOPMENTAL TOXICITY

The subject of testing is both complex and controversial. Because of this, various questions remain to be answered, but not all are purely technical. Some are perhaps matters of opinion and tend to be determined by logic or circumstance rather than purely established fact.

1. Adequacy of Current Standard Tests

a. More attention might profitably be paid to the issue of test sensitivity. It appears that the recommendations regarding adequate numbers of animals to use in current developmental toxicity tests are based more on cost considerations than on concern for test sensitivity (cf., Nelson and Holson, 1978). This is especially true of studies using rabbits. Admittedly, cost is an important consideration, but if a given test is so insensitive as to give meaningless results, what is gained by doing it at all?

One approach to this issue would be to test coded samples of known human teratogens in comparison with relatively less hazardous agents by the standard test protocols. Each compound should be tested in at least three laboratories. If a reassuringly high percentage of known developmentally toxic agents are revealed as hazardous, and if they are adequately distinguished from the compounds of lower toxicity, the test procedures should be considered relatively useful. If not, modifications would obviously be required. *High priority.*

b. A modification that should be investigated would be the a priori calculation of numbers of test animals needed per dosage group based on the variability observed in historical or preliminary data. The desired

TABLE 3-1. OPPORTUNITIES FOR PHARMACOKINETIC RESEARCH IN
REPRODUCTIVE AND DEVELOPMENTAL TOXICOLOGY

A. Model Development
  1. Development of models of maternal physiological and pharmacokinetic adaptation to pregnancy across species.
  2. Development of models of fetal physiology and pharmacokinetics across species and during gestation.
  3. Development of models of placental physiology and pharmacokinetics during pregnancy and across species.
B. Data base Development
  1. Develop data bases of physiological and pharmacokinetic parameters for the maternal compartment across species during pregnancy.
  2. Develop data bases of fetal physiological and pharmacokinetic parameters across species during pregnancy.
  3. Develop data bases of placental physiological and pharmacokinetic parameters across species during pregnancy.
C. Model Validation
  1. Validation of in vivo and in vitro models of maternal physiological and pharmacokinetic adaptation to pregnancy across species.
  2. Validation of in vivo and in vitro models of fetal physiology and pharmacokinetics across species and during gestation.
  3. Validation of in vivo and in vitro models of placental physiology and pharmacokinetics during pregnancy and across species.

---

level of precision for each parameter might be derived from the data obtained from the suggested blind tests of known human developmental toxicants. *High priority.*

  c. A further possible goal is the determination of whether only moderately inbred strains, highly inbred strains, or strain crosses could be superior animal models. This consideration is probably only of concern when using the mouse, however, as other species are not generally available as highly inbred strains. Thus it is of lower priority. *Low priority.*

2. End Points

A number of end points are assessed in attempts to measure maternal and developmental toxicity. To a considerable extent, these seem to be based on what is readily observable, but there seems to have been inadequate consideration of how predictive each end point really is.

  a. It could be useful to evaluate individual end points and indices made up of combinations of such values. This would allow determination of whether some end points could be omitted or if certain parameters could be grouped to provide more sensitive or meaningful indicators, especially relative to prediction of possible human effects. Such evaluations should be done in the common test species (at least rat and rabbit) to determine if there are significant species differences, and could be further refined by comparing strains among species. Development of indices that would allow cross-species comparisons is a possible goal (Hogan and Hoel, 1982). During this process of end point evaluation, it must be kept in mind that some end points, such as death and malformation, are sometimes interrelated. *High priority.*

b. At least some effort should be made to assess readily available and relatively inexpensive biochemical end points, especially for maternal toxicity. For example, clinical chemistries might provide a useful measure of toxicity to the dam. The major drawback would be the need for obtaining blood samples during the treatment period, a procedure that could itself influence test results. Even if such tests could not be used routinely, they might be helpful in cases where additional testing was required to assess whether maternal toxicity had been achieved in a test protocol. *Medium priority.*

3. Test Conduct

One aspect of test conduct on which agreement is needed but definitive data appear to be lacking is the question of whether chronically dosed pregnant test animals should be given a constant amount per animal or a constant dosage, adjusted for changes in body weight. It has been suggested (U.S. EPA, 1986a) that adjustment of dosage may be important for chemicals with a steep dose-response curve (a characteristic of many developmental toxicants). The optimal amount of adjustment may not be linearly correlated with increase in body weight, however, because various other factors could influence response. These could include lack of proportional distribution across the placenta, so that maternal levels of the test chemical or its metabolites would rise disproportionately to the increase in total weight of maternal body plus uterine contents. Another such factor would be maternal capacity-limited biotransformation, especially if combined with low rates of placental transfer. This could influence the observed dose response, depending on whether the parent compound or one or more metabolites were critical for production of maternal or developmental toxicity. *Medium priority.*

4. In Vitro Tests and Other Prescreens

A large number of possible short-term tests for developmental toxicity have been proposed and subjected to some degree of attempted validation. The current need in this area is probably not for additional proposed tests but evaluation of the more promising of those already suggested.

a. Further developmental work should be done on the Chernoff-Kavlock assay (Chernoff and Kavlock, 1982; Gray and Kavlock, 1984), primarily to assess the value of longer-term postnatal assessment protocols. *Medium priority.*

b. An effort should be made to assess the status and potential of the currently suggested prescreens and to assure that the most promising are put through a well-thought-out validation procedure. Such a procedure should involve tests of a priori criteria, and should be done blindly in more than one laboratory with a range of test chemicals. These must include compounds that yield somewhat ambiguous results in standard mammalian tests, as well as definite positive and negative agents.

Tests should be planned so that their results could then be evaluated comparatively among the competing test systems. Criteria should include cost and time factors as well as test validity. Care should be taken in interpretation of the results so as to avoid screening systems that cannot distinguish merely cytotoxic agents from those that are selective developmental toxicants (Neubert, 1985; Neubert et al., 1985). Also, the role of metabolism in determining developmental effects and test outcome must be carefully assessed (Kimmel, 1985). *High priority.*

MALFORMATIONS vs. VARIATIONS AND 'MINOR DEFECTS'

1. It should be useful to obtain a consensus on categorization of each of the numerous possible effects on developing offspring. Publication of such a categorization of anomalies could aid in making data from different laboratories more comparable. Each malformation, minor defect, variation, and manifestation of delayed development should be adequately described and even illustrated when necessary. Such a publication could become a valuable reference for developmental toxicologists, in addition to its usefulness as an aid to standardization of terminology. *High priority.*

2. Investigation of the significance and utility of the various end points is described in the discussion of tests for developmental toxicity, earlier in this chapter.

ANIMAL MODELS OF EFFECTS OF PRENATAL INSULT

1. Much has been said regarding the desirability of pharmacokinetic data for developmental toxicity risk assessment, especially in terms of selecting

the best animal model for extrapolation to humans. Nevertheless, such data are often lacking at the stage in the testing process when test species are to be selected. Also, there is only a modest amount of data in the literature that relates results in humans to those in animals on the basis of similarity or dissimilarity in pharmacokinetic parameters. Thus, it would be desirable to examine the available literature and to develop appropriate new data that would allow a comparison of developmental toxicity outcomes in test animals and humans on the basis of pharmacokinetic parameters. If such data can be shown to consistently allow significantly more accurate risk extrapolation, more emphasis could be placed on its use in routine testing. In order to justify the increased cost and time involved, the improvement in predictive ability would have to be substantial. For example, if it allowed testing in one species rather than two, such use of pharmacokinetics could be cost-effective as well as intrinsically useful. For further discussion and prioritization of research needs in this area, see the section on fetal pharmacokinetic and psychological models, earlier in this chapter.

2. The presumed influence of placental type on response of the conceptus has often been invoked as of possible importance in choice of animal models or in interpretation of experimental outcomes. This has occurred despite the fact that only a few developmental toxicants are believed to act by specific effects on a particular placental type (e.g., trypan blue on the rodent visceral yolk sac). It is likely that most direct-acting agents can readily penetrate any placental type at any developmental stage and enter the embryo/fetus, so relative barriers are not likely of significance (Brown and Fabro, 1983). In order to decide the issue on an empirical basis, data should be obtained by use of representative classes of developmental toxicants in terms of (1) their relative abilities to cross different placental types at various stages of placental maturation, and (2) their effect, if any, on placental function. Such data should then be correlated with effects on the embryo/fetus, taking developmental stage and maternal pharmacokinetic parameters into consideration. Doses should be adjusted so as to obtain relatively similar maternal blood levels of the active compound (i.e., parent compound or metabolites, depending upon which is believed to be the ultimate developmental toxicant). *Medium priority.*

3. The possibility of the use of strain crosses and the determination of interspecies comparability of developmental toxicity end points have been mentioned in the discussion of tests for developmental toxicity.

USE OF HUMAN DATA

1. Registries

The utility of birth defects registries for identifying developmental hazards could be increased by ensuring that information on exposure is available, either through interviews or by linkage with other data sources. In addition, it is important to expand the number of registries and to extend registration to developmental outcomes other than congenital malformations (e.g., fetal loss, low birth weight, developmental disabilities). *High priority.*

2. Case Reports/Clusters

Obstetricians, pediatricians, other health workers and patients should be encouraged to report suspected associations, "new" syndromes, and "unexpected" concentrations to a central source. The reports should be cross-indexed by exposure history and effect and merged with existing toxicologic data. The computerized data base should be reviewed regularly by central staff for testable hypotheses; it should also be available for review by outside researchers.

Limited initiatives along these lines have been made by the Food and Drug Administration, by the Reproductive Toxicology Center in Washington, D.C., and by the Birth Defects Information System at Tufts-New England Medical Center, but further development of the approach is needed. *High priority.*

3. Record Linkage

Better use could be made of available data on developmental outcome and toxic exposure if a means could be found to facilitate record linkage. A unique health record number system has been proposed (Dixon, 1984) and should be supported. *High priority.*

4. Epidemiologic Approaches

While initial per-project costs may be high, in-depth research targeted on a few compounds should ultimately prove cost-effective. Techniques such as meta-analysis might be used to identify likely toxins in the existing experimental and epidemiologic literature. These target compounds should be studied with the following specific aims: confirmation of hazard in humans; development of dose-response data; investigation of process. The design(s) to be used in studying human populations is best suggested by the circumstances of exposure, but should be guided by certain general principles:

• Populations selected for study should have relatively well-defined exposure, and should include a proportion exposed at relatively high concentrations. If a case-control design is used, the possibility should exist for more accurately measuring exposure.

• To improve resolving power, efforts should be made to refine the description of exposure (timing, dose, duration). Environmental and biological measures of exposure should be used. Where appropriate, measures should be carried out in both parent(s) and in the placenta/embryo/fetus/offspring.

• An explicit biological rationale (or alternative rationales) should be developed regarding critical periods of exposure and relevant outcomes.

• In order to gain precision in characterizing outcome, special diagnostic studies (e.g., subtyping of childhood leukemias, karyotyping of miscarriages) should be conducted as needed.

• Biomarkers of response/effect should be developed and applied. Implicit in these general guidelines is an attempt to improve the precision of measurement of variables, since measurement error usually has the effect of attenuating results. Specific recommendations along these lines are contained in the next section. *High priority.*

5. Improved Measurement of Variables

a. Support should be available for studying the natural history of end points which may ultimately prove useful to environmental research (e.g., infertility, behavioral disorders). *Medium priority.*

b. Investment in special diagnostic studies is needed in order to develop data on the mode of action of developmental toxicants in humans. Human placenta is readily available and can be examined in a variety of ways, from routine pathology to cell phenotyping (e.g., analysis of decidual cells). *Medium priority.*

c. Biological markers of exposure and subclinical effect should be developed, validated, and appropriately utilized in human studies of developmental toxicity. Samples of placental and fetal tissue, cord blood, and amniotic and breast fluids are obvious candidate materials for such an enterprise. Materials available through in vitro fertilization or organ donor programs may be useful in developing markers and in the crucial step of validation in humans. *Medium priority.*

6. Coordination of Experimental and Human Research

Mechanisms should be sought for promoting regular exchange of research questions and findings, as well as actual collaborations between epidemiologists, clinical researchers, and toxicologists. *Medium priority.*

7. Research Opportunities and New Directions That May Contribute to Risk Assessment of Developmental Toxicity in Humans

a. Taken together, the results of studies of the relationship of head circumference to CNS damage (e.g., Otake and Schull, 1984) indicate that it may be fruitful to (i) examine the association of exposure to CNS-damaging agents and reduced head circumference in other cohorts, (ii) examine directly the relationship of decrements in head size to performance measures of cognition, and (iii) support efforts to ensure that head circumference data are systematically collected and recorded so that they are available for future research. *Medium priority.*

b. Other end points that merit attention include minor physical anomalies (MPAs) and functional and behavioral outcomes. For MPAs to be useful in research, efforts must be made to see that they are comprehensively and uniformly recorded. Development and application of measures of adverse functional and behavioral outcomes is an active area of research that deserves support. *High priority.*

c. Under pressure of malpractice legislation, obstetric routines are changing in ways that may ultimately redound to the benefit of researchers. For example, in one state a comprehensive uniform perinatal record has been instituted, mainly for the purpose of standardizing and documenting level of care but with obvious advantages for perinatal epidemiologists. In some hospitals, collection and pathological review of placentas are now mandatory for all deliveries. It will be important to discover, support, and exploit the research opportunities presented by such changes in medical practice. *Medium priority.*

d. Finally, in designing clinical or epidemiologic research on developmental toxicity, consideration should be given to uses of:

- Cases available through surveillance programs for follow-up hypothesis-testing studies
- Cohorts known to have experienced unusual prenatal exposures
- Populations potentially available through the federal Agency for Toxic Substances and Disease Registry
- Exposed cohorts enrolled in ongoing medical surveillance programs (e.g., residents living near toxic waste sites)

- Infertility patients, who may be particularly motivated to participate in research
- Existing national health surveys, particularly those involving exposure histories and physical exams as well as reported illness (e.g., the National Health and Nutrition Examination Survey) *Medium priority.*

STRUCTURE-ACTIVITY RELATIONSHIPS

The sections that deal with the biological aspects of teratogenicity address the problem of defining specific biological end points in terms of a spectrum of well-characterized biological processes. Therefore, only the approaches that can be subsumed under the topic of structure-activity relationships (SARs) will be addressed here. An essential component in causal SAR is the proper definition of parameters that represent the relationship between chemical structure and molecular reactivity. This can be achieved by using the methods of theoretical chemistry, which will be discussed below in relation to SAR. Since quantitative structure-activity relationship (QSAR) is a useful method for predicting biological activity and, when properly formulated, can also become a tool in constructing a mechanistic hypothesis, this approach will be discussed initially.

1. QSAR

Two distinct approaches can be identified under the topic of QSAR: One is an approach that addresses data sets composed of compounds with diverse structures that have the same, or apparently the same, biological end point; the other is an approach that correlates biological activity for chemicals with similar structures.

a. The aim of the first approach is to classify the compounds in the data set into two major classes — active and inactive — and then establish more detailed subclassifications. In this approach, large data sets are required because of the structural diversity of the chemicals, and consequently, causal relationships are very difficult to establish. The methods that are of major use in this approach are discriminant analysis, pattern recognition, cluster analysis, correlations, and regression analysis.

A set of descriptors is either defined or generated for the data set and then processed with one of the appropriate methods. Definition of descriptors can be done based on chemical substructures usually associated with functional groups. This has certain advantages, because the correlation generated appears as related to chemical structure. However, a word of caution is necessary here because these correlations have, in fact, only a small affinity to the actual structure and the chemical entities to which they are associated.

Another method of generation of descriptors is based on techniques that automatically select the substructural descriptor that is most appropriate for the discriminant analysis and for the subsequent regression analyses. One example is the Computer Automated Structure Evaluation (CASE) technique.

These methods are very important for quick identification of toxic compounds, and they should therefore be developed further. Because they depend strongly on large data sets, the development of such data sets is of great importance. Furthermore, care should be taken to include in the data sets homogeneous data that have similar or identical biological end points with widely varying activities to help in formulating statistically significant regression analyses.

Methods for generation of descriptors based on structure should also be improved. Of special interest would be the pursuit of the relationship between the descriptors and chemical reactivity. Such a formulation will facilitate the connection of the statistically derived SAR to causal SAR that will eventually lead to the identification of biological mechanisms of developmental toxicity. *Medium priority.*

b. The major advantage in QSAR of structurally related compounds is that it can be performed on smaller data sets. The most commonly used method is the classical Hansch QSAR type, in which linear relationships are sought between a set of molecular parameters and biological activity. The underlying principle is the linear free energy relationship that was originally formulated by Hammet. In addition to the electronic parameters defined by Hammet, additional parameters (such as the hydrophobic parameter in its various forms) have been introduced in the biological correlations. Also, the well-defined but rather limited steric parameter of Taft has proven to be too restricted in the biological correlations, and the definition of a proper steric parameter is greatly needed. A related method is ADAPT, in which the parameters used for the correlation or the discriminate analysis are derived computationally. However, since the method is not based on a mechanism, the choice of the appropriate parameters is left to the statistical procedure. The result is always in doubt as to whether some other relevant parameter has been left out. Both methods would benefit greatly from a clearer definition of the relationship between the parameters (experimentally or computationally derived) and molecular reactivity.

The molecular superposition method is almost entirely devoted to the steric properties of molecules. In this approach, the volume associated with the stable form of the investigated molecules is calculated. The superposition volume is obtained as the union of the superimposed volumes of active molecules. The residual volume occupied by the inactive compounds is called excluded volume and is related to the steric restrictions imposed by the biological site of action. Attempts are being made to present other properties that could be relevant to molecular interactions on the molecular surface, e.g., the electrostatic potential. The method is not very automated, and there is a great degree of arbitrariness in the superposition techniques.

The physical basis for the relationship between the molecular connectivity graphs generated with Graph Theoretical Techniques and biological activity is rather skimpy. This topological approach is basically an empirical ranking of structures based on their similarity.

The usefulness of these methods, like those described in the previous section, is in the rapid formulation of correlations or other mathematical relationships between a set of parameters and the observed biological activity. The predictive power of these methods is their greatest asset, and they could be used for this purpose with some confidence. The strength of these methods would increase if the relationship between the parameters and specific molecular reactivities were defined.

Perhaps the most promising would be the approach that will take advantage of the molecular superposition techniques in combination with the depiction of the properties related to the parameters that are found to correlate structure and activity. This will combine spatial relationships and the notions associated with reactivity of substructures (e.g., electrostatic, dipolar, hydrophobic) that had been expressed as parameters. This approach would bring QSAR closer to a formulation of the causal relationship between structure, molecular reactivity, and the molecular mechanisms of action of toxic compounds. *Medium priority*.

2. Causal Molecular Parameters

As has been emphasized before, the most difficult part in a SAR study is the definition of molecular parameters that will reflect molecular reactivities related to the causal relationship between molecular structure and the resulting biological activity. Methods of theoretical and computational chemistry are very well suited to provide not only the parameters but also the methodology for simulating molecular mechanisms. These could shed light on the discriminating properties of molecules in relation to biological activity. The major shortcoming of such computational simulations is the relatively large investment of time and computational resources to produce a significant result. A systematic approach is therefore needed to limit the number of molecules that will be investigated in great depth without effectively losing the important information about the remaining molecules.

a. In such an approach the first step can be the grouping of compounds according to elements of similarity that also correlate with activity. This can be achieved by one of the statistical methods described above. Examples of such groupings could be substituted aromatic amines, halogenated hydrocarbons, nitroso compounds, etc. *Medium priority*.

b. The next stage of the procedure is selection of a small subset of these groups, usually a few molecules that have distinct quantitative differences in their activity but share the same biological end point. Examples of such end points are teratogenicity, embryotoxicity, mutagenicity, etc. It is important to emphasize that greater specificity of the biological end points will lead to more precision of the computational simulation and to conclusions of better quality. *Medium priority*.

c. The third stage in this procedure is the most time-consuming but also should yield the most valuable information regarding the definition of molecular descriptors that are relevant to reactivity. At this stage, a detailed computational simulation of the molecular interactions would be performed, based on a proposed mechanism of action. The result of such simulations would be the identification of the molecular properties that are of primary importance to the mechanism of action and that discriminate between molecules with different biological activities. *Medium priority*.

d. These discriminant properties can now be formulated as parameters that will become useful in the next stage. In this stage, the parameters defined, based on the computational simulations, will be calculated for other molecules from the data sets that were obtained in stage one. Then an attempt to correlate biological activity with these parameters will be undertaken. This is a crucial step, because it tests whether the computational procedure identified the proper parameters relevant to the biological activity. *Medium priority*.

The test can be performed with QSAR methods or through experimental testing of new compounds. In either case, if the test is successful, the chosen parameters provide a rapid and reliable tool to predict biological activity based on causally determined parameters. A failure of the test would indicate that the parameters were not discriminant, in which case they should be reexamined for their mechanistic relevance. Also, the methods used to produce these parameters should be examined and reevaluated.

e. The methods of theoretical and computational chemistry are inherently capable of producing both the mechanistic simulation and the proper formulation of the parameters. With these methods, structural and electronic properties of isolated molecules can be calculated to a high degree of precision. For example, molecular structures can be optimized, conformational energies can be calculated, and the accessibility of conformers can be estimated on this basis. Charge distribution, dipole, and higher moments can be calculated from the wave functions obtained from quantum mechanical calculations. Ionization potentials and electron affinities as well as electrostatic potentials and electric fields can be obtained from the same source. Simulation of molecular interactions and calculations of potential energy surfaces can be done to investigate the energetics of crucial mechanistic steps. These calculations can be performed with ab initio methods or, when the systems become too big, with semi-empirical methods. *Medium priority.*

f. Molecular dynamics methods can be used to explore the conformational changes that a flexible molecule undergoes, and with the recent development of Brownian dynamics, bimolecular interactions can be studied. The interaction of a molecule with a specific biological target can be investigated by the optimization of the structure of the interacting complex. For example, enzyme-inhibitor or drug-receptor models can be calculated, and under certain approximations their relative geometries can be optimized. The analysis of the forces that hold these complexes and direct their interaction can be translated into parameters for recognition. The investigation of the changes in the properties of the targets upon interaction can suggest mechanisms of activation or response of the target.

Of special importance are the recently developed empirical calculations that are coupled directly with a graphic display system. These "real time" simulations allow one to execute "docking" experiments of compounds into their binding sites, inhibitors with the active sites of enzymes, or intercalating agents with DNA molecules. These studies help in the simulation of the fundamental molecular processes that give rise to toxic effects and prepare the ground for the definition of parameters relevant to toxicity. *Low priority.*

Clearly, the advantages of the theoretical computational approach outweigh the difficulties that may be encountered in the research process. Following the systematic steps outlined above will ensure the formulation of meaningful parameters. These will have the capability of rapidly predicting biological activity within the QSAR approach as well as the causal relationship that is so important for a mechanistic understanding of the association between structure and biological activity.

In summary, emphasis should be placed on the development of causal relationships between the parameters used in predictive methods (QSAR) and the molecular properties of compounds exhibiting developmental toxicity. The theoretical-computational multistage approach is suggested as the most promising one because of its ability to produce meaningful parameters and its testability with respect to the significance of these parameters.

Because it is difficult to single out specific areas for targeted research support, it is essential that as many as possible of the promising studies proposed by knowledgeable investigators be funded. As areas of research begin to appear especially promising, they can be emphasized, but this emphasis must be based on significant findings rather than on a priori assumptions. *High priority.*

STATISTICAL ANALYSIS OF DEVELOPMENTAL TOXICITY DATA

1. Although many statisticians currently are leaning to the beta-binomial probability model for analyzing developmental toxicity data, this does not mean that it has been universally accepted. One disturbing note is the discrepancy in its performance that has been observed in various simulation studies. As mentioned earlier, the boundary conditions on the correlation parameters and the different simulation models used for data generation could be the culprits. Another possibility is the particular parameterization chosen to represent the beta-binomial model. Some forms of expressing the beta-binomial parameters lead to very unstable maximum likelihood estimates. The most stable approach appears to be that recommended by Kupper et al. (1986), in which the correlation parameter θ and μ = logit(θ) = log[$\theta(1-\theta)$] are used. Many of the authors who conducted simulation studies did not indicate how they parameterized the beta-binomial model. A more exhaustive simulation, in which various parameterizations and data-generating models are employed, is needed to clarify the capabilities and limitations of the beta-binomial model.

Other aspects yet to be developed for a beta-binomial likelihood analysis include goodness-of-fit tests to determine when the beta-binomial might be a poor model and diagnostic criteria for identifying influential observations. Such methodology is available for regression and analysis of variance (ANOVA) with a continuous variable and is starting to appear in the literature for a logistic regression model with a dichotomous variable. *High priority.*

2. Extensions of the beta-binomial model for situations encountered in developmental toxicity studies are needed. First of all, the implications of Prentice's (1986) results on a negative bound for the correlation parameter require investigation. More importantly, generalizations of the beta-binomial that allow for random litter sizes would provide more efficient and less biased estimates.

There are a number of ways to approach this. A probability model for the litter size, such as a Poisson or a negative binomial, can be assumed, and then the marginal distribution of the number of affected fetuses can be derived. Some generalizations of the beta-binomial of this type have been investigated in other contexts. A statistical review of this class of models is provided by Johnson and Kotz (1969, Chapter 9). Unfortunately, the probability functions for many of these models do not have closed-form solutions, and parameter estimation is extremely difficult. A simplification could result for developmental toxicity data if the probability distribution of the litter size is taken to be finite valued rather than infinite. Candidates include a truncated Poisson, a truncated geometric, a truncated negative binomial, or a discrete uniform.

Assuming that a model or class of models is found to be tractable, two major concerns arise. First of all, is it necessary to model for random litter sizes if the litter size distributions are relatively homogeneous across groups? Secondly, if the litter size distributions differ significantly across groups, is it worthwhile even to statistically compare the treatment groups with respect to the number of affected fetuses? As mentioned earlier, statistical research is also needed for the inclusion of random litter sizes in analyzing a continuous variable. *High priority.*

3. Parametric modeling, such as use of the beta-binomial or its generalizations, is important in developmental toxicity studies because it provides a basis for a low-dose extrapolation and threshold models — otherwise, we could concentrate on hypothesis testing and some of the nonparametric and transformation approaches discussed earlier. Nevertheless, statistical methods for performing rank tests and ANOVA on transformed data that adjust for random litter sizes would be extremely useful. *High priority.*

4. Many scientists who conduct developmental toxicity studies believe that threshold doses exist. However, most of the statistical models used in the analysis and risk assessment of developmental toxicity data do not incorporate a threshold effect. One form of a threshold model is to model the probability of response at dose d as

$$P[d] = \begin{array}{ll} P_0 & d_T \quad ; d < d_{TH} \\ P_0 + (1 - P_0) \, F \, (d - d_{TH}); & d > d_{TH} \end{array} \qquad [3\text{-}1]$$

where

$F(\cdot)$ = any nondecreasing function mapping the positive real line onto the [0, 1] interval,

d_{TH} = the threshold dose, and

P_0 = $F(d_{TH})$.

If such a model were to be used within a beta-binomial framework, i.e., θ = P[d] in equation [20-2] from Chapter 20, then more dose groups than the usual four or five are needed to estimate all the parameters of the model. Statistical research in this area, in terms of model feasibility, goodness of fit, choice of the function F, etc., could prove fruitful in terms of developmental toxicity screening and risk assessment. *Medium priority.*

5. All of the above concerns have focused on one particular dichotomous end point in a developmental toxicity study. Before statistical decision rules can be developed for handling all the dichotomous end points measured in these studies, a general consensus is needed among statisticians as to an appropriate statistical model or class of models. (This has occurred in carcinogenicity studies, in which the binomial distribution is widely accepted as an adequate model.) For the model, researchers and statisticians should remain aware of inflating the overall false-positive rate when too many statistical tests are conducted. A temporary solution is to employ a smaller significance level—say, 0.01—as is done with common tumors in carcinogenicity studies (Haseman, 1983). *Medium priority.*

MATHEMATICAL MODELING OF TERATOGENIC EFFECTS

1. Development of Additional Models

It seems clear that new models for developmental toxicity data should incorporate the biology of development and mechanisms of action for toxic agents known to affect fetal development. Such models would permit a systematic evaluation of classes of compounds having similar mechanisms of action.

Highly specific mechanisms of action are unknown for most teratogens, but general mechanisms can often be postulated with a reasonable degree of confidence. Agents might be classified on the basis of the following four general categories of response:

1. Acute but reversible toxic response, such as death of cells that have the capacity to replicate

2. Chronic reversible response, such as cholinesterase inhibition

3. Molecular biological effect, such as irreversible change in the information coded in DNA

4. Chronic, irreversible accumulation of many small events, such as neuron cell death

Classification of this sort can lead to a simple paradigm that yields a mathematical model for the class of agents that acts in one of these four postulated manners.

To illustrate this approach, we have postulated several simple sets of biological assumptions and generated mathematical models based on them.

Example 1: Molecular Biological Effect Model

We assume:

- Exposure is continuous during the one-cell stage.

- The teratogenic effect will occur if one of two genes at a critical locus on homologous chromosomes is deactivated and is not repaired before replication.

- If both genes at the critical locus on homologous chromosomes are deactivated at the same time, death will occur.

- The transition rate for each gene deactivation is constant over time and proportional to exposure.

- The repair rate is constant over time.

These assumptions may be diagrammed as below:

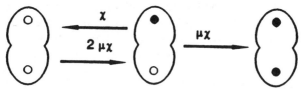

where

μ = the gene transition rate per unit of exposure,

χ = the exposure level,

λ = the repair rate, and

- denotes a deactivated gene and o an active gene.

This simple paradigm yields the mathematical model below:

$$P(t, \chi) = 1/2R\{e^{r1+} [(\lambda - \mu\chi) + R] + e^{r2+} [-(\lambda - \mu\chi) + R]\} \quad [3\text{-}2]$$

where
$$R = (\lambda^2 + 6\lambda\mu\chi + \mu^2\chi^2)^{1/2},$$
$$r_1 = [-(\lambda + 3\mu\chi) + R]/2,$$
$$r_2 = -[(\lambda + 3\mu\chi) + R]/2, \text{ and}$$
the value t is the length of exposure.

Example 2: Multiple Effect Model

An embryo contains a large number of critical sites defined as groups or clusters of cells. We assume:

- The number of cells that make up a critical site is variable, with a few large clusters and many small clusters.
- The relative frequency of cluster size is proportional to a constant between zero and 1, raised to the power of the number of cells in the cluster. This constitutes a logarithmic series distribution as described by Fisher et al. (1943).
- The probability of an agent deactivating a cell is proportional to the amount of exposure.
- If two[4] or more cells in any single cluster are deactivated, a birth defect will occur.

Using these assumptions, the probability of a birth defect is:

$$P(x) = 1\{ - \frac{-\ln(1-Te^{-Sx}) \, TSxe^{-Sx}/(1-Te^{-Sx})}{-\ln(1-T)} \}^N \quad [3\text{-}3]$$

where
N = the number of critical sites or clusters,
S = the cell deactivation transition rate per unit of exposure,
x = the exposure level, and
0 < T < 1 = the cluster size frequency proportionality constant.

---

4. This number can be varied to obtain different functional forms.

In a number of situations, crude estimates for N and T might be obtainable from anatomical observations alone, or might be fixed in advance based on past experience. In such a case, only one parameter S would have to be estimated from the other teratogenicity dose-response data, where the end point was one or more birth defects. *High priority.*

2. Other Considerations in Model Development

Several other factors need to be explored in the development of new mathematical models. Feasibility studies might be conducted to look at in vivo and in vitro test systems, using information from the same species and strains in which delivered doses are related using pharmacokinetic models. Other models, such as Cox's ordered logistic model (1966) might be explored for use in examining series of end points that suggest continuous progression of fetal damage. Models could be developed based on certain deficiencies that result from deprivation of vitamins, minerals, and other nutrients. Other models, based on continuous variables, such as birth weight or reflex time, could be investigated. Finally, whether a teratogen acts at an early or late stage should be investigated in relation to the resulting dose-response curve, and the implications of this on mechanisms of action should be explored. *High priority.*

3. Validation of Models

New mathematical models for use in developmental toxicology will require verification. One task crucial to verification will be sorting out and evaluating the available information from human and animal dose-response studies. In every situation where information exists for both human and animal studies, the relationships between results should be carefully documented and compared. A particularly interesting and potentially fruitful subject for this kind of inquiry may be the relationship between radiation and microcephaly in animals and humans.

A number of epidemiologic studies have been conducted on the relationships between certain agents and birth defects. Unfortunately, in many such studies the exposures are ill-defined, a limited number of end points are evaluated, and the sample sizes are too small to detect low probability defects. As a result, many of these studies do not demonstrate rates elevated above the control levels that are associated with agent exposure. It is possible that useful information could be gleaned from certain of these studies in the form of "upper-bound" rate estimates for a given exposure; these upper-bound estimates could be based on conservative exposure values and statistical confidence limits on elevated rates. Such values would constitute important benchmarks in validating mathematical extrapolations from animal dose-response data to low-level responses. Figure 3-1 illustrates this concept.

To obtain an upper-bound estimate of the increased probability of a birth defect occurring, it is necessary to have the following information:

• The population background birth defect rate.

• The number of individuals in the study cohort.

• The number of birth defects in the study cohort.

• An estimate of the exposure of the cohort to the toxic agent.

The upper-bound estimated value is plotted on a birth defect exposure graph. Various models are used to extrapolate to a 1×10^{-5} risk level. These values can then be compared to the no-observed-effect level (NOEL)/lowest-observed-effect level (LOEL) safety factor approach. Models that predict more response than the upper bound can be viewed as conservative. If multiple exposure information is available, upper-bound estimates of parameters in postulate models could also be obtained using negative data. Although this approach would be mathematically complex, it would make the most efficient use of the available information. *High priority*.

4. Use of Simple Systems to Delineate Shape of Dose-Response Curve

Independent verification of the general shape of dose-response curves could be achieved using simple test subjects, such as adult Hydra attentuata and artificial "embryos" derived from hydra cells (Johnson and Gabel, 1983) or Pacific oyster (*Grassostrea gigas*) larvae prior to the two-cell developmental stage (Nelson, 1972). These systems can be employed to delineate mechanisms by the use of multiple exposure scenarios that can be carried out quickly and without great expense. *Medium priority*.

5. Extrapolation between Species

One criticism of using animal data to extrapolate to humans is that inbreeding of laboratory animals causes too homogeneous a response. To avoid the homogeneity problem, it is possible to assume equal sensitivity between the average human and laboratory animal. Then human variability assumptions can be imposed on the animal model. *Medium priority*.

Example:

a. The animal slope parameter in the probit model would be replaced by the reciprocal of the standard deviation of an enzyme level in the human population, where that enzyme is critical to the expected toxic effect.

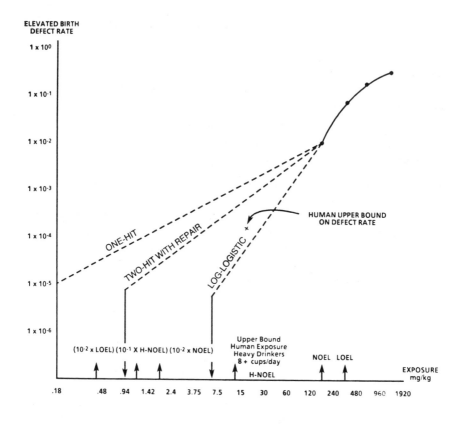

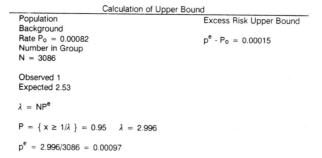

Figure 3-1. Hypothetical example of the relationship between safety factor approach model extrapolation and negative human data.

b. Mixed populations of individuals carrying critical genes might be postulated to define sensitive subpopulations, where the sensitivity was proportional to some phenotypical expression of the gene. This would yield (for nonlinear dose-response relationships) a variation on the variable threshold model.

APPLICATION OF EXPERIMENTAL DATA IN RISK ASSESSMENT

Although a few additional areas of interest were reviewed in this chapter, no obvious research projects were apparent.

4.

MECHANISMS OF DEVELOPMENTAL TOXICITY

Ronald D. Hood

MOLECULAR vs. CELLULAR vs. TISSUE OR ORGAN LEVEL MECHANISMS

In the following discussion, the term *mechanism* as it pertains to developmental toxicity will be applied to key events at any of various levels of organization, beginning with changes at the molecular level and progressing to alterations at successively more complex levels of the affected developmental pathways. Since much is yet to be learned about mechanisms at any level of organization, all are important targets for further study. It is generally believed that a thorough understanding of mechanisms is essential if we are ever to effectively regulate developmental toxicants (e.g., Skalko, 1981; Wolkowski-Tyl, 1981; Johnson, 1983a). Wilson (1973) properly stated that the most important such event is the initial effect in the series leading to abnormal development, and he therefore reserved the term *mechanism* for such initial effects. Wilson (1973) proposed a variety of basic teratogenic mechanisms at the molecular level and updated his discussion in 1977 (Wilson, 1977a). Mechanisms proposed by Wilson include mutation, mitotic interference, altered nucleic acid integrity or function, lack of precursors and substrates needed for biosynthesis, altered energy sources, enzyme inhibition, osmolar imbalance, and (possibly) altered membrane characteristics. Although many of these are likely to be valid, problems arise in attempts to determine which event was actually the first to occur following toxic insult, and additional categories could be proposed, such as interaction with cellular receptors (Kimmel, 1981b).

1. Molecular Mechanisms

A number of studies have attempted to establish specific mechanisms of developmental toxicity at the molecular level. Since Wilson (1977a) and others (e.g., Juchau, 1981; Skalko, 1981; Williams, 1982; Beckman and Brent, 1984) have reviewed many such studies, only a few examples will be given here. Also, it must be kept in mind that, as Skalko (1981) has commented, unequivocal evidence for the mechanism of action of any of the many agents studied has proven exceedingly difficult to obtain. Even thalidomide, one of the most studied developmental toxicants, is yet the subject of controversy with regard to its mechanism of action (Shull, 1984; Koch and Czejka, 1986; Stephens, 1988).

Among the categories of possible teratogenic mechanisms, the concept of interaction of developmental toxicants with cellular receptors has received considerable attention and has been thoroughly reviewed (Kimmel, 1981b; Salomon, 1983; Pratt, 1984). It has been assumed that such teratogens as concanavalin A, insulin, glucocorticoids, sex steroids, and 2,3,7,8-tetrachlorodibenzo-p-dioxin (TCDD) act via mechanisms initiated by binding to specific receptors. For example, in the cases of glucocorticoids and TCDD, sensitivity to induction of cleft palate in mice is positively correlated with the levels of specific receptors in the cells of the palatal primordia that are most affected by each (Pratt, 1985). In the case of glucocorticoids, palatal mesenchyme appears to be the primary target, while for TCDD, the medial palatal epithelium is most affected. Gupta et al. (1984) have proposed an additional step in the pathway of cleft palate production by glucocortoids. They suggest that dexamethasone induces the formation of a protein capable of inhibiting the synthesis of phospholipase A_2, thereby preventing programmed cell death in the medial edge epithelium of the palatal shelves and preventing their fusion during palatogenesis. More recent results from the same group indicate that both cleft palate and failure of neural tube closure in offspring of diabetic rats could be alleviated by treatment with arachidonic acid, a compound dependent on phospholipase A_2 for its release in the cell (Goldman et al., 1985). Similar results were seen in the case of neural tube closure in mouse embryos cultured in a hyperglycemic medium and supplemented with arachidonic acid.

As a further example, Jurand (1985) reported that the effects of certain opiates that can produce malformations of the central nervous system (CNS) in mice can be blocked by the opiate antagonist naloxone hydrochloride. Also, Sterz et al. (1982; 1985) described the production of wavy ribs by treatment with beta-sympathomimetic drugs and prevention of the effect by use of a blocker of beta-receptors.

A possible mechanism that has recently been proposed is interference with intercellular communication (Trosko et al., 1982). Evidence in support of this has been provided by Welsch and Stedman (1984), who found that a number of structurally different teratogens could interfere with the exchange of a metabolite of 6-thioguanine between cultured cells, apparently by interfering with gap junctions. Alteration of intracellular pH is another newly proposed mechanism that is currently under investigation (Nau and Scott, 1987).

2. Cellular and Tissue Mechanisms

In addition to elucidating mechanisms at the fundamental level of biochemical effects, it is also important to understand the effects of developmental toxicants on higher levels of organization in the embryo. Again, there have been reviews that, at least in part, attempted to address this issue. These included, among others, Bergsma (1975), Langman et al. (1975), Saxen (1977), Scott (1977), Yamada (1977), Wilson (1977a), Johnston and Sulik (1979), Kallen (1979), Melnick (1979), Kameyama (1985), Danes (1980), Pratt and Christiansen (1980), Bernfield (1983), and Skalko (1985a).

A variety of alterations in cellular properties have been proposed as possible contributors to abnormal development. For example, alterations in the normal pattern of cell migration, adhesion, or changes in cell shape are presumed to contribute to teratogenesis (Yamada, 1977; Bernfield, 1983; Pratt et al., 1987). Additional cell behaviors that may be involved in a teratogenicity response include changes in the rates of cell proliferation (Bernfield, 1983) and cell death (Scott, 1977; Wise and Scott, 1982).

Tissue interactions, such as embryonic induction, have been implicated (Saxen, 1977; Kollar, 1985). Nieuwkoop (1985) proposed that induction may actually involve relatively nonspecific inducers and that the specificity of the induction resides within the responding tissue. This might explain how a variety of teratogenic agents could interfere with the same process. Further, it has been suggested that alterations in developmental fields (a topic often ignored) are important in dysmorphogenesis and may form a basis for the ability of disparate teratogens to cause the same or a similar syndrome of malformations (Opitz, 1979).

Another concept of importance in understanding effects at the cellular level was discussed by Skalko (1985a), who stated that developmental toxicants interacted with populations of "target cells," just as do other classes of toxic agents. These cells may be in either the embryo, the placenta, or the dam, and may act as the primary site of action or as a secondary site contributing to the overall effect on the offspring. It has been further proposed that defects in specific cellular events, such as the normal process of shape changing in neural plate cells, are presumed to lead to events such as failure of neural fold elevation followed by lack of neural tube closure and finally by CNS malformations (Copp, 1983).

3. Mechanisms at Higher Levels of Organization

Additional mechanisms of developmental perturbation have been proposed at increasingly complex organizational levels in the embryo. It must be kept in mind, however, that these "mechanisms" tend to be merely succeeding events in aberrant morphogenetic pathways that were set in mo-tion by toxicity at the biochemical level. Proposed mechanisms have included abnormalities of vascularization of specific organ primordia (e.g., Fraser and Travill, 1978). More recently, Graham (1983) postulated that certain limb reduction anomalies, especially those occurring in otherwise normal children, may be due to a spatially restrictive uterine environment. He suggested that such an environment can be due to factors such as uterine myomas or uterine malformation (e.g., bicornuate uterus). He stated that early amniotic rupture may also produce such effects, in addition to the constriction or amputation defects caused by amniotic bands, citing Kennedy and Persaud's (1977) study of the rat conceptus following amniotic puncture as supporting evidence. Although mechanical causes were cited as the initial mechanisms in Graham's (1983) report, he commented that production of the anatomical defects observed was likely to have been mediated by extrinsic vascular compression or intrinsic vascular occlusion followed by localized tissue destruction.

A number of more purely mechanical mechanisms have been suggested. In mice that are homozygous for a gene that prevents muscle contraction, craniofacial skeletal development has been found to be altered, presumably due to a lack of normal muscular tension (Herring and Lakars, 1981). Additionally, weakness of only some of the muscles controlling movement of a given joint and unopposed contraction of the remaining musculature may be responsible for the abnormal fixation of affected joints in human offspring with congenital contractures (Swinyard, 1982). Mechanical causes involving early rupture of the chorion and/or yolk sac have also been put forth. According to Kaplan et al. (1985), this might lead to ectopia cordis and sternal clefting.

SPECIES- AND STRAIN-SPECIFIC vs. GENERALIZED MECHANISMS

It is widely known that a given developmental toxicant may greatly affect one animal species, while having a strikingly different effect or little effect in another. A commonly used example is thalidomide, a drug that readily produced limb reduction defects and other malformations in primates and lagomorphs, while rodents were significantly less sensitive in this regard (Stern, 1982).

Species or strain differences in response to developmental toxicants have been attributed to differences in maternal metabolism. Although factors such as elimination rates and levels of plasma-binding proteins may differ considerably among species, maternal absorption, distribution, and xenobiotic metabolizing pathways are often similar (Nau, 1986). In some cases, dissimilarities may be due to intrinsic differences in the embryo.

These differences in response may be associated with disparities in the metabolism of a teratogen, according to data on the murine Ah locus and benzo[a]pyrene metabolism from Nebert's laboratory (e.g., Shum et al., 1979; Nebert and Shum, 1980; Nebert, 1983), but individual variation in the cytosolic receptor for polycyclic aromatic compounds is believed to be the basic mechanism involved. Differences in TCDD-induced cleft palate in mice have also been attributed to disparities between affected and normal fetuses in the levels of this same receptor (Dencker and Pratt, 1981).

The foregoing studies involving genetically mediated inter-strain differences in inducible levels of xenobiotic receptors indicate only one of the ways that genotypic variation influences developmental toxicity. Additional possibilities have been reviewed previously, and include a number of examples of gene-teratogen interaction and strain or species differences in response (e.g., Kocher, 1977a,b; Biddle, 1981).

SINGLE vs. MULTIPLE MECHANISMS

As Skalko (1981) reminds us, a given developmental toxicant may act by more than one mechanism. Obviously, this greatly increases the complexity of experimental systems involving such agents used in attempts to elucidate mechanisms and exacerbates the difficulty of interpreting their results. Unfortunately, there is a general tendency to interpret the outcomes of virtually all types of experimentation involving biologically active chemicals in the light of a single activity of the agent used. This is a carryover from Erlich's concept of the "magic bullet," and is untenable in view of the multiple actions of most biologically active substances.

DIRECT vs. INDIRECT MECHANISMS

It is believed that in some cases adverse developmental effects following maternal intoxication are indirect and result from interference with essential maternal contributions to the welfare of the developing conceptus. This concept will not be discussed at this point, however, as it will be dealt with in Chapter 7.

ROLE OF THE PLACENTA IN MECHANISMS OF TERATOGENICITY

According to Beck (1981), the possible influence of the placenta on response to developmental toxicants has been relatively neglected by researchers, and this is so despite our awareness of large species variations in structure and function, a view echoed by Goodman et al. (1982). It has been suggested recently, however, that species-related differences in morphology of the mature placenta may not be as relevant as similarities in early placental function (U.S. EPA, 1986a). As pointed out in Environmental Health Criteria 30 (1984), it is believed that humans depend on the yolk sac as a source of nutrition for around one month. Our knowledge of the influence of the placenta on developmental toxicity is yet relatively meager, although reviews are available detailing what we do currently believe regarding comparative placentation (e.g., Benirshke, 1975; Juchau, 1982; Enders, 1982; King, 1982; Benirschke, 1983; Chao and Juchau, 1983; Winick, 1983; Jollie, 1986)

Interest in the placental role does appear to have sparked several studies in recent years. Juchau (1982) states that the placenta may play a role in developmental toxicity in at least four ways:

1. Impairment of placental physiological capacities may lead to damage to the conceptus and/or the dam.

2. Alterations in maternal physiology due to normal placental function may influence the toxicity of chemical agents and such chemicals might also interact with the products of placental metabolism.

3. The placenta plays a significant role in determining which agents reach the embryo/fetus and in what quantities. Such effects are due to placental anatomy and, in some cases, placental biotransformation capabilities.

4. It may even be possible for placental enzymes to activate compounds to more reactive and harmful intermediates.

Impairment of the function of the visceral yolk sac of the rat has been shown by Brent and coworkers to have teratogenic effects. In a series of experiments, antisera to the visceral yolk sac have been shown to cause abnormal development both in vivo and in vitro, presumably due to inhibition of nutrient uptake (Freeman et al., 1982). A similar mechanism has been proposed for the teratogenicity of trypan blue, based on observations of dye uptake by the visceral yolk sac rather than the embryo and evidence that it can inhibit pinocytosis in the yolk sac (Williams et al., 1976; Beck, 1979). Further, trypan blue is effective only when the source of nutrition is primarily associated with visceral yolk sac function in the rat (Gulamhusein et al., 1982), and similar histiotrophic nutrition in the ferret (Beck, 1981) and the pig (Rosenkrantz et al., 1970). Additionally, Freeman and Lloyd (1983) caused malformations in cultured rat embryos by addition of leupeptin, an inhibitor of lysosomal proteinases, to the culture medium. They postulated the mechanism to be inhibition of proteolysis in the visceral yolk sac. It has been pointed out that much discussion of differences in late placental morphology may be irrelevant, in that early placental function may be similar across species, allowing teratogens such as trypan blue to affect ferrets as well as rodents (U.S. EPA, 1986a). Adequate experimental evidence is lacking on this point.

Reduction of nutrient transport by microvilli of the chorioallantoic placenta has also been speculated to be a possible mechanism of developmental toxicity. For example, metals and metal compounds such as cadmium, methylmercury, and inorganic mercury have been said to decrease placental amino acid transport (Goodman et al., 1982). Decreased placental blood flow is also thought to be a cause of undernutrition of the developing offspring, and may occur due to incomplete placental vascularization caused by maternal undernutrition (Winick, 1983). Toxic insult can directly influence placental blood flow, according to results such as those of Levin and Miller (1981) with cadmium. It was not clear, however, if the observed decrease in placental perfusion was the cause or the result of the placental necrosis that accompanied it. According to Goodman et al. (1982), a number of other agents can decrease placental blood flow, apparently by acting directly on the vessels involved.

Although the ability of placental tissue to metabolize a variety of compounds is now established (e.g., Chao and Juchau, 1983), the significance of this finding with regard to placental mediation of developmental toxicity remains obscure. Of particular concern is the ability of human placental microsomes to activate xenobiotics to reactive intermediates with carcinogenic or mutagenic potential. In general, the biotransforming ability of placental tissue is considerably less than that of adult liver, but there appear to be some exceptions, such as glucuronyltransferase activity (Goodman et al., 1982).

Another possible mechanism of developmental toxicity based on placental compromise involves the alteration of placental endocrine function, an area that has received little attention. For example, it has been suggested that the cytochrome P450 induced by polycyclic aromatic hydrocarbons in cigarette smoke is the form that catalyzes hydroxylation of 17 beta-estradiol in place of the P450 type that metabolizes cholesterol to pregnenolone (Goodman et al., 1982).

MECHANISMS OF PATHOGENESIS OF DEVELOPMENTAL EFFECTS

According to Wilson (1977a), the pathogenesis of malformations tends to be reduced to one or more of at least five manifestations. These included:

1. Excessive or reduced cell death
2. Failed cell interactions
3. Reduced biosynthesis
4. Impeded morphogenetic movement
5. Mechanical disruption of tissues

Wilson (1977a) further proposed that these events all tended to converge in common pathways that involved either "too few cells or cell products to effect localized morphogenesis or functional maturation," or "other imbalances in growth and differentiation," resulting in production of the final defect. The final manifestations of developmental toxicity were then said to be death, malformation, retarded growth, and functional deficits.

In a further discussion of pathways, Bixler et al. (1979) remind us that we must also consider the problem of pleiotropy, where multiple defects are manifested in the same individual. Thus, the same or different mechanisms may act by Wilson's (1977a) final pathways in different structures developing concurrently. Alternatively, according to Bixler et al. (1979), expression of a given pathway of dysmorphogenesis may secondarily result in a defect in some other structure of the embryo/fetus. Interpretation of experimental findings is made more difficult because, according to the concept of common pathways of pathogenesis, similar defects do not necessarily share the same initial causal mechanism.

5.
CHEMICAL INTERACTIONS

Ronald D. Hood

WHAT ARE THE BASES FOR INTERACTIVE EFFECTS IN DEVELOPMENTAL TOXICITY?

Murphy (1981) (quoted by Moskowitz et al., 1983) described a toxicologic interaction as a "condition in which exposure to two or more chemicals results in a qualitatively or quantitatively altered biological response relative to that predicted from the action of a single chemical. Such multiple chemical exposures may be simultaneous or sequential in time, and the altered response may be greater or smaller in magnitude."

Interactive effects on the conceptus due to multiple chemical exposures have been known for over 25 years (Wilson, 1964; Schumacher et al., 1969; Wilson et al., 1969). Numerous examples, including additive, synergistic, and antagonistic combinations, can be found in the literature (Fraser, 1977; Skalko et al., 1978; Skalko and Kwasigroch, 1983; Skalko, 1985b). Examination of the literature suggests that most of the tested combinations resulted in some type of apparent interactive effect, although at least some did not (Ritter, 1984). Such an apparent preponderance of interactive effects may be misleading, in that negative results often are not pursued or go unpublished even if an experiment is completed. Also, combinations of agents are often chosen with some logical a priori reason for expecting interactive effects, though this does not always appear to be the case (e.g., Gale, 1984). On the other hand, timing and dose appear to greatly influence some interactive effects, and some instances of apparent negative results may therefore be due to lack of an effective protocol (Skalko and Kwasigroch, 1983; Ritter, 1984).

In many cases, experiments involving treatment of experimental animals with multiple compounds have the stated purpose of investigating developmental toxicity (e.g., Ritter, 1984). Among the remainder are evaluations of the possibility of extra hazard arising from multiple exposures. These are based on the premise that pregnant women are typically exposed to a variety of agents, including adverse environmental factors, rather than single chemicals in an ideal environment (e.g., Lee, 1985). Another purpose of testing for interaction is the development of strategies for prevention or alleviation of the effects of known developmental toxicants (e.g., Hood and Pike, 1972; Hood and Vedel-Macrander, 1984).

Relatively few studies of chemical interactions in developmental toxicity appear to have been planned with regard to the appropriate pharmacokinetic considerations. In efforts to address this problem, Skalko and coworkers (e.g., Skalko and Kwasigroch, 1983; Kwasigroch and Skalko, 1985) performed a series of studies designed to evaluate the influence of chemical interactions on such factors as maternal biotransformation, uptake and retention of the test compounds by the conceptus, and how effects on such parameters related to observed alterations in the offspring. For example, combined treatment with 5-diazouracil and 5-fluorouracil (5-FU) resulted in decreased 5-FU catabolism with a resultant increase in levels and persistence of 5-FU in the embryo. Such effects were associated with greatly enhanced prenatal mortality. Others have investigated such phenomena with additional pairs of compounds (e.g., Lum and Wells, 1986).

Other approaches have looked at the role of alteration in binding to specific receptors for keys to interactive effects. Such work has been done by Yoneda and Pratt (1981), who found that vitamin B_6 decreased the incidence of cortisone-induced palatal clefts in mice by inhibiting the binding of the hormone to its cytosolic receptor. Similarly, Birnbaum et al. (1986) investigated the synergistic effect of combinations of 2,3,7,8-tetrachlorodibenzo-p-dioxin (TCDD) and hydrocortisone on cleft palate induction in mice and speculated that such results were likely to have been caused by an increase in number or affinity of glucocorticoid receptors in the palatal mesenchyme. Shared target receptors were suspected in the mechanism of the joint effects of TCDD and 2,3,7,8-tetrachlordibenzofuran (TCDF) on mouse embryos (Weber et al., 1985).

It must also be remembered that any effects of single or multiple chemicals on developing systems take place against the background of both the parental and embryonic genomes (Fraser, 1977). Accounts of interactive effects between chemical agents and specific genetic backgrounds have frequently been published, particularly with inbred mice as animal models. Such studies have investigated the bases for strain differences (Biddle and Fraser, 1977) as well as interactions with mutant genes (Lary et al., 1982; Seller et al., 1983; Trasler et al., 1984).

HOW CAN INTERACTIONS BE ASSESSED?

It is assumed that toxic interactions can be categorized as either pharmacodynamic or pharmacokinetic (Fraser, 1977). Pharmacodynamic interactions occur when one agent modifies the action of another with regard to receptors or physiologic control mechanisms that are involved in its mechanism of toxicity. Pharmacokinetic interactions are involved if one agent affects the time course of absorption, distribution, biotransformation, or elimination of another. Obviously, interactions often may be reciprocal as well as unidirectional.

In a related approach, toxicant interactions have been divided into two basic types:

(1) Those in which the quantity of the active form of a chemical available to the critical cellular macromolecules is altered by the current or past presence of one or more other chemicals. This case involves uptake and "sites of loss," such as pathways of excretion and storage sites. (2) Those in which the reactivity of the critical macromolecules with the active forms of the chemical(s) is altered by the current or past presence of one or more other chemicals which may or may not be capable of producing a response by themselves. This case considers "sites of action," such as vital target sites and target enzymes. (Murphy, 1981, as seen in Moskowitz et al., 1983).

Studies of chemical interactions affecting the conceptus at times appear to have been designed on an ad hoc basis, with little thought given to pharmacokinetic or pharmacologic principles. Although we currently have only a very modest ability to predict interactive effects even when we know a great deal about the agents involved, we should still be able to use study designs based on basic pharmacologic principles. An effort in this direction has been made by Skalko and Kwasigroch (1983). They designated one member of each pair of test chemicals as the "primary" developmental toxicant and the other as the "secondary" toxicant. In their protocol, the primary agent is given at a wide range of dose levels in a pilot study. Then a minimally effective dose level is selected and combined with a subthreshold level of the secondary agent. Treatment is given when the test animals (mice) are at a susceptible stage of gestation. The sequence of treatment requires administration of the secondary agent at one of the following times in relation to dosing with the primary agent: 3 hours or 1 hour before, concurrently with, or 1 hour or 3 hours after.

Little is yet known regarding the relative sensitivity of such timing for testing a broad range of combinations. Different combinations may require different test protocols (cf., Ritter, 1984), but we currently lack the knowledge to tailor protocols for individual combinations. Nevertheless, use of a protocol such as that proposed by Skalko and Kwasigroch (1983) may allow detection of a variety of possible interactive effects.

The outcome of exposure to more than two chemical agents (or to chemicals plus adverse environmental factors, such as dietary deficiencies, e.g., Singh and Hood, 1985, 1986) has received very little attention. Specific protocols for such tests remain to be developed, but the likelihood of obtaining useful information from studies of multiple factors decreases in proportion to the numbers of possible combinations examined. Such studies are likely to be employed only in specific cases of great interest, but there is evidence that simultaneous exposure to three developmental toxicants could result in a high incidence of malformed offspring (21 percent), even when the individual agents given separately at these dose levels were associated with no more than 1 percent malformations (Wilson, 1964).

6.
PREIMPLANTATION EFFECTS

Ronald D. Hood

It has been widely accepted that in the majority of cases when embryos are exposed to toxic insult prior to implantation, they either die or they recover and develop normally (Wilson, 1973, 1977a; Bell and Glass, 1975; Miller, 1983; Karkinen-Jaaskelainen, 1985; Persaud, 1985). It has also been assumed that this all-or-none type of response is due to the regulative abilities of mammalian embryos and the relative similarities and totipotency of their cells in the earliest stages of development. An insult occurring prior to implantation would thus be likely to damage many or all of the embryo's cells to a similar degree. If the damage is too great, the embryo loses all or at least too many of its cells and is killed; if not, it recovers. Surviving embryos repair their damaged cells and replace dead cells with counterparts that still have the potential to develop into replacements for those that are missing. Even the embryo's size can be regulated, so that an embryo that is too small may assume a normal size during further development.

There is evidence that preimplantation exposure to at least some developmental toxicants can result in abnormal development or fetal or neonatal death (Spielmann, 1976; Generoso et al., 1988, 1989). In experiments with rabbits, treatment with triethylenemelamine resulted in delivery of dead offspring, but this outcome may have been due to an adverse effect on the dam's reproductive tract. Treatment with 6-mercaptopurine caused early fetal death, but the cause was unclear. In the case of 5-bromouracil, the offspring were born but died as neonates. In none of these cases were malformations seen, but numbers of litters observed were small (Adams et al., 1961). Malformations were induced in the offspring of mice exposed to high doses of vitamin A (10,000 to 30,000 International Units) 60 hours after copulation, and the high dose was associated with increased resorptions and fetal mortality (Pillans et al., 1988). When blastocytes were examined 81 hours after parental mating, no effects were seen in their visible chromosome structure or in their viability, cell number, or mitotic index. Such findings lead the authors to conclude that the treatment effects observed may have been due to actions of maternally retained vitamin A and occurred at a later developmental stage.

Malformations have been attributed to preimplantation exposure of rabbits to cyclophosphamide, nitrogen mustard, and thalidomide (Gottschewski, 1964). Similar results were seen with cyclophosphamide in rats by Brock and von Kreybig (1964), but their results could not be reproduced by Spielmann et al. (1977). The presumed malformations reported by Brock and von Kreybig (1964) may have merely been severe developmental retardation as seen in the later study, as the embryos in both studies were examined at mid-gestation. According to Spielmann et al. (1979), the effects seen may have been due to an effect on the embryo proper or on the developing placenta.

Preimplantation irradiation with x-rays has been claimed to result in malformations in some studies. Inman and Markivee (1963) reported such effects in rabbit embryos examined on gestation day 9.5. They stated that the severely affected embryos would probably not have survived for examination at term. According to Rugh and Grupp (1959), the incidence of exencephaly was elevated in term mouse fetuses from x-irradiated dams, but Russell (1950, 1956) and Russell and Montgomery (1966) failed to find such effects. Increased prenatal mortality was seen in some of the studies with irradiated mice. Gibbons and Chang (1973) found decreased prenatal survival, as well as developmental delay, in offspring of x-irradiated rats, but observed no increase in malformations either at mid- or late gestation. Brent and Bolden (1968) failed to find any effect on development or survival of offspring of irradiated rats.

Recently, Takeuchi (1984) observed fetal deaths, decreased fetal weights, and malformations (particularly exencephalies, cleft palates, and tail anomalies) in the offspring of mice treated on gestation days 2.5, 3.5, or 4.5, but not those treated on days 0.5 or 1.5 with methylnitrosourea (MNU). The effects appeared to be dose-related and were observed in near-term fetuses, a finding later confirmed by Vogel and Spielmann (1986), who also exposed preimplantation mouse embryos to MNU. Other mutagenic compounds have been investigated by Generoso and his colleagues. Among these was ethylene oxide, which was found to induce increases in resorptions (presumably due to dominant lethal mutations) when treatment of mated female mice occurred prior to mating or at 9 or 25 hours after mating (Generoso et al., 1987). In addition to such resorptions, fetal malformations, edema, and mid- or late-gestation deaths of the offspring were seen when the agent was administered either 1 or 6 hours after mating (Generoso et al., 1987; Rutledge and Generoso, 1989).

Three additional chemical mutagens, ethyl methane-sulfonate (EMS), ethyl nitrosourea (ENU), and triethylenemelamine (TEM), were administered to female mice before mating or at 1, 6, 9 or approximately 25 hours after mating (Generoso et al., 1988). This timing corresponded to treatment of preovulatory oocytes, oviducal eggs and sperm, early pronuclear stage zygotes, pronuclear DNA synthesis stage zygotes, and two-cell embryos, respectively. ENU and TEM exposures were associated with increased death of the conceptus mainly before or around the time of implantation, regardless of the timing of exposure. Conversely, EMS treatment was effective only when exposure was primarily to oviducal eggs and sperm or early pronuclear stage zygotes and resulted in mid- and late-gestation death in addition to early resorptions. Thus, the results with EMS were similar to those found earlier with ethylene oxide. EMS, ENU, and TEM also induced "fetal defects" (not described), but EMS was said to have been considerably more effective than the latter two agents.

The studies discussed above tend to support the assumption that preimplantation embryos are vulnerable to toxic insult. They also suggest that such embryos may or may not exhibit the generally accepted all-or-none response. In some cases it appears that they may live for a portion or the whole of gestation and die at some point, or they may survive with decreased growth and/or morphologically abnormal delayed development.

Suggested mechanisms by which chemicals may cause developmental toxicity in the embryo can be found in the recent literature. According to Generoso et al. (1989), nocodozole, a compound known to induce aneuploidy by interfering with tubulin polymerization, caused high levels of peri-implantation embryonic mortality when mated mice were treated with the agent around the time of fertilization. Conversely, maternal exposure within 4 days prior to mating or between 6 and 31 hours after a 30-minute mating period had no such effect, suggesting that the metaphase II stage was uniquely susceptible. The assumption that the observed embryolethality was related to aneuploidy was supported by the finding of abnormal chromosome number in the cells of cleavage stage embryos.

Katoh et al. (1989) investigated the mechanism by which EMS and ethylene oxide caused malformations and mid- and late-gestation fetal deaths in mice. Maternal toxicity was eliminated as a factor by zygote transplantation. Cytogenetic analysis revealed no structural chromosomal abnormalities or aneuploidy, indicating that the effects seen in the conceptus may have been due to nonlethal mutations. This view was similar to that of Iannaccone et al. (1987) regarding the outcome of preimplantation exposure to methylnitrosourea. According to the results of a specific locus test, ENU exposure of mouse zygotes derived from dams carrying mutant marker genes resulted in a relatively high rate of mosaic offspring in comparison to those seen following ENU exposure of parental spermatogonial stem cells (Russell and Stelzner, 1988). This increased incidence of mutations was presumed due to either altered single strands of the maternal double helix or to copy errors. However, neither ethyl nitrosourea nor x-rays, both of which induce specific-locus mutations, result in high frequencies of mid- or late-gestation offspring mortality as seen with EMS and ethylene oxide. Thus, Katoh et al. (1989) propose that the late manifestations of developmental toxicity seen with the latter two compounds were caused by an as yet unknown genetic lesion.

Examination of surviving offspring indicated that, in some cases, malformations were induced by exposure to chemical (but probably not to physical) agents prior to implantation. Thus, although effects experimentally induced by toxic agents before implantation are often only embryo- or fetotoxic but not teratogenic, this is obviously not always the case. In either case, such effects cannot be ignored, as they would be considered a significant hazard if they occurred in humans, and potent mutagens appear to be of special concern in terms of hazard to the preimplantation conceptus.

7.
MATERNAL vs. DEVELOPMENTAL TOXICITY

Ronald D. Hood

VALIDITY OF THE CONCEPT

The possibility of maternally mediated effects on the conceptus has been experimentally investigated for a number of years. Interest in the concept, and particularly in its implications for regulation of developmental toxicants, has been heightened recently. The publication of reviews on the subject by Khera has been a major cause of both the renewed interest and some controversy over both his proposals and their practical significance (cf., Palmer et al., 1987; Schardein, 1987; Schwetz et al., 1987; Skalko et al., 1987).

In Khera's (1984b) initial paper, he proposed that increased resorption rates, low fetal body weights, and a number of common malformations and variations in mice occurred as a secondary result of maternal toxicity. Khera (1985) soon expanded his hypothesis to include similar effects in rats, hamsters, and rabbits. He arrived at these conclusions upon reviewing a number of articles from the literature in which at least some information regarding maternal toxicity was provided. According to Khera, the above-mentioned defects were rarely seen at doses that were apparently not maternally toxic, were species-specific in some cases, and often did not appear to be dose-related.

More recently, Khera (1987a,b) followed his original reviews on the topic with evaluations of the literature on human pregnancy outcomes following maternal toxic insult or endogenously caused alterations of maternal metabolism (e.g., phenylketonuria, diabetes mellitus, toxemia of pregnancy). Khera stated that maternal drug toxicity data were lacking in most of the studies he reviewed in the human literature. He nevertheless concluded that the literature supported (though only weakly) his hypothesis that mortality of the conceptus is causally related to maternal toxicity. He further proposed that because a number of the syndromes ascribed to maternal metabolic disorders and intoxications shared certain features, these features may well have a common cause. Khera suggests that this common cause is maternally mediated, although he admits that some agents that can cause significant maternal effects (e.g., methylmercury) may fail to produce the commonly seen fetal defects. He further mentions that some outcomes of maternal disease states or drug intoxications (e.g., fetal hemorrhage leading to perinatal mortality) may be specific to the disease or chemical agent. Khera also describes obviously selective developmental toxicants, such as androgens, diethylstilbesterol (DES), and thalidomide, that can act on the conceptus even in the absence of maternal toxicity.

Khera's (1984b, 1985, 1987a,b) proposal has been criticized as showing a possible association but not proving a cause-and-effect relationship. Because of the retrospective nature of Khera's studies as well as the bias against negative data in the open literature, it would be difficult to avoid a selection bias (Palmer et al., 1987). It has been further suggested that the defects Khera listed should not be used at this time as specific evidence of maternally mediated effects on the conceptus (U.S. EPA, 1986a). It can also be contended that there are possible alternative explanations for the fact that certain relatively species-specific defects are most commonly seen in association with maternal toxicity. For example, the embryo/fetus may be as resistant (either intrinsically or as the result of lower absorbed doses or insufficient levels of activating enzymes) as the dam to the adverse effects of a majority of toxic chemicals, so detectable effects on the offspring would often occur only at maternally toxic doses.

There is another possible explanation for some of Khera's findings. Certain kinds of teratogenic effects depend on interaction of the toxicant with specific receptors in the conceptus (e.g., 2,3,7,8-tetrachlorodibenzo-p-dioxin [TCDD]-induced cleft palate). Such agents are described by Khera (e.g., 1987b) and may produce defects at doses that are not maternally toxic. Cytotoxic agents, however, comprise the majority of known developmental toxicants. Such compounds are more likely to produce both maternal and developmental toxicity at similar doses, because their mechanisms of toxicity are less selective. If, as seems likely, cytotoxins are also less specific in the types of defects they cause, this could lead to results such as those of Khera (1984b, 1985, 1987a,b). Further, each species or strain tends to have certain weak links in its developmental sequences, and thus each is likely to display certain specific defects as a response to any of a wide variety of toxic insults (e.g., Palmer et al., 1987).

As a test of Khera's (1984b) hypothesis, Kavlock et al. (1985) treated pregnant mice with maternally toxic doses of ten relatively disparate compounds. There were a variety of responses seen in the offspring, but only increased incidences of supernumerary ribs (SNR) were found to be associated with maternal toxicity across a majority of the agents tested (70 percent). No such association was seen for the other end points predicted by Khera (1984b). Although the work of Kavlock et al. (1985) was not definitive, it strongly suggested that an experimental approach could be used to answer the interesting questions posed by Khera's (1984b, 1985) studies. In addition to such a priori studies, analysis of data bases collected in individual laboratories by an appropriate common protocol could be of value in addressing the issue.

In more recent studies, Chernoff and his coworkers have also addressed the issue of the role of maternal effects (Beyer and Chernoff, 1986; Chernoff et al., 1987). These workers investigated the possibility that the presence of SNR might be a useful indicator of maternal stress in the mouse and rat. They found that high doses of a chemical, sodium salicylate, were effective at inducing SNR when given on gestation day 9 to pregnant CD-1 mice or on day 10 to Sprague-Dawley rats. When gravid females were subjected to stress by physical restraint plus food and water deprivation on the above gestation days, SNR, fused ribs, and exencephalies were seen in the offspring of stressed mice, but no effects were observed in litters from similarly treated rats. The presence of SNR and extra ossification sites in fetal mice was significantly correlated with maternal weight loss during treatment. Interestingly, a slightly different method of restraint that allowed somewhat greater maternal mobility resulted in induction of SNR in mice but failed to produce exencephaly or rib fusion (Chernoff et al., 1987, description of unpublished data).

Analysis of studies such as those described above indicates that maternal toxicity may be seen with or without obvious accompanying effects on the offspring, including prenatal mortality and decreased size. This contention is supported by others as well (e.g., Francis and Farland, 1987; Hardin, 1987; Palmer, 1987; Seidenberg and Becker, 1987). It appears that a key to determining the true relationship between maternal and developmental toxicity is the use of prospective rather than retrospective approaches. Such relationships also seem to be species- and even treatment-specific, making broad generalizations difficult.

Although the topic has controversial aspects, there is little doubt that maternally mediated effects on the conceptus can be important (DeSesso, 1987). The controversy appears to be largely over such matters as their prevalence and significance (e.g., Neubert and Barrach, 1983), as well as how they can be distinguished from direct effects. In the following section, a number of additional examples of apparently maternally mediated effects will be given.

EVIDENCE FOR MATERNALLY MEDIATED EFFECTS AND PROPOSED MECHANISMS

A number of possible mechanisms for maternally mediated effects have been suggested (e.g., Beyer and Chernoff, 1986), and the following discussion will present only a few examples:

Stress-induced cleft palate in mice has been attributed to increased maternal corticosterone levels. Hemm et al. (1977) measured plasma corticosterone levels in chronically food-deprived mice and found amounts apparently adequate to induce cleft palates. Barlow et al. (1975) also reported corticosterone elevations in pregnant mice that were restrained, chilled, and food-deprived for 24 hours, and they found a positive correlation between plasma corticosterone level and incidence of cleft palate in the offspring of individual mice. Inexplicably, however, mice that were food-deprived without restraint had fetuses with a higher incidence of cleft palate than those that were both food-deprived and restrained. Also, in this group there was not a significant correlation between maternal steroid levels and fetal cleft palate. Previously, it had been reported that the fetuses of mice that were either deprived of both food and water for 48 hours or both deprived and restrained had a relatively high incidence of cleft palate (56 percent to 69 percent) (Rosenzweig and Blaustein, 1970). Those from dams restrained but fed lab diet (plus being supplied with some moisture from potatoes) had 37 percent clefting.

In a further test of the hypothesis that endogenous corticosterone elevation might be the cause of cleft palate in offspring of stressed mice, Barlow et al. (1980) found no interaction of diazepam treatment with either maternal food deprivation or corticosterone injection. Diazepam or corticosterone were also given alone. Doses of either agent causing similar incidences of palatal clefting were associated with similar maternal plasma levels of the steroid at 6 hours posttreatment, although the hormone level at 1 hour was almost twice as high in the corticosterone-injected mice.

As discussed above, Beyer and Chernoff (1986) reported that maternal immobilization (with food and water deprivation) for a specific 12-hour period during gestation could result in an increased incidence of supernumerary ribs, fused ribs, and exencephaly in their offspring. No such effects were seen in food- and water-deprived controls or in similarly treated rats.

Maternal restraint during pregnancy has also been said to have adverse effects on the postnatal growth and development of rat pups whose dams were allowed to deliver (Barlow et al., 1978). Such effects were attributed in part to maternal effects during pregnancy, as well as to effects of being reared by a stressed mother, according to data from cross-fostering experiments. In a subsequent report, the same workers described similar effects in rats, as well as decreased learning ability (Barlow et al., 1979). That such effects were stress-related was supported by the finding that restrained mothers concurrently treated with diazepam gave birth to apparently normal offspring.

Maternal restraint has also been associated with feminization of male offspring of treated rats (Ward and Weisz, 1984). This effect was attributed to decreased steroidogenic enzyme activity in the fetal testes, resulting in a lack of testosterone during the critical period for behavioral masculinization. Similar results with rats have been found in male (but not female) offspring of dams subjected to crowding, malnutrition, and other stressors (Ward, 1984). In the case of mice, maternal restraint plus heat and bright light was also said to result in behavioral effects on their offspring, but both sexes exhibited some effects (Politch and Herrenkohl, 1984). Interestingly, the demasculinization of such male offspring could be prevented by perinatal treatment with testosterone propionate (Dorner et al., 1983).

Other forms of stress have also been related to adverse fetal outcomes. Geber (1966) exposed pregnant rats to intermittent noise and visual stimuli and recorded increases in malformations and developmental delays. Similar results were reported for mice subjected to audiogenic stress by Ward et al. (1970). In a study by Briese et al. (1984), however, noise and cage vibration caused increases in retarded development, hematomas, and resorptions but no malformations. Also, Kimmel et al. (1976) failed to find evidence of developmental toxicity in mice or rats exposed at various times during gestation to high noise levels, with the exception of an increased incidence of resorptions in litters of treated mice.

Additional effects of maternal stressors that have been investigated include induction of cleft palate in mice by shipping stress (Brown et al., 1972) and a variety of adverse outcomes in several species following maternal hyperthermia (Khera, 1985). In the latter case, however, there is a controversy regarding whether or not the treatment is a direct or an indirect teratogen (Brent, 1986; Edwards et al., 1986 ; Khera, 1986).

Maternal stress has been combined with chemical teratogens in tests for potentiative effects. When immobilization of pregnant rats was combined with vitamin A intubation, the teratogenic effect of the chemical agent was apparently enhanced, but the number of litters in the group given the combined treatment was small (Hartel and Hartel, 1960). In a test using more adequate numbers of rats, Goldman and Yakovac (1963) also found potentiation of teratogenicity by maternal restraint. In this study, as little as 4.5 hours of restraint plus an otherwise sub-teratogenic dose of sodium salicylate produced litters with 29 percent malformed fetuses, and the types of malformations differed from those seen with salicylate alone. These results suggest that maternal stress may modify the effect of a direct-acting teratogen, leading to a greater incidence of defects and at times modifying their types.

Additional studies have been published with particular relevance to elucidation of mechanisms. For example, Clark et al. (1984) found that diflunisal, a nonsteroidal antiinflammatory drug, was teratogenic in rabbits, although it had not been so in rats or mice in previous studies (Nakatsuka and Fujii, 1979; Winter et al. 1981). Clark and coworkers determined that drug treatment resulted in severe hemolytic anemia in pregnant rabbits, an effect not seen in other species. Even when diflunisal was given to the does on gestation day 5, they developed an anemia that lasted for more than 10 days, although the drug was cleared by about 4 days after dosing. Under these circumstances, the offspring were found to have the same type of axial skeletal defects (fusion, misalignment, or partial agenesis of vertebrae, fusion and partial or complete agenesis of ribs) seen when treatment was given during organogenesis. Since the drug was cleared prior to the time when these defects would be expected to be initiated (day 9), and because there was little transfer of diflunisal to the embryo, it was concluded that the malformations seen following day 5 dosing were induced as a result of maternal toxicity.

In another study from the same laboratory (Clark et al., 1986), developmental toxicity was observed in rabbits treated with the antibiotic norfloxacin. As is common with rabbits dosed with antibiotics, norfloxacin-treated does typically ate less and lost body weight, presumably due to interference with the intestinal flora essential for digestion in that species. When additional groups of rabbits were given restricted diets, their offspring also exhibited effects similar to those from antibiotic-treated does. In addition, no adverse effects on the conceptus had been seen in studies with mice or rats, even at norfloxacin doses five to eight times higher than those given to the rabbits (Irikura et al., 1981; Tesh et al., 1982).

In another recent study, Moriguchi and Scott (1986) adrenalectomized pregnant mice and prevented a considerable proportion of the malformations expected when these mice were dosed with caffeine. They proposed that caffeine teratogenesis may be due to catecholamines released from the maternal adrenal glands. Their contention is supported by previous data showing that beta-adrenergic blocking agents decrease the developmental toxicity of caffeine, while pargyline (a monoamine oxidase inhibitor) or cocaine (an inhibitor of uptake of norepinephrine at the synaptic cleft) increased the effects of caffeine (Fujii and Nishimura, 1974; Fujii, 1976; Hayasaka and Fujii, 1977). Also, caffeine has been shown to increase catecholamine release (Robertson et al., 1978). A puzzling aspect of the study was the fact that while adrenalectomy greatly diminished their incidence, it failed to completely eliminate the malformations attributed to caffeine treatment. The authors postulated several explanations for this outcome. They suggested that the most likely rationale was that caffeine and maternal catecholamines had an additive effect on the limb primordium that resulted in the typical defects seen.

Further evidence for a possible role of endogenous maternal catecholamines in developmental toxicity comes from the work of Ugen and Scott (1986). They found that concurrent treatment with phenylephrine, an alpha-adrenergic agonist, enhanced the ability of acetazolamide to induce right forelimb ectrodactyly. Conversely, pretreatment with alpha-adrenergic antagonists (phenoxybenzamine or prazosin) prevented the effect of phenylephrine, and treatment with the antagonists alone decreased acetazolamide-induced ectrodactyly. The authors proposed that decreased uterine blood flow, with a consequent increase in carbon dioxide levels and a decrease in embryonic intracellular pH, may have been the mechanism by which alpha-adrenergic agents were acting.

DISTINGUISHING BETWEEN MATERNALLY MEDIATED AND DIRECT EFFECTS ON THE CONCEPTUS

In many cases it is difficult to be certain whether or not a specific example of developmental toxicity is maternally mediated. Further confounding the issue is the likelihood that in some proportion of studies the effects observed resulted from a combination of maternotoxicity and direct effects (DeSesso, 1987).

Specific biochemically or physiologically based strategies for investigating possible maternal influences have been devised, as can be seen from examples in the preceding section. Other techniques have been used, such as the intraamniotic application of test agents, in attempts to avoid maternal influences (e.g., Dostal, 1977; Dostal and Jelinek, 1979). Hassoun et al. (1984) used crosses between sensitive and insensitive strains to determine the relative degree to which the embryo and the mother influenced the developmental toxicity of a TCDD congener, and other studies have employed embryo transfers to the same end. In additional studies, involvement of specific receptors in the embryo appeared to be critical for the expression of toxicity (e.g., Pratt, 1984; Jurand, 1985).

A number of studies involving specific nutritional deficiencies have been proposed as examples of maternally mediated developmental toxicity (Clark et al., 1986). In such cases, the question remains whether the conceptus was affected by some alteration in maternal physiology or biochemistry secondary to the nutrient deficit, or whether the offspring was displaying a direct effect of the shortage of the deficient nutrient in its own tissues. In cases of overall food deprivation where specific defects (such as cleft palate) are produced, maternally mediated effects may well be at work (e.g., Hemm et al., 1977). When nonspecific end points (such as fetal weight) are altered, the fetus is likely to have been directly affected, but this is not definitive, and species or strain differences can play a role in the outcome as well.

Khera (1984b, 1985, 1987a,b) has proposed that most cases of certain malformations and variations seen in fetuses from intoxicated dams are secondary effects of some not clearly understood alteration in the maternal economy, but the case is far from proven (Kavlock et al., 1985; U.S. EPA,

1986a). Although Kavlock et al. (1985) found that supernumerary ribs were common in offspring of maternally stressed mice, and that finding has been confirmed in the mouse (Chernoff et al., 1987), similar studies in other species are essential to determine if specific end points can be discovered.

Clearly, untangling the relationships between direct effects on the embryo/fetus and placenta and indirect effects resulting from toxicity to the dam is not a simple task (DeSesso, 1987; Rogers, 1987; Skalko et al., 1987). Furthermore, it may be difficult to obtain the needed answers with one or a few standard procedures. Instead, such questions often may have to be addressed on an individualized basis.

One particular need is for better data on maternal toxicity (Schwetz and Moorman, 1987; Schwetz et al., 1987). Published studies in the field of developmental toxicology often lack information essential to the evaluation of the maternal health status. Further complicating the matter is our lack of understanding in terms of exactly which maternal toxicity end points are meaningful indicators. We also are uncertain of the relative importance of specific end points and even how often specific end points should be measured. Indeed, use of certain parameters (e.g., histopathology or weight of specific target organs) may require evaluation on a case-by-case basis (U.S. EPA, 1986a).

IMPLICATIONS OF MATERNALLY MEDIATED vs. DIRECT EFFECTS ON THE OFFSPRING

The practical implications of the presence or absence of maternally mediated effects are somewhat controversial. Several points of view have been expressed. On one hand, there is the assumption that toxicants that have developmental effects only at exposure levels that are also maternally toxic are of little consequence or concern except on the basis of their adult toxicity. The opposite opinion holds that any agent with an adverse developmental effect should be viewed with great alarm and regulated accordingly. Perhaps a more realistic point of view contends that whether or not a particular agent should be regulated as a developmental toxicant depends on two factors: (1) the significance of any long term or permanent effects on the offspring, and (2) the amount of the agent to which a pregnant mother is likely to be exposed. Thus, participants at the EPA-sponsored Consensus Workshop on the Evaluation of Maternal and Developmental Toxicity expressed the opinion that all agents found to be associated with developmental toxicity should be subjected to a hazard assessment, regardless of the presence or absence of detectable maternal toxicity (Kimmel et al., 1987).

Some agents, (e.g., ethanol, isotretinoin) can cause serious permanent effects such as mental retardation or malformation in the offspring under conditions that may cause some toxicity but little or no serious permanent damage to the mother. It seems obvious that such chemicals should be considered as developmental toxicants. Also, if the level of a given chemical to which pregnant women may be exposed is high enough to cause developmental toxicity, such an effect may be important even if there is concurrent toxicity to the mother. Again, the key question is, "What are the relative effects on mother vs. offspring?" Certainly those compounds to which the conceptus is uniquely susceptible are of major significance (Johnson, 1980b, 1984), but they are not necessarily the only agents of concern.

A further question remains: In terms of the regulator, how important is it to know whether a chemical is a direct- or indirect-acting developmental toxicant? There has been some tendency to view indirectly acting agents as of no concern. This may be reasonable in cases where it is definitely established that there are no adverse significant effects on the conceptus at exposure levels that are not maternally toxic and where pregnant women are highly unlikely ever to be exposed to toxic doses. It is also reasonable when the maternal toxicity is clearly due to species-specific effects not seen in humans. Where it is not a valid concept is the case where pregnant women will likely be exposed to doses that are adequate to cause significant developmental toxicity. Then, it matters not at all to the offspring whether it was harmed directly or indirectly; only the outcome is important in such a case.

8.
PATERNALLY MEDIATED EFFECTS

Ronald D. Hood

ARE THERE PATERNALLY MEDIATED
DEVELOPMENTAL TOXICANTS?

The possibility of effects on the conceptus following exposure of the male parent to toxic agents has been somewhat controversial and has received much less attention than have effects following exposure of pregnant females. In recent years, however, there has been increasing interest in paternal effects. This has been reflected in reviews, such as those of Schardein (1976a), Soyka and Joffe (1980), Joffe and Soyka (1981), Pearn (1983), and Brown (1985).

A number of reports of male-mediated effects have appeared in the literature over the decades, implicating a variety of toxic agents. Among the earliest were those dealing with lead. Cole and Bachuber (1914) and Weller (1915) found decreased birth weights and survival in offspring of lead-intoxicated male rabbits and guinea pigs, respectively. Stowe and Goyer (1971) reported effects on numbers of pups per litter, birth weight, and pup survival to weaning of rats following either paternal or maternal chronic lead exposure (1 percent lead in the diet) and additive effects when both parents were lead exposed. Leonard et al. (1973), however, found no such effect on the offspring of mice given lead in their drinking water at levels up to 1 g/L.

Ethanol has also received consideration as a possible paternally mediated developmental toxicant. In an early paper, Stockard (1913) described fetal and neonatal loss in the offspring of alcohol-treated male guinea pigs, but his results were not replicated by others in guinea pigs (Durham and Woods, 1932) or mice (MacDowell et al., 1926a,b; MacDowell and Lord, 1927). More recently, Badr and Badr (1975) found increased prenatal death in the offspring of ethanol-treated male mice, while Randall et al. (1982) found no such effects.

Pfeifer et al. (1977) reported increased pup deaths occurring in rats sired by alcohol-treated males. Klassen and Persaud (1979), also described increased early prenatal mortality in litters sired by alcohol-exposed male rats, but the number of litters from treated males was small (6), and the sire's body weight was considerably decreased in the treated group. Tanaka et al. (1982) found decreased fetal weight and litter size of rats mated to alcohol-treated males, but again the treated males gained considerably less body weight than did the controls. Male rats were also exposed to ethanol by Mankes et al. (1982), who reported more embryonic mortality and decreased pup weights in litters from the treated males (whose body weights were not decreased). Additionally, they reported malformations, such as microcephaly, microphthalmia, cranioschisis, and hydronephrosis. According to Nelson et al. (1988), rat pups from sires exposed by inhalation to ethanol had altered brain norepinephrine levels, while changes were found in 5-hydroxytryptamine and Met-enkephalin levels in the brains of offspring if either parent was ethanol-exposed. No behavioral effects were seen in this study.

These results suggest a considerable variability in response of the conceptus to paternal alcohol exposure. The effects may have been influenced by a number of factors, such as species, strain, and treatment mode and dose, but there are enough positive results to indicate that real treatment effects were likely.

Lutwak-Mann (1964) reported decreased fertility and offspring survival in rabbits sired by thalidomide-treated males. Two malformed offspring were sired by one of the test males. Only six males were evaluated, and the results may have been confounded by the males' ages, but they are suggestive of an adverse effect. Conflicting results in two rat strains were reported by Husain et al. (1970), who used small numbers of litters and observed high death rates even in control litters.

Cyclophosphamide has also been used in efforts to produce male-mediated effects. For example, Trasler et al. (1985, 1986) and Hales et al. (1986b) found increased pre- and postimplantation loss, malformations, and decreased fetal weight in litters sired by treated rats. Hales et al. (1986b) also reported that the effect was reversible following cessation of treatment. Other tests with cyclophosphamide focused on behavioral effects in the progeny, and positive results were reported by Adams et al. (1984) and Auroux and Dulioust (1984), both using rats.

Decreased pup survival in rats has also been seen in the case of paternal treatment with methadone or morphine, and methadone also resulted in decreased pup weights (Soyka and Joffe, 1980; Joffe and Soyka, 1981). Similar findings with regard to pup weight were reported for morphine in mice by Friedler (1985). Soyka and Joffe suggested that the effects of exposure of males to narcotics on survival of their offspring may be caused by a treatment-related decrease in testosterone levels. Soyka et al. (1980) supported this hypothesis with the finding that concurrent administration of testosterone to methadone-treated male rats increased the survival of their offspring.

Urethane (Nomura, 1982) and x-rays (Kirk and Lyon, 1984) have been said to induce malformations in mouse embryos following exposure of the sire. On the other hand, when male mice were exposed to low doses of cadmium, no effects were seen on the offspring (Zenick et al., 1982). This was also true of mice exposed to mixtures of 2,4-dichlorophenoxyacetic acid (2,4-D), 2,4,5-trichlorophenoxyacetic acid (2,4,5-T), and 2,3,7,8-tetra-chlorodibenzo-p-dioxin (TCDD) (Lamb et al., 1981). An epidemiologic study of TCDD-exposed male workers also failed to find significant effects on their offspring (Townsend et al., 1982).

POSSIBLE MECHANISMS OF ACTION

Studies such as those described above substantiate the belief that exposure of the male parent to toxicants can result in deleterious effects on the offspring. Such effects are most often manifested as decreased survival or growth, but malformations have been observed in some cases following treatment with genotoxic agents. The cause of paternally mediated effects is not well established (Joffe and Soyka, 1981). Nevertheless, it is assumed that most such effects are due to mutations or chromosomal aberrations induced in male gametes (Brown, 1985). In support of this, Friedler (1985) reported heritable decrements in the body weight and maturation of offspring of morphine-treated male mice.

Epigenetic effects appear to be a less likely cause, but they may be acting in cases involving nongenotoxic agents, such as ethanol (Brown, 1985). Although other mechanisms, such as transfer of chemicals in semen, have been proposed (Joffe and Soyka, 1981; Mann and Lutwak-Mann, 1982), there is little evidence in their support (Brown, 1985). Hales et al. (1986a) found an increase in preimplantation loss in litters sired by male rats that had been given cyclophosphamide immediately prior to mating, and radiolabel from [^{14}C]cyclophosphamide was found in the semen and in the mated females. Nevertheless, the effect seen may have been due to damage to the ejaculated sperm rather than to ova or early embryos. What is clear is that paternal effects deserve more attention from researchers until they are much better understood and their relative importance is established.

9.
EVALUATION OF BEHAVIORAL EFFECTS

Charles V. Vorhees

The relative importance of postnatally measurable functional effects caused by pre- and/or perinatal toxic insult has become increasingly evident. Such end points can be broadly categorized as behavioral effects, which result from damage to the nervous system, and other functional effects, such as compromised function of the heart, kidneys, lungs, and immune system and diminished reproductive capability. Behavioral effects have been studied to a much greater extent, a fact that is reflected in the amount of material available for the current review. Nevertheless, it must be realized that other functional effects may prove to be of considerable importance as well.

IMPORTANCE OF BEHAVIORAL TERATOLOGY

The recent report by the Federation of American Societies for Experimental Biology on "Predicting Neurotoxicity and Behavioral Dysfunction from Preclinical Toxicologic Data" (FASEB, 1986) noted that behavioral analyses offer several noteworthy strengths, including that (1) "alterations in behavior provide a relatively sensitive indicator of exposure . . . ," (2) "are important because they provide information on the integration of several underlying processes and neurofunctions including motor, sensory, attention, motivation, and reactivity," and (3) "because they are noninvasive and can be used repeatedly in longitudinal studies of chronic exposure, or to study persistent effects following acute exposure" (p. 14).

The report notes evidence from Japan that has also been discussed at length previously in the United States (see review by Vorhees, 1986), that behavioral teratology testing has "indicated that [the] dose causing behavioral effects is frequently lower than that inducing teratogenicity and that behavioral disorders in the offspring of rats can be more sensitive indicators of developmental toxicity . . ." (pp. 31-32). The National Academy of Sciences report on "Toxicity Testing: Strategies to Determine Needs and Priorities" (NAS, 1984) concluded that the greatest testing needs across all classes of chemicals were "chronic studies, inhalation studies, and more complex studies . . . , e.g., neurotoxicity, genetic toxicity, and effects on the conceptus" (p. 99). For pesticides and chemicals in commerce, testing on developing animals and tests for neurobehavioral toxicity were consistently identified as the most urgently needed and for which the least data are available for health hazard assessment. The NAS (1984) report found the need for neurobehavioral toxicity testing to be the top priority for pesticides and cosmetic ingredients and third in need for chemicals in commerce. These rankings were based on lists of 12 to 30 test types identified in the various use categories.

It is clear from the FASEB (1986) report to the Food and Drug Administration on the value of behavior in toxicology and from the NAS (1984) report on the need for behavioral toxicity data for purposes of hazard assessment, that neurobehavioral toxicity research is a pressing need on the national agenda for toxicity information, and that it is particularly acute for pesticides, chemicals in commerce, and cosmetic ingredients, the first two of which are within the direct purview of the U.S. Environmental Protection Agency.

EVALUATION OF BEHAVIORAL EFFECTS

Functional teratology embraces the abnormal development of any organ or system, but the utility and importance of functional assessment has had its greatest impact in the area of neurobehavioral effects. This is because of the complexity of the nervous system and the difficulty of developing appropriate anatomical and biochemical tests that adequately survey the integrity of this organ system. The FASEB Panel noted that, at present, adequate neurochemical methods for screening the nervous system for damage are not available, nor is the functional significance of many neurochemical changes that can be detected well understood. The Panel further concluded that behavioral methods are the most appropriate for screening for nervous system injury, along with selected follow-up neuropathological examinations. With this in mind, the following summarizes the current state of the science in behavioral teratology.

Recently, the National Collaborative Behavioral Teratology Study was completed (Buelke-Sam et al., 1985b). This multiyear effort addressed a number of important issues related to evaluation of behavioral testing procedures. What follows is a summary of this large and complex project. The reader is referred to the full report for details (Buelke-Sam et al., 1985b).

1. How Useful is Behavioral Testing? Questions Addressed in the National Collaborative Behavioral Teratology Study

The questions basic to the applicability of behavioral teratology testing, as perceived when this project was planned, were formulated by Kimmel and Buelke-Sam (1985, Table 1, p. 542) as follows:

a. How reliable/reproducible are the test methods used in behavioral teratology and the data resulting from these both within and across laboratories?

b. Can the methods used detect alterations produced by known behavioral teratogens at doses below those producing other forms of toxicity?

c. Are any or all of the positive test compounds selected good candidates for use as positive control agents during further methods clarification and/or for use as positive controls in on-going screening systems?

d. How do early behavioral testing and/or multiple test interactions influence behavioral evaluation? This is a critical economic aspect of screening, i.e., can animals be scheduled for one or for all behavioral tests within a given test battery?

e. Can a behavioral test battery of five or six methods adequately sample major CNS sub-system functions, e.g., motor function, sensory system function, reactivity, learning abilities, memory, etc.?

2. Further Objectives of the National Collaborative Behavioral Teratology Study

Since not all issues could be fully addressed in a single study, questions a, b, and d became central to the Collaborative Study. From these main study goals, a series of subordinate objectives were developed. These included:

- Testing the effects of vehicle controls against untreated controls as a means of determining whether manipulations per se had significant effects on postnatal behavior, and, of crucial importance, if such effects interacted significantly with an experimental treatment to either accentuate or attenuate apparent treatment-related effects

- Testing the intralaboratory reliability of behavioral methods in terms of (1) reproducibility within laboratories across replicates within a given study (four in this protocol) and (2) reproducibility across studies (two in this project); this could be evaluated as replicate comparisons either (a) among control groups, or (b) among treatment groups.

- Testing the interlaboratory reliability of behavioral methods in terms of (1) consistency of control groups from one laboratory to the next, (2) the consistency of treatment effects from one laboratory to the next. Each of these comparisons could be made in identical studies with d-amphetamine sulfate (Study a) and methylmercuric chloride (Study b).

- Evaluation of the sensitivity of the test methods employed in the project in order to estimate the inherent variability of such tests and to use this information as a basis for calculating the magnitude of effects these tests would be likely to require if used in future test settings to detect the effects of agents of unknown behavioral teratogenicity
- Evaluation of the interactions, if any, between experimental and control groups for changes in postweaning behavior as a function of whether they did or did not receive preweaning testing, and the attendant extra handling experience such testing requires
- Evaluation of the contribution to explained experimental variance of individual progeny compared to the contribution accounted for by litter membership
- Evaluation of the inherent variability, baseline performance, and experimental responsivity of male compared to female progeny. Is one sex preferable to the other in reflecting prenatal central nervous system (CNS) injury?

These subordinate objectives are further discussed in Adams et al. (1985). A discussion of the statistical methods used to extract objective answers to these questions has been presented in detail by Nelson et al. (1985).

3. Results of the National Collaborative Behavioral Teratology Study— Answers to the Initial Questions

The results of this project will be summarized as briefly as possible.

a. How reliable/reproducible are the results?

The results showed that the behavioral data were reliable and had a degree of reproducibility that equaled or exceeded some measures of physical development.

b. Can the methods detect effects at nonovertly toxic doses?

The results with methylmercury clearly showed that behavioral methods could detect effects at doses that produced no significant overt toxicity in the progeny.

c. Are there adequate positive control test agents available?

This point will be discussed below in greater detail.

d. Do early tests influence later behavior?

The answer to this question will be discussed below in detail, but the overall answer was that early testing did not interact with treatment effects to produce experience x drug interactions. Since this is potentially the most troubling aspect of this question, the answer is reassuring in that early testing does not appear to mask or unmask drug-related effects on later tests based on the Collaborative Study findings.

e. Can a test battery of five or six tests adequately sample major CNS sub-system functions?

The Collaborative Study was not able to address this question in any direct way because it was not feasible within one project to attempt the complex task of trying to compare different test batteries against one another. Such an approach is needed to adequately address this point. The adequacy of particular tests only has meaning when compared to alternative tests. It is possible to compare tests within the Collaborative Study test battery, but it is not possible to compare tests outside of the study.

4. Results of the National Collaborative Behavioral Teratology Study – Findings from the Additional Objectives

The answers to the subordinate objectives outlined above are as follows:

a. Comparisons among Control Groups

The Collaborative Study found that vehicle controls and untreated controls are not identical in their postnatal behavior. Prenatal vehicle exposure, whether it be by subcutaneous injection of saline on days 12-15 of gestation or by gavage of water on days 6-9 of gestation, produces enough stress to alter postnatal performance on some tests.

These differences were most notable on tests such as startle, and were generally small for other tests. The Collaborative Study did not, however, support the need for use of untreated controls in routine behavioral teratology studies.

b. Intralaboratory Reliability

Each laboratory showed a number of significant replicate main effects, i.e., instances in which the test animals' performance baselines shifted significantly over time. Of greater importance, however, is that there were almost no cases of replicate x treatment interaction, demonstrating that such modest changes in baselines between replicates generally had no impact on treatment-related effects, and they did not confound the experimental findings.

c. Interlaboratory Reliability

The Collaborative Study found many significant main effects due to laboratory, indicating that even with attention to procedural uniformity, different labs with different personnel can be expected to observe small, but reliable, baseline performance differences. Of greatest importance, however, is that the Collaborative Study found almost no laboratory x group interactions, demonstrating that small baseline differences between labs did not alter treatment-related effects and did not constitute an important source of experimental confounding. Both in Study a, where no treatment effects were seen, and in Study b, where effects were seen, laboratory was not an interactive variable. This indicates that lab-to-lab comparisons of behavioral data can be made, provided that there is reasonable standardization.

d. Test Sensitivity

Test sensitivity was defined as the amount of change in mean behavioral performance on a task required to be detected as significant, primarily in terms of calculation of coefficients of detection (CD). The CD is defined as the standard error of the mean of the saline control group multiplied by the value of t at a predetermined alpha level (0.05) and divided by the sample mean, with the entire quantity multiplied by 100 (Vorhees, 1985a). Using this method, it was estimated that tests of preweaning development had CDs of 9 percent-16 percent, for tests of activity values were 5 percent-25 percent, for startle values were 9 percent-38 percent, and for operant learning (correct responses) values were 3 percent-12 percent. While CD values must be adjusted for estimating differences required in multigroup studies, they demonstrate, at least in descriptive terms, that tests of behavior have sensitivities that are generally quite good, as good as those seen with measures of morphological and biochemical end points.

e. Interaction with Test Experience

The Collaborative Study demonstrated unequivocally that early testing can significantly alter postweaning behavioral performance. This was demonstrated both on the test of activity and operant conditioning. It was not surprising that some experience effects would be found—there is a vast literature in developmental psychobiology demonstrating the existence of such effects. The Collaborative Study confirmed this finding by showing significant experience main effects in the analyses of variance. What was unexpected in the outcome of the Collaborative Study analyses was (1) that so few experience main effects were found, and (2) that even fewer experience x group interactions were found. The latter constitutes the crux of the Study's findings on experience effects by demonstrating that early testing does not confound the later detection of treatment-related effects. This is a very profound finding, as it indicates that the use of expensive and complex crossover experimental designs for the detection of behavioral teratogenesis may be unnecessary.

f. Litter vs. Subject as the Unit of Analysis

One of the major conclusions to emerge from the Collaborative Study was a virtually definitive resolution of this long-standing controversy. The Collaborative Study found that the litter term was uniformly a significant source of variance on all physical, ponderal, and preweaning behavioral measures, where it could reasonably be expected. More importantly, it was also a reliably significant factor on all postweaning measures of behavior. This lays to rest this debate and shows that the litter must be statistically taken into account in all behavioral teratology experiments. This can be done by treating litter as a nesting variable within a hierarchical analysis of variance model or by using litter as the unit of experimental analysis in a standard analysis of variance or equivalent nonparametric model.

g. Male vs. Female Variability

The Collaborative Study demonstrated that for the methods used in this project, both sexes showed comparable variability, and hence, comparable detection sensitivity. Some of the treatment-related findings in fact suggested that females exhibited greater responsivity to treatment than males under certain circumstances, e.g., Study b, the startle findings. Moreover, in this example, the clearer experimental effect seen among the female progeny could not have been predicted based on simple considerations of sex-dependent baseline performance differences, i.e., those related to potential "floor" and "ceiling" effects. Thus, the Collaborative Study showed that use of only one sex of offspring is inadequate. The data clearly support the practice widely followed among behavioral teratologists of evaluating both sexes.

From the previous discussion, it should be clear that the Collaborative Study resolved many important issues relevant to the use of behavioral techniques in the detection of developmental neurotoxicity. Studies conducted in parallel with the Collaborative Study confirmed a number of the major findings of the Collaborative Study (Vorhees, 1985b,c; data from West German laboratory cited in Buelke-Sam et al., 1985a). Despite these advances, it is clear that a number of major issues in the field were not addressed by the Collaborative Study or its parallel projects. In addition, as with any good experimental investigation, the Collaborative Study raised many questions as a result of the findings obtained.

10.
ISSUES OF EXTRAPOLATION IN BEHAVIORAL TERATOLOGY

Donald E. Hutchings

ISSUES OF EXTRAPOLATION

A major consideration in attempting to extrapolate from lower organisms to humans is the recognition of fundamental species-specific differences in biobehavioral processes. For example, borrowing from an interpretive issue in teratology, Skalko (1985a) has emphasized that our current risk assessment strategy is predicated on the assumption that homologous pharmacokinetic mechanisms exist between humans and commonly used test species. Yet evidence to support this assumption is generally lacking. Thus, for a given test compound, studies in comparative pharmacokinetics are essential to determine similarities and differences between the test species and man with respect to the way in which the compound or active metabolite is delivered to the putative site of action.

Similarly, many behavioral processes are tacitly assumed to be homologous between species but may, in fact, be controlled by entirely different mechanisms. For example, both humans and rats attach to the mother's nipple in order to suckle and ingest milk. Attachment in the human infant is largely under the control of tactile stimulation, whereas in the rat, olfactory cues predominate. Another component of suckling is the amount of sucking pressure the infant is able to produce which, in turn, determines the amount of milk ingested over time. Possibly, for both rat and man, as well as other mammalian species, the motor component governing suckling pressure shares a common central nervous system (CNS) motor control mechanism, thereby affording more direct and relevant comparisons.

COMPARISON OF NEUROBEHAVIORAL EFFECTS IN HUMANS AND ANIMALS

The accumulated and emerging evidence from both human and animal observations suggests that there are certain neurobehavioral outcomes that can and cannot be produced by exposure to xenobiotics during pregnancy. With respect to the serious, chronic psychotic disorders of childhood, including infantile autism, schizophrenia, and major depression, the available epidemiologic data have yet to implicate any prenatal chemical exposure as causal. Of course, it is possible that adequate clinical or epidemiologic studies with thorough and accurate prenatal drug histories have yet to be carried out. Therefore, we can only say that, to date, the evidence fails to support such a relationship. But it is essential to appreciate that animal studies are highly unlikely to model or predict frank psychotic outcomes— or at least those that include delusions, hallucinations, and thought and language disorders.

Of the kinds of outcomes that can be produced by prenatal exposure to drugs, alcohol, and the opioids, those caused by heroin and methadone afford the most interesting comparisons between human and animal findings. Because each of these compounds has been reviewed in detail elsewhere (Hutchings, 1983, 1985; Hutchings, 1987; Hutchings and Fifer, 1986; Meyer and Riley, 1986), only a brief synopsis will be presented here.

The most serious and debilitating neuropsychiatric effects associated with prenatal drug exposure are the generalized cognitive deficits collectively referred to as "mental retardation." This disorder typically includes markedly delayed developmental milestones, significantly below average intellectual functioning with limited speech, and inability to comprehend abstract questions. Associated problems include impaired adaptive functioning, particularly in areas of learning and social interactions.

Of several prenatally administered compounds that can produce mental retardation, alcohol (causative agent in the fetal alcohol syndrome or FAS), has been the most thoroughly studied. The data indicate that alcohol exerts a continuum of developmentally toxic effects, ranging from mild to severe. These include hyperactivity, distractibility, deficits in attention and reaction time, reduced speed of performance, and mild to severe cognitive deficits.

The more recent studies with animals have clearly demonstrated that prenatal administration of alcohol is developmentally toxic, producing, as in humans, both dysmorphogenesis and long-term neurobehavioral impairment. Moreover, the behavioral effects described in the offspring resemble effects observed clinically in affected children: developmental delays, hyperactivity, and inhibitory deficits.

Heroin and methadone provide particularly interesting comparisons, because, unlike alcohol, neither appears to be teratogenic; that is, the combined animal and human data indicate that none of the opioids produce dysmorphogenesis. They do, however, produce in humans a neonatal abstinence syndrome that appears to reflect a nonspecific increase in CNS arousal. This syndrome includes hyperactivity, hyperexcitability, hyperacusis, sleeplessness, tremors, and prolonged high-pitched crying. Though these acute symptoms subside within 3-6 weeks, they are followed by a secondary or subacute withdrawal that persists for 4-6 months and includes restlessness, agitation, tremors, and sleep disturbance. Long-term follow-up studies of children who were exposed prenatally to methadone tend to find that on developmental scales, they score within the normal range. At four years of age, no consistent differences were found on several standard measures of cognitive performance. Studies do suggest, however, that these children are at risk of developing an attention deficit disorder accompanied by impaired fine motor coordination. Though they are described as being restless and impulsive when performing structured tasks, they are not, by contemporary diagnostic criteria, hyperactive. Thus, comparing relative risk of alcohol and the opioids, alcohol produces far more serious and debilitating chronic neurobehavioral impairment.

In rats prenatally exposed to methadone, our laboratory found a prolonged sleep disturbance analogous to the subacute withdrawal described among human neonates. Though the interpretation of adult animal data derived from behavioral studies is extremely controversial (Hutchings and Fifer, 1986), our laboratory found no remarkable neurobehavioral effects that persisted into adulthood. Thus, the clinical observation that prenatal alcohol exposure poses more developmental hazard than does maternal abuse of opioids clearly correlates with the animal findings.

11.
NONBEHAVIORAL FUNCTIONAL EFFECTS

Ronald D. Hood

Many of the initial studies of the postnatally observable consequences of pre- or perinatal toxic insult were behavioral evaluations, but a number of other areas have been investigated. These include a wide variety of physiological parameters, such as reproductive, neurological, renal, cardiac, hepatic, and immunological functions, as well as various biochemical end points. A number of these areas will be discussed below.

REPRODUCTIVE FUNCTION

Reproductive toxicology is a broad research area in its own right, and it would require an extensive review, comparable to the current document, to do it justice. The state-of-the-art in assessment of reproductive toxicity and our current knowledge of reproductive toxicants have received several recent reviews (e.g., McLachlan et al., 1981; Rao et al., 1981; Christian and Voytek, 1983; Dobson and Felton, 1983; Koeter, 1983; Mattison, 1983; Mattison et al., 1983; Meistrich, 1983; Nisbet and Karch, 1983; Smith, 1983; Hendrickx, 1984; Overstreet, 1984; Prasad, 1984; Wyrobeck et al., 1984; Yanagimachi, 1984; Mattison et al., 1985; Steinberger and Lloyd, 1985; U.S. Congress, Office of Technology Assessment, 1985; Amann, 1986; Clegg et al., 1986; Lamb, 1986; Witorsch, 1986; Zenick and Clegg, 1986; Ewing and Mattison, 1987; Hirshfield, 1987; Rao and Gibori, 1987).

Relatively few chemical substances have been unequivocally shown to adversely affect the developing reproductive system (Steinberger and Lloyd, 1985). This is especially true in the case of prenatal exposure alone, but this may be due in large measure to a lack of appropriate studies (McLachlan et al., 1981). Additionally, the number of possible end points to be monitored is relatively large in the case of reproductive toxicity, especially considering that testing would be required in both sexes.

It has been established that pre- or perinatal exposure to physical agents can adversely affect reproductively related functions in both sexes. Ionizing radiation, which acts by destroying oocytes, is an example. The period of sensitivity appears to vary by species and by developmental stage. Some species, such as the squirrel monkey, are sensitive prenatally. Others (e.g., mice and rats) are more sensitive postnatally, while still others (e.g., macaques and man) fail to show germ cell loss unless exposed to relatively high doses of X- or gamma rays (Dobson and Felton, 1983).

Oocyte loss in mice has been seen following administration of toxic chemicals, and in some cases (e.g., with methylcholanthrene or benzo[a]pyrene), exposure during pregnancy resulted in greater effects on the fetus than on the mother (Felton and Dobson, 1982). That such effects can result in decreased adult fertility of transplancentally treated mice has recently been shown in the case of lead by Wide (1985). Destruction of oocytes or blockage of their production in the fetus can apparently lead to premature ovarian failure (Mattison et al., 1983).

Prenatal human exposure to diethylstilbestrol (DES) has been found to alter structure and function of both the female and male reproductive systems, presumably due to its estrogenic properties (Steinberger and Lloyd, 1985). These authors point out that although the evidence for decreased fertility in prenatally DES-exposed women is ambiguous, they clearly have been shown to be at significantly greater risk for ectopic pregnancy, spontaneous abortion, or premature delivery. Their offspring experience an increased incidence of perinatal death. Animal studies cited by Steinberger and Lloyd (1985) give further evidence of the adverse effects of DES on reproductive structure and function in both sexes following either transplacental or neonatal exposure.

Exposure of female rats, either pre- or postnatally, to the estrogen agonist-antagonist clomiphene has been found to cause alterations in the reproductive tract (e.g., Clark and McCormack, 1977; McCormack and Clark, 1979; Morishita et al., 1979). Persistent estrus has also been reported following exposure of the neonatal rat (Leavitt and Meisner, 1967; Gellert et al., 1971). It is also well known that pre- and perinatal exposure to any of a number of other synthetic sex hormones can result in masculinization of female and feminization of male offspring. Such agents include danazol, cyproterone, and medroxyprogesterone acetate (Steinberger and Lloyd, 1985).

A variety of additional chemical agents have also been found to affect development of the reproductive system and in some cases cause abnormal reproductively related functions (e.g., altered gonadotrophin levels) or sterility in man or laboratory animals. Examples include lead (Wiebe et al., 1982), cyclophosphamide (Parra et al., 1978; Pennisi et al., 1975), procarbazine (McLachlan et al., 1981), alkane sulfonates (Hemsworth, 1968), including busulfan (Ehling and Malling, 1968; Gaulier and Roux, 1970), and various herbicides, fungicides, and insecticides (McLachlan et al., 1981), including 1,2-dibromo-3-chloropropane (DBCP) (Lui and Wysocki, 1987).

RENAL FUNCTION

Alteration of the function of the developing kidney has received a modest degree of attention, beginning with the studies of Zeman and coworkers (Hall and Zeman, 1968; Zeman, 1968; Allen and Zeman, 1973). These studies dealt with the effects of maternal protein deprivation, however, rather than toxic insult (Zeman, 1983).

More recently, the effects of chemical toxicity on kidney development have been investigated (Kavlock and Daston, 1983). A variety of approaches were used in pregnant rodents. These resulted in detection of effects on: the fetal renal pelvis due to methyl salicylate (Woo and Hoar, 1972); organic anion uptake and capacity to bind phlorizin in renal tissue slices from pups following treatment with 2,3,7,8-tetrachlorodibenzo-p-dioxin (TCDD), dinoseb, and paraquat (Gibson, 1976); excretion of polycyclic aromatic hydrocarbons (PAHs) in neonates due to glycerol and potassium dichromate exposure (Braunlich et al., 1979); renal functional capacity after dinoseb treatment (McCormack et al., 1980); ability of pups to respond to exogenous antidiuretic hormone following maternal chlorambucil exposure and their renal structure and ability to concentrate urine after prenatal nitrogen treatment (Kavlock and Gray, 1983); and the ability of pups to clear creatinine, retain water and sodium, and excrete acids following prenatal exposure to adriamycin (Kavlock et al., 1986).

Exposure of neonates has also resulted in altered kidney structure and function. Examples include effects on a variety of renal functions in the rat due to lead (Johnson and Kleinman, 1979) or methylmercury (Chang and Sprecher, 1976) and development of polycystic kidneys due to exposure of rabbits and rodents to glucocorticoids (Crocker et al., 1983).

From the previously mentioned studies, it seems clear that both treatment of the pregnant mother and treatment of the growing pup can result in changes in the structure and function of the kidneys. Functional changes have been seen in the absence of overt structural damage, suggesting that current screening procedures for developmental toxicants will miss some cases of renal damage (Kavlock and Gray, 1983). Interestingly, it was also found in at least one instance that the critical periods for inducing defects of renal function and morphology were not completely identical (Kavlock et al., 1986). These authors also suggested that tests that strain the renal functional reserve capacity were especially useful in detecting functional toxicants and that combining tests of basal clearance with tests of concentrating ability might be advantageous in screening for effects on the developing kidney.

CARDIAC FUNCTION

The possibility that prenatal toxicity could adversely affect the developing heart was first explored experimentally by Grabowski and his colleagues. Initially, Grabowski and Tunstall (1977) reported that treatment of pregnant rats with trypan blue could result in functional anomalies that were in some cases detectable only by examination of fetal electrocardiograms. The finding of trypan blue-associated cardiac dysfunction was later confirmed by Watkinson et al. (1983). Similar studies from Grabowski's laboratory employed the fetuses of rats given Mirex in their diet (Grabowski and Payne, 1980; Grabowski and Payne, 1983a), and functional abnormality was detected in the absence of lesions detectable by either gross morphological examination or microscopic inspection of stained serial sections of the heart. Heart damage was, however, highly correlated with the incidence of fetal edema (Grabowski and Payne, 1983a).

When Mirex-treated dams were allowed to deliver, offspring that had second-degree heart block at birth invariably died within the hour, and several of the newborns with first-degree blocks died within the first day (Grabowski and Payne, 1983b). Other neonates from treated litters appeared to die from respiratory failure. Perinatal deaths were inducible if treatment was administered during late gestation, even at doses that appeared to be innocuous when given during organogenesis (Grabowski, 1983; Grabowski and Daston, 1983). Additional compounds found to be positive for effects on the electrocardiogram of neonatal rats following prenatal treatment included ethylenethiourea and sodium salicylate, while Dipterex had no such effect, even at levels lethal to 29 percent of treated dams (Grabowski, 1983).

In the neonatal rat, early lead exposure was also said to be cardiotoxic, resulting in increased likelihood of developing arrhythmia in response to norepinephrine and increased incidences of bradycardia when challenged with ouabain or procainamide (Williams and Abreu, 1983). Interestingly, these effects were seen primarily in mature rats, although lead exposure occurred via the dam's milk during lactation. Further, chemically induced changes in the timing and degree of cardiac sympathetic innervation appeared to have deleterious effects on the development of heart function, and possibly its structure as well (Slotkin, 1983).

PULMONARY FUNCTION

The lung is another major organ whose function as well as structure has been found to be vulnerable to chemical damage during development. Agents such as phenobarbital given to pregnant rabbits can apparently decrease pulmonary surfactant production in their fetuses (Karotkin et al., 1976). Both zinc deficiency (Vojnik and Hurley, 1977) and cadmium excess (Daston, 1983) have been shown to cause lung damage along with altered surfactant production in the pups of treated pregnant rats. At least in the case of cadmium, treatment doses that were not associated with other observed toxic effects were able to decrease phosphatidylcholine accumulation in fetal lungs (Daston, 1983).

Newman and Johnson (1983) reviewed the effects of prenatal vitamin A excess on rat lung development and stated that although lung structure and function were compromised, surfactant production, secretion, and composition appeared to be normal. Additionally, postnatal studies with rat pups tested up to 6 weeks following treatment of their pregnant dams with nitrogen revealed that lung function was apparently normal at 3 weeks but had become compromised by 6 weeks of age (Raub et al., 1983).

A number of tests of pulmonary function have been used to assess the possibility of perinatal toxicity. These include measurement of lung compliance, oxygen consumption, respiratory rate, and the ability to produce normal amounts of surfactant with the typical composition (Daston, 1983; Newman and Johnson, 1983). The wide range of "normal" values and the ability of the lung to compensate modest damage make detection of toxic effects difficult if only functional criteria are employed (Newman and Johnson, 1983).

IMMUNE FUNCTION

The immune system has drawn increasing interest as a possible target of chemical effects, including developmental toxicity. This newly emerging field has recently been reviewed by Schmidt (1984), and only a representative sample of pertinent studies will be discussed in the current document.

Among the first workers to state the need for immunotoxicological studies in developing systems was Pinto-Machado (1970). He treated pregnant mice with busulfan and found that the thymus glands of their offspring were hypoplastic.

DES has also been found to alter the immunocompetence of the offspring of mice treated during gestation (Luster et al., 1978, 1979) and that of individuals treated neonatally (Kalland, 1980a,b; Ways et al., 1980). Urso and Gengozian (1980) found a decreased plaque-forming cell response in the offspring of mice treated during gestation with benzo[a]pyrene, while Luster et al. (1980) reported that pre- plus postpartum treatment with TCDD compromised immune function in mice according to various criteria, including susceptibility to infection. Such a seemingly innocuous agent as corn oil has been shown to decrease the lymphocyte responsiveness of the offspring of dams treated during gestation (Schmidt and Abbott, 1983), while in utero chlordane exposure altered the immune function of mice by decreasing the nonspecific delayed hypersensitivity response (Barnett et al., 1985).

Nutrient deficiency has been said to influence the developing immune system. For example, according to Beach et al. (1982), maternal zinc deprivation throughout gestation resulted in a depressed immune response. This occurred not only in the F_1 offspring but also for two subsequent generations kept continually on a diet adequate in zinc. No mechanism for the reported carryover in response to subsequent generations is currently known (Schmidt, 1984), and further work is needed to confirm this finding.

Sufficient evidence to establish the ability of toxicants to compromise the developing immune system has already been reported. The studies to date, however, have examined a number of different end points and treatment protocols, making a coherent understanding of the implications difficult.

OTHER FUNCTIONAL EFFECTS

Functional deficits other than those discussed above have been reported in offspring following treatment of their pregnant dam with a variety of agents. For example, Christian (1983) described alteration of gastrointestinal tract para-meters, such as rectal emptying, transit time, or gastric emptying in offspring whose dams had been treated with agents such as actinomycin D, hydroxyurea, methotrexate, and Vitamin A. Such effects were attributed to possible changes in the intramural nerve plexuses of the gut, effects on the mucosal lining, or altered response of the young rats to the stress of undergoing tests of gastrointestinal function. Christian (1983) also reported results of evaluation of other functional parameters from the same study (originally reported by Christian and Johnson, 1979). They found transient anemia, an increase in nucleated erythrocytes, hypo- or hyperglycemia, increased blood urea nitrogen, and altered urine parameters.

BIOCHEMICAL PARAMETERS

Although changes at the molecular level presumably precede both functional and structural alterations in developing systems, testing for such effects is not required by regulatory guidelines. Nevertheless, a large number of studies have looked for changes at the biochemical level in animals subjected to toxic insult during development. Such research has been aimed primarily at elucidation of teratogenicity mechanisms and will not be discussed herein.

A few workers have, however, attempted to use measures of biochemical alterations as tools for detecting developmental toxicants. For instance, periodic acid-Schiff staining was used by Highman et al. (1979) to detect retardation of fetal kidney development. Andrew and Lytz (1981) briefly described a procedure for testing rats for changes in enzyme activities during the period between birth and weaning. No data were given, but a rationale for the possible utility of such tests as indicators of developmental toxicity was presented. Even such factors as differences in intrauterine environment may affect biochemical indices, however, and must be controlled if test results are to be meaningfully interpreted (Wechman et al., 1985).

12.
TRANSPLACENTAL AND PERINATAL CARCINOGENESIS

Ronald D. Hood

Transplacental carcinogenesis is a significant area of developmental toxicology. Ample evidence is available from animal models and the human experience with diethylstilbesterol (DES) to demonstrate that the fetus is at risk from chemical carcinogens. A recent study has been reported suggesting an association between maternal cigarette smoking and childhood cancers, such as Hodgkin's lymphoma, acute lymphoblastic leukemia, and Wilm's tumor (Stjernfeldt et al., 1986). Childhood brain tumors have also been associated with a number of parental chemical exposures in several studies. The relevant human and animal data have been reviewed by Rice (1973, 1976, 1979, 1981), Tomatis and Mohr (1973), Miller (1977), Mohr et al. (1980), Grice et al. (1981), Kleihues (1982), Bolande (1984), and Anderson et al. (1985). According to Anderson et al. (1985), however, we still lack the ability to quantitatively predict human risk of transplacental carcinogenesis from experimental animal data.

TRANSPLACENTAL AND PERINATAL CARCINOGENS

A variety of agents have been shown to be capable of inducing tumor formation in the offspring of laboratory animals treated during gestation. Some are much more potent than others in this regard, but the majority share an ability to bind covalently with intracellular nucleophiles, most importantly to nucleic acids. These irreversible reactions occur because of formation of electrophilic intermediates. According to Rice (1981), the greatest hazard is associated with direct-acting alkylating agents, such as methylnitrosourea (MNU). These compounds do not require enzymatic activation but spontaneously decompose under physiological conditions to yield proximate and/or ultimate carcinogens (Kleihues, 1982). Rice (1981) further states that even compounds that are among the majority of chemical carcinogens, in that they require metabolic conversion to attain carcinogenic activity, can be transplacental carcinogens. Compounds such as 7,12-dimethylbenz[a]anthracene (DMBA) are apparently activated by maternal enzymes, but their carcinogenic metabolites are stable enough to enter the fetus and initiate tumorigenesis. Maternal enzymatic activation of some carcinogens results in intermediates that are so reactive that they cannot reach the fetus. These compounds (e.g., dimethylnitrosamine, DMN) make relatively poor transplacental carcinogens, as they require activation by fetal enzymes that tend to be present at relatively low levels, if at all.

According to Kleihues (1982), N-nitrosamides, aryldialkyltriazenes, hydrazine derivatives, and DMBA are the most effective transplacental and perinatal carcinogens in animal tests. Other compounds have been evaluated as transplacental carcinogens in animals, including the N-nitrosamides, aromatic amines, and a number of polynuclear aromatic hydrocarbons. They seldom induce malignant neoplasms, but some of these agents do significantly increase the occurrence of benign tumors in mice.

In addition to activation, another element of importance in transplacental carcinogenesis is the ability to reach fetal tissues in sufficient quantities. Increased lipid solubility, which allows greater placental transfer, tends to enhance carcinogenic activity (Rice, 1976).

FACTORS INFLUENCING TRANSPLACENTAL AND PERINATAL CARCINOGENESIS

Chemical carcinogenesis is greatly influenced by developmental stage at the time of exposure. Exposure between conception and the implanting blastocyst stage results in either death or no detectable carcinogenic effect, a characteristic shared with most teratogens. During the remainder of the embryonic period, treatment of pregnant rodents with carcinogens tends to result in developmental toxicity, including malformations, but usually not neoplasia (Rice, 1981). Some studies show tumor induction due to treatment at this time (Anderson et al., 1985), but the types of tumors observed may differ from those associated with treatment with the same chemical at later stages (Rice, 1973). After about gestation day 11 or 12, however, exposure of the offspring to carcinogens becomes increasingly effective at tumor induction, producing greater numbers of tumors with decreased latency (Rice, 1981; Kleihues, 1982).

The factors that enhance the sensitivity of the fetus to chemical carcinogens are not established. Anderson et al. (1985) proposed that the high rate of cell division, the lack of complete differentiation, and the inefficiency of detoxification and immunosurveillance during the fetal stage probably contribute to susceptibility. They also mention possible initiating factors, such as lack of activating enzymes in the fetal cells and maternal and placental factors that may decrease exposure to at least some carcinogens.

These temporal relationships can be altered, as in the case of ethyl-nitrosourea (ENU) in a nonhuman primate, the Old World monkey *Erythrocebus patas* (Rice, 1981). When ENU was given to pregnant monkeys beginning on day 30 of a 170-day gestation period, it was considerably more tumorigenic to their offspring than a similar treatment given even 30 days later. If man responds like this nonhuman primate, risk may be greatest early in gestation rather than late, as is the case with rodent models. Indeed, according to Herbst et al. (1979), DES exposure did not cause vaginal tumors in women unless their transplacental exposure occurred prior to the eighteenth week of gestation. The temporal responses of primates vs. rodents are not surprising, however, if their relative states of maturity are compared.

Neonatal rodents, particularly mice, are more susceptible than adults to certain carcinogens, even though the young have lower levels of xenobiotic metabolizing enzymes (Rice, 1976, 1981; Mohr et al., 1980; Kleihues, 1982). Some test compounds, such as furylfuramide and alkyl-methanesulfonates, have been shown to be carcinogenic primarily by the transplacental route, and the same is true of DES in humans (Kleihues, 1982).

Concern has been expressed regarding the possibility of exposure to carcinogens via the mother's milk. Apparently, transfer of carcinogens and tumor production in their offspring have been observed with a variety of agents given to lactating rodents. When maternal carcinogen exposure ceases prior to delivery, there is little if any effect on the offspring (Mohr et al., 1980). This is apparently due to lack of transfer of carcinogen to the pups once maternal exposure ceases. In the case of ^{14}C-diethylnitrosamine (DEN), no radioactivity is detectable in the milk by 2 hours after treatment (Spielhoff et al., 1974).

In some cases, postnatal exposure to chemical agents following transplacental treatment with a carcinogen decreased tumor incidence. For example, chinchilla rabbits exposed in utero to ENU, followed postnatally by MNU, had fewer tumors than those given ENU alone (Dimant and Beniash-vili, 1978). Also, either *N*-butylbiguanidine or nerve growth factor given to adult rats reduced the tumor incidence expected from transplacental exposure to MNU (Alexandrov et al., 1980; Vincres and Koestner, 1982).

Conversely, transplacental or neonatal exposure to various chemicals may have effects on the outcome of postnatal exposure to carcinogens. When mice were exposed to polychlorinated biphenyls transplacentally and while nursing, they were partially protected against the tumorigenicity of postnatal exposure to DMN (Anderson et al., 1983). They appeared, however, to have a higher incidence of hepatic tumors. According to Rustia and Shubik (1979) and Boylan and Calhoon (1981), transplacentally administered DES resulted in a greater susceptibility of rodents to the carcinogenic effect of DMBA.

The mechanism(s) involved in developmental stage specificity of transplacental carcinogenesis is unknown. The differential effects seen do not result from lack of carcinogen transfer to the embryo (Kleihues, 1982), but could require that cells attain a stage of sufficient differentiation (Mohr et al., 1980). It has been suggested that rapidly proliferating tissues are more susceptible to carcinogens (Rice, 1979). Embryonic tissues also often divide rapidly, but the presence of greater numbers of potential target cells in the fetus may be important. Actually, the apparent insensitivity of the embryo vs. the fetus or neonate may at least in part be due to a lack of studies in which carcinogens are given chronically at subtoxic doses early in gestation (Anderson et al., 1985).

Lack of the embryo's ability to metabolically activate carcinogens is also an unlikely cause of refractoriness to tumor initiation. During embryogenesis, even those carcinogens that are either spontaneously activated or that are enzymatically activated by the mother prior to transfer to the offspring are as inactive transplacentally as those with highly reactive metabolites requiring in situ activation to ultimate carcinogens.

Some experimental results appeared to show an increase in the incidence of tumors in the unexposed offspring of transplacentally carcinogen-treated rats or mice. In some cases, the male or female parent alone had been exposed, while in others, both parents seemed to require carcinogen exposure (Mohr et al., 1980; Anderson et al., 1985). In certain studies, the effect appeared to extend to a second generation as well. Such events indicate a genetic alteration in immature germ cells (Kleihues, 1982; Anderson et al., 1985), a finding supported by evidence of increased tumor incidence in offspring of male rats that had been treated with ENU prior to mating (Tomatis et al., 1981).

Of further concern with regard to exposure to carcinogens during pregnancy is the possibility that the mother could have an enhanced susceptibility to carcinogens, although the evidence to date is derived from animals. Pregnant rodents given ENU or MNU had increased incidences of tumors, especially those of the reproductive organs and mammary glands (Alexandrov, 1969; Ivankovic, 1969). Perhaps, more importantly, Rice (1979) reported an increased incidence of highly malignant trophoblastic tumors that led rapidly to death in patas monkeys exposed to ENU in early pregnancy. According to Rice, "The disease resembles human choriocarcinoma both clinically and histologically, and is one of the most rapidly progressive chemically induced neoplasms ever reported in a primate." Nonpregnant females given similar ENU treatments did not develop such tumors.

CARCINOGEN BIOACTIVATION

A major factor influencing both transplacental and perinatal carcinogenesis is the ability of mother and/or offspring to metabolize those carcinogens requiring enzymatic activation. In comparison with the adult, the fetus and neonate have a relatively modest ability to enzymatically activate carcinogens (Rice, 1979), although the human fetus tends to have higher biotransforming enzyme activities than those of rodents. This should result in a lower carcinogenicity potential for compounds that are maternally biotransformed to highly reactive intermediates, although considerable variation has been seen in the ability of human fetal tissue to biotransform carcinogens (Anderson et al., 1985). In some cases, maternally activated proximate or ultimate carcinogens cannot reach the fetus before reacting with nearby molecules or spontaneously decomposing. The parent compound reaching the fetus or neonate may largely fail to be bioactivated.

Since a number of chemicals are maternally bioactivated to carcinogens that are stable enough to be transported to the fetus or the nursing offspring in their active form, such compounds can be relatively hazardous. Also, carcinogens that do not require enzymatically catalyzed activation are hazardous in proportion to the dose reaching the fetus or neonate.

The carcinogenicity of enzymatically activated (or inactivated) compounds can be influenced by the levels of the required enzyme activities. In rodents, certain biotransforming enzymes can be induced in both mother and offspring. Such induction can result in more rapid biotransformation of carcinogens to which the organism is subsequently exposed and either increase or decrease the levels of proximate or ultimate carcinogen. Exposure of pregnant mice on gestation day 15 to β-naphthoflavone, an inducer of arylhydrocarbon metabolism, decreased the transplacental tumorigenicity of 3-methylcholanthrene applied 48 hours later (Anderson and Priest, 1980). This presumably occurred because the activated carcinogen was rapidly further metabolized to inactive forms. There is no good evidence, however, that carcinogen biotransforming enzymes can be induced in the human fetus (Anderson et al., 1985).

Exposure to promoters can be a factor increasing tumor incidence in developing individuals (Rice, 1981). Tumor promotion was observed when a phorbol ester was given postnatally to mice that had been transplacentally exposed to DMBA or urethane (Goerttler and Loehrke, 1976). Using DEN and DMBA in a Solt-Farber (1976) protocol, Ogawa et al. (1982) rapidly induced altered hepatic foci in rats whose treatment was begun transplacentally. Promotion has also been shown to be of importance in the expression of transplacentally initiated skin tumors (Anderson et al., 1985).

SPECIES, ORGAN, AND AGENT SPECIFICITY

All species tested have shown susceptibility to transplacental carcinogenesis, so man is presumed to be susceptible as well (Anderson et al., 1985). Different species exposed to transplacental carcinogens tend to develop specific tumor types, but this can at times be modified by choice of strain and treatment timing (Anderson et al., 1985). Rats often have increased incidences of malignant gliomas of the central nervous system and malignant neurinomas of the peripheral nerves, with lesser numbers of nephroblastomas. Mice develop benign tumors, such as hepatomas and respiratory tract adenomas (Kleihues, 1982).

A point of conjecture is the mechanism responsible for the organ specificity of response. There appears to be a positive correlation between both the timing of appearance and the relative levels of carcinogen activating enzymes in fetal tissues and the susceptibility of such tissues to carcinogens that require bioactivation (Anderson et al., 1985). Even in the case of a carcinogen such as ENU that does not require enzymatic activation and is evenly distributed among the fetal tissues, however, tumors appear primarily in the nervous system of transplacentally exposed rats (Rice, 1981). Conversely, in neonatal mice, ENU induces tumors of the liver, kidney, and ovary, as well as the nervous system (Rice, 1976).

Relative proliferation rates have been proposed as being of significance in at least some organ-specific responses. If this is the case, other factors must account for species differences, unless relative organ proliferation rates vary considerably among various species even when gestation lengths are relatively similar (e.g., rat and mouse).

Differences in the relative abilities of various fetal organs, such as liver and brain, to repair DNA damage induced by carcinogens have been suggested as another possible mechanism to account for differing susceptibilities. The lack of a consistent correlation between lack of repair ability and tumorigenesis has, however, weakened the case for such a mechanism (Anderson et al., 1985).

Specific agents also tend to induce particular tumor types, at least within a given species. For example, while transplacental exposure of rats to ENU results mainly in gliomas and schwannomas, DMN and DEN largely induce renal tumors (Rice, 1973). The types of tumors induced in the fetus are often the same types commonly seen in the carcinogen-exposed neonate (Mohr et al., 1980) and the adult (Anderson et al., 1985), and the time to tumor is approximately the same for a given type of neoplasm in fetus, neonate, or adult (Rice, 1976). At times, however, tumor types induced by a particular agent in adults may differ considerably from those seen after exposure of the fetus or neonate (Kleihues, 1982).

Although the question has apparently not been adequately addressed in epidemiologic studies, it has been suggested that at least some tumors seen in adults may have originated due to transplacental or neonatal exposure. There is suggestive evidence to this effect from studies of emigrants: Individuals who emigrate as young adults have been found to have similar types and incidences of tumors to those of their native country, while their children are more like those of their new country (Anderson et al., 1985).

CARCINOGENESIS vs. TERATOGENESIS

The possibility that carcinogenesis is related to teratogenesis has frequently been considered in the literature since the report of Miller in 1966. The case for such a relationship is based on observations that specific neoplasms are associated with certain malformations and teratologic syndromes. Additionally, neoplasms at times arise within such developmental anomalies as vestigial structures and heterotopias. They particularly occur in hereditary hamartomas and in dysgenic gonads of individuals with abnormalities of the sex chromosomes (Bolande, 1984).

Kleihues (1982) pointed out that although many teratogens are probably not carcinogens, all known transplacental carcinogens are teratogenic. The significance of that relationship is obscure. Although both carcinogens and a number of teratogens appear to affect dividing cells, they probably act by different mechanisms. Teratogens often interfere with mitosis, but if carcinogens permanently interfered with proliferation, tumorigenesis would not result. Both carcinogenesis and teratogenesis may be responses to specific types of cell damage (Bolande, 1984), but the types are likely to differ. Further, Bolande proposes that teratogenesis may in some way predispose an individual to oncogenesis, but the mechanism is unknown. More recently, Loch-Caruso and Trosko (1985) suggested that the link between teratogenesis and carcinogenesis may involve inhibition of intercellular communication by affecting gap junctions.

13.
PHARMACOKINETIC CONSIDERATIONS IN DEVELOPMENTAL TOXICITY

Elaine M. Faustman and Paul Ribeiro

Pharmacokinetics (PK) is the study of the factors that govern the time course of the concentrations of biologically active form(s) of a compound at the active sites of target cells and involves the relationship of these concentrations to the incidence and magnitude of the biological/toxicologic response (Gillette, 1987). Four basic factors that are the fundamental determinants of the action of compounds on living tissues are absorption, distribution, biotransformation, and elimination. In this chapter, we will first highlight variables or changes in these processes that are important in the specific consideration of the pharmacokinetics of developmental toxicants. The processes and considerations critical to the formulation of models for the dynamics of events occurring during gestation will be addressed next. Specific examples of models formulated for developmentally toxic compounds will be highlighted, including a discussion of the incorporation of pharmacokinetic parameters into in vitro systems.

PHYSIOLOGICAL CHANGES DURING PREGNANCY

The pregnant state itself may alter pharmacokinetics (Juchau and Faustman-Watts, 1983; Hytten, 1984; Krauer, 1987). Our examination will discuss chemical disposition in the unborn human being. Particular attention will be focused on early changes occurring during the embryonic period (organogenesis), as it is the period of gestation that has the highest susceptibility to teratogenesis. Table 13-1 (modified from Hytten and Leitch, 1971; Hytten and Chamberlain, 1980; Juchau and Faustman-Watts, 1983; Levy, 1984; Krauer, 1987) lists the physiological variables that are known to change during pregnancy. Some of the significant changes that occur during the first trimester are footnoted.

TABLE 13-1. THE PHYSIOLOGICAL VARIABLES IN
PREGNANCY

System	Parameter	Change	Nonpregnant Adult Value (%)
Gastrointestinal	Motility	−	
	Gastric		
	Acid secretion	−	30-50
	Mucous secretion	+	
	Vomiting[a]	+	
Respiratory	Respiratory minute volume	+	
	Alveolar ventilation	+	
	Tidal volume	+	40
	Residual volume	−	20
	Pulmonary blood flow	? +	
Cardiovascular	Cardiac output	+	30-40
	Rate	+	0-20
	Stroke volume	+	10
	Peripheral blood flow	+	
	Perpiheral resistance	−	
	Skin/mucosa/epidural perfusion	+	
Renal	Plasma flow[a]	+	85[b]
	Glomerular filtration rate	+	70[b]
Metabolism	Oxygen consumption	+	15
	Body temperature	+	(0.5°C)
	Hepatic metabolism[a]	+/−	
	Extrahepatic metabolism	+	
	Placental and fetal[a]	Present	
Blood	Total volume	+	35-40
	Plasma volume	+	50
	Red cell mass	+	18
	Hemoglobin	−	
	Phospholipids	+	
	Cholesterol	+	
	Free fatty acids	+	
	Protein concentration		
	Albumin concentration[a]	−	30
	Globulin concentration	+	
	Creatinine concentration[a]	−	55
	Urea concentration	−	40
Body water	Total	+	(~7-8 L gain)
Body fat[a]		+	(~3-4 kg)

[a]Early changes occurring within first trimester.
[b]Values range up to indicated percentage.
Source: Modified from Hytten and Leitch, 1971; Hytten and Chamberlain,
1980; Juchau and Faustmann-Watts, 1983; Levy, 1984; Krauer, 1987.

110

1. Absorption

a. General

The estrogen-mediated gastrointestinal (GI) disturbances that often occur during early human pregnancy have been suggested as a potential factor in the alteration of drug absorption from the gastrointestinal tract. Nausea and vomiting can reduce translocation of compounds from the upper tract to the maternal circulation. It also results in an empty stomach, which could cause increased absorbance of subsequent compounds to which the mother is orally exposed. Pregnancy also results in reduced gastric secretions and motility (leading to constipation). Decreases in gastric hydrochloric acid secretion can result in an increase in the pH of the upper GI tract and possibly cause a decreased rate of absorption of weak acids (e.g., aspirin). Increased rates of absorption of weak bases (e.g., narcotic analgesics) due to decreased ionization would also be predicted. The observed decreases in motility could enhance absorption because of the lengthened time for complete transit.

Because absorption is dependent upon the degree of ionization of compounds, the pH of the embryo/fetal blood can be important in determining the amount of transfer of acidic and basic compounds. Studies have shown that the pH of fetal blood is less than that of maternal blood; thus concentrations of basic compounds (e.g., anesthetic agents) would be greater in fetal than maternal blood. On the other hand, lower concentrations of acidic compounds (e.g., valproic acid) would be observed in the fetal versus maternal blood (Nau, 1986a). In mammalian embryos, the pH of embryonic tissue is higher than that of maternal plasma, and this could result in accumulation of acidic drugs during the sensitive period of organogenesis (Scott and Nau, 1987). Examples of teratogens that accumulate in embryos include valproic acid, dimethadione, salicylic acid, methoxyacetic acid, and thalidomide (Scott and Nau, 1987).

Respiratory changes also occur during pregnancy, primarily in the later stages (see Chapter 14). Increases in the volume of air inspired per minute seem due to both an increase in tidal volume and an increase in alveolar ventilation. These changes, along with increased pulmonary blood flow, might enhance the absorption of inhaled substances. However, little documentation is available to substantiate these postulates or the potential effects of these factors.

b. Exposure Routes

Some consideration of exposure route differences should be included in a discussion of the pharmacokinetic considerations of absorption. Intraperitoneal (i.p.) administration of compounds has been shown to result in significantly higher embryo/fetal concentrations than most other exposure routes (Nau, 1986a). Examples of agents that show such kinetics are 2,3,7,8-tetrachlorodibenzo-*p*-dioxin (TCDD), alkylating agents, piperacillin, ethanol, and methadone (Nau, 1986a). With i.p. injection, some of the compound can enter the systemic circulation directly, while the remainder will pass through the liver (first-pass effect) prior to entering the systemic circulation. With oral routes of exposure, the majority of the compound will have a first pass through the liver. These first-pass effects, because of their dependence on hepatic metabolism, can exhibit significant species differences (Nau, 1987). In general, interspecies differences in the extent and rate of absorption are not very dramatic, because diffusion of chemicals is primarily based on physiochemical properties of an agent, resulting in similar diffusion across epithelial membranes for most species.

Dencker and Danielsson (1987) have discussed the distribution of radiolabeled, highly lipid-soluble compounds (e.g., xylene, toluene, benzene, tetrachloroethylene, trichloroethylene, halothane, chloroform) to the fetus following maternal exposure via inhalation. In these studies, the uptake of volatile radioactivity in embryonic and fetal tissues was surprisingly low compared with that of maternal organs and was shown to disappear rapidly after inhalation was discontinued. However, if the nonvolatile metabolites of the halogenated solvents were examined, these derivatives were shown to accumulate and be retained in amniotic and fetal body fluids.

Inhalation absorption kinetics were found to be very compound-specific. For example, immediately after inhalation, agents such as carbon disulfide were shown to be taken up in higher amounts in fetal tissue than in maternal brain tissues. This is in contrast to the patterns observed for the solvents discussed above (Dencker and Danielsson, 1987). Such compound-specific differences should also be observed for dermal exposure. Mattison (see Chapter 14) has discussed the pharmacokinetic considerations of dermal absorption.

The timing of gestational exposure to potential teratogens is a critical factor in determining whether a chemical will produce an effect on the embryo or fetus. Most of the attention has focused on exposure during organogenesis, undeniably the most sensitive point in the gestational period with respect to dysmorphogenesis. Much less attention has been devoted to the possible effects of exposure at much earlier and later gestational times. Recent papers have discussed the possible effects of paternal exposure prior to mating on reproductive success as well as the developmental outcome of the pregnancy (Dixon and Hall, 1982; Brown, 1985; Trasler et al., 1985). Potential routes of exposure prior to implantation could include presence of the teratogenic agent in semen (Hales et al., 1986a) or in the uterus and fallopian tubes (Spielmann and Vogel, 1987).

Significant exposure to developmental toxicants during the first week after fertilization most commonly results in the termination of the pregnancy. At this time, substances readily enter the embryo by simple diffusion. Studies with rabbit blastocysts have demonstrated that lipid-soluble drugs with a molecular weight of less than 600 daltons can rapidly traverse the membranes of the blastocyst. Studies with a number of drugs and chemicals have shown that many of them reach the blastocyst within a matter of minutes following maternal administration (Spielmann and Vogel, 1987). These findings are significant for humans, since pregnancy is usually not detected for several weeks. Such rapid equilibration of the levels of compound in the uterine fluids may lead to decreased implantation success.

At the end of gestation, exposure to the neonate can continue through direct exposure (therapeutic or environmental) or indirectly via the ingestion of breast milk (Aranda and Stern, 1983). With respect to the latter route, many environmental agents have been shown to pass readily from the maternal circulation into the breast milk. The high lipid content of the milk serves as a sink for lipid-soluble compounds.

2. Distribution

a. Protein Binding

The distribution of chemicals from the maternal circulation into organs and tissues is primarily a function of the physiochemical properties of the chemicals. However, some changes, such as decreases in plasma albumin concentrations during gestation, can increase the availability of free compound for transport. Examples of such compounds are phenylbutazone, warfarin, and salicylates. Because of this change in available protein binding sites, increased problems of drug or chemical interactions are possible, and normally nontoxic exposures could thus become highly toxic doses. Lovecchio et al. (1981) examined the binding affinity between salicylate and serum albumin during human gestation and found that the binding affinity decreased for females during pregnancy. The mean value for the association constant (k') for nonpregnant controls was 40. This constant was 32, 28, 26, 15.5, 18.4, and 37.6 for the first, second, and third trimester, labor, 4 days postpartum, and 6 weeks postpartum, respectively. Levy (1984) identified decreased serum binding for other drugs in pregnant women, including weak acids, such as sulfisoxazole and phenytoin, the weak base diazepam, and the steroid dexamethasone. Reduction of protein binding was evident at 8 to 15 weeks of gestation, became more pronounced through 26 to 29 weeks, and then remained constant for the remainder of gestation. Dexamethasone binding showed the least differences from nonpregnant binding values. Binding of valproic acid to serum proteins during pregnancy has also been investigated, and the amount of free drug was found to be almost 1.6 times that in nonpregnant controls (Nau, 1986a).

Plasma protein binding would affect the availability of compounds for transport across the placental membranes. The concentration of albumin (the predominant binding protein) has been shown to fall by approximately 10 g per liter of blood during the first half of pregnancy (Hytten, 1984). This change represents almost two-thirds of the nonpregnant level. Since only free drug is available for transport, decreased protein binding would increase the potential of compound transport. Levy (1984) discussed in detail the pharmacokinetic and pharmacodynamic implications of decreased maternal serum binding for fetal drug concentrations.

Plasma protein binding can also affect transport in the opposite direction. Binding of compounds to proteins in the fetal circulatory system would limit the elimination of compounds from this compartment and yet would theoretically maintain the concentration gradient for the diffusible form. Relative binding rates on the maternal versus embryo/fetal side are critical factors in identifying placental transport. Krasner has cited examples of how such differential protein binding can affect transplacental movement of drugs (Krasner, 1972). Nau (1986a) has extended this discussion and cites differences in valproic acid protein binding that may explain differences in species sensitivity to this teratogen.

b. Placental Considerations

In the study of environmentally induced teratogenesis, attention has been given to the possible contribution of interspecies differences in the placenta to the teratogenic outcome. Due to obvious ethical considerations, data on the effects on the human conceptus and the involvement of the maternal embryo/fetal exchange are either generally not available or limited to information obtained just prior to delivery and postpartum. These circumstances provide the impetus for studies in laboratory animals concerning the comparison of the structure and function of the placenta among animal species and how those differences relate to the teratogenicity response. Knowledge obtained from such studies may help to explain interspecies variation in teratogenic outcome and contribute to the formation of improved predictive models for human teratogenesis (Beck and Lloyd, 1977; Mattison and Jelovsek, 1987).

During most of gestation, the placenta acts not only as a support system for the endocrine and nutritional maintenance of pregnancy but also as a lipoidal impedance to the transport of compounds from maternal to embryo/fetal circulations. Transfer of compounds is thus dependent upon the physiochemical properties of the compound and especially its lipid solubility. Transfer most typically occurs via simple, passive diffusion along a concentration gradient. The outdated concept of the placenta as a "placental barrier" is misleading, since most lipid-soluble compounds will have access to the embryo/fetal compartment. However, it cannot be assumed that the rate of absorption is dependent solely on lipid solubility. Placental membranes contain several layers of cells, requiring that the substance pass through not only lipoidal phases but also aqueous phases before reaching capillary beds within the membranes. Thus, the final rate of diffusion depends on the rates for each type of phase. The rates of diffusion of substances with very high oil/water partition ratios could be limited by concentration and decreased transfer through the aqueous phases (Gillette, 1987) (Fig. 13-1).

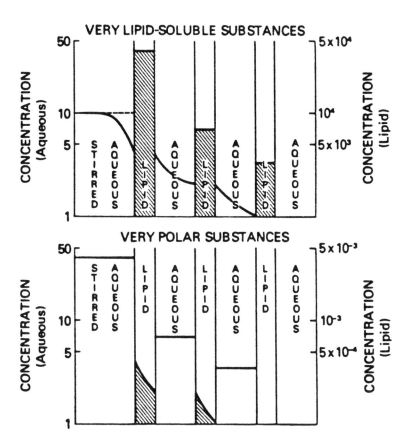

Figure 13-1. Diffusion through multilayer cell membranes. Source: Gillette, 1987.

Examples of three developmental toxicants whose placental transport is not dependent solely upon lipid solubility are valproic acid, TCDD, and retinoic acid. In the mouse, valproic acid at physiological pH is 99 percent in the ionized form, yet it rapidly crosses the placenta, and equilibrium with maternal plasma is established within 30 minutes (Nau, 1986a). In contrast, the highly lipid-soluble compound TCDD reached very low levels in both mouse embryos and fetuses (Nau, 1986a). This may be due to the low fat content of the developing organism. For another teratogen, retinoic acid, specific binding proteins have been postulated for its rapid transport across the mouse placenta (Dencker and Danielsson, 1987; Kochhar et al., 1987).

In most mammalian species, two types of placentas exist during the normal course of gestation, the yolk sac placenta and the chorioallantoic placenta. Both of those placental types provide separate and important functions during particular times of embryo/fetal development. The predominance of either placental type may be a critical determining factor in the susceptibility of the embryo to certain agents (Beck and Lloyd, 1977). During early gestation, particularly during early organogenesis, the yolk sac is the predominant organ for the exchange of nutritive materials between the mother and fetus (Garbis-Berkvens and Peters, 1987). Morphological studies have demonstrated large interspecies differences in placental type. In the rat, the yolk sac serves as a primary nutritional source up through the limb bud stage, when the chorioallantoic placenta begins to take over the majority of the nutritive functions (Beck and Lloyd, 1977; Waddell and Marlowe, 1981). Nevertheless, the rat yolk sac remains and continues to function throughout the duration of the pregnancy in a supporting role. In humans, the yolk sac degenerates at the end of the first trimester, and the chorioallantoic placenta has presumably become the primary nutritive source by the limb bud stage (Beck and Lloyd, 1977; Waddell and Marlowe, 1981; Garbis-Berkvens and Peters, 1987). Unfortunately, not much is known about the functional aspects of the human yolk sac. Such information is vital because, as in the rat, this organ may be the predominant source of nutrition to the human embryo during the early portion of organogenesis (Dencker and Danielsson, 1987; Garbis-Berkvens and Peters, 1987).

Marked species differences exist in the structural design and histology of the chorioallantoic placenta (Waddell and Marlowe, 1981). Histologically, the chorioallantoic placentas of both rats and humans have been classified as hemochorial, in that the maternal tissues are completely eroded by the invading fetal trophoblast. On the other hand, the organs of both species differ in their geometry with respect to blood flow. The human placenta is a villous type, whereas that of the rat is a labyrinthine type. Throughout most of pregnancy, the human placenta is hemomonochorial (no maternal layers, three fetal layers, including a single trophoblast layer, a mesoderm, and a capillary endothelium); during early pregnancy, however, the human organ is actually hemodichorial due to the presence of an additional trophoblastic layer, which eventually dissipates by the end of the first trimester (Miller et al., 1976; Beck, 1981; Ramsey, 1982). In the case of the rat, the placenta can be classified as hemotrichorial (three trophoblast layers, mesoderm, and capillary endothelium) throughout the major portion of gestation; in the later stages of pregnancy, one of the trophoblastic cell layers attenuates (Beck, 1981; Miller et al., 1976; Ramsey, 1982). The number of cell layers does not necessarily reflect the true distance that the substances must traverse to go from the maternal to the fetal circulation or vice versa (Waddell and Marlowe, 1981). This is especially evident in the gradual thinning of the placental membranes observed as term is approached. The human placental membrane tissues undergo a 10- to 12-fold reduction in thickness between the first trimester and term (Juchau and Faustman-Watts, 1983; Mattison and Jelovsek, 1987). This process may also differ between species.

Other transgestational changes in the placenta that should be considered are the parallel changes in surface area and fetal and maternal blood flow (Juchau and Faustman-Watts, 1983; Mattison and Jelovsek, 1987). From midgestation to term, the human placenta undergoes a 10-fold increase in surface area. Studies with pregnant sheep have demonstrated that the perfusion rate of this organ increases throughout the latter part of gestation and may amount to as much as 15 percent of the total maternal cardiac output by the latest stages. Parallel changes in membrane thickness, surface area, and perfusion rate suggest increased facilitation of transport of substances across the placental membranes as gestation approaches term. This idea has been validated in the case of the human placenta, but surprisingly, the opposite result was found in the rat. The placenta as a target organ is another area of interest (Garbis-Berkvens and Peters, 1987): The majority of the studies mentioned here have centered on the role of the placenta primarily as a barrier to the passage of xenobiotics; much less attention has been given to the valid question of how these agents may directly affect the normal functions of this organ, with special regard to nutrient transport (Beck, 1981; Miller et al., 1983; Mattison and Jelovsek, 1987). Several studies have suggested that the teratogenic substances trypan blue and cadmium may both act predominantly by affecting these functions (Williams et al., 1976; Juchau and Faustman-Watts, 1983; Miller et al., 1983). These findings are of interest in that they suggest that some xenobiotics may produce a teratogenic outcome without direct interaction with the fetus.

Care must be exercised to guard against preoccupation with anatomical differences, since few correlations have been made between functional and anatomic differences (Waddell and Marlowe, 1981; Nau, 1986a). Parallel comparison of placental transfer of drugs in different species and at comparable gestational ages are necessary to correlate observed structural differences with possible functional differences.

In a discussion of distributional factors during pregnancy, it is important to realize that some chemicals can accumulate in specific fetal tissues and organs. Examples of such compounds include the following: acetaminophen, diethylstilbestrol, and retinyl acetate, which localize in fetal liver of rats; polyhalogenated biphenyls, DDT, and diphenylhydantoin, which concentrate in fetal adrenal glands; mercury, arsenic, and L-dopa, which accumulate in the optic lens; heavy metals and tetracyclines, which incorporate into fetal bones and teeth (Ullberg et al., 1982). Most of this accumulation information is from rodent studies, and little information is available for humans. One generalization that is made for chemical accumulation is that levels tend to be higher in the fetal brain compared to the maternal brain, possibly due to the undeveloped blood-brain barrier in prenatal life.

3. Biotransformation

a. Maternal

Both increases and decreases have been reported in maternal hepatic biotransformation during pregnancy. Each compound must be examined individually. Blake et al. (1978) have shown a significant pregnancy-dependent increase in the microsomal production of a diol metabolite during early gestation. These observations are important since the early generation of reactive and potentially toxic intermediates would coincide with the times of greatest sensitivity. Data also point to the possibility that the rates of maternal biotransformation may vary as a function of the length of gestation in different species (Juchau and Faustman-Watts, 1983).

Extra-hepatic biotransformation has also been shown to change during pregnancy. Devereux and Fouts (1975) have reported that the rates of demethylation and N-oxidation of dimethylaniline and the cytochrome P450 concentrations measured in pulmonary microsomes of rabbit fetuses at the twentieth and twenty-eighth days of pregnancy were 2 times as high as the analogous preparations of adult female nonpregnant rabbits. No changes in hepatic parameters were detected. These studies suggest that not only compound-specific but also organ-specific changes during pregnancy must be determined to evaluate contributions of biotransformation to developmental toxicity. There are also important species-related differences in biotransformation (Juchau and Faustman-Watts, 1983). For example, rats have been shown to exhibit profound sex differences in metabolism, and they may be a poor model species for the study of the effects of pregnancy on drug metabolism.

b. Embryo/Fetal

Determining the capability of the embryo or fetus to biotransform xenobiotics has been the aim of many recent investigations. Generation of reactive intermediates within target tissues would obviously have important toxicologic consequences. Studies in rodents comparing fetal enzyme activities to adult enzyme activities have usually suggested that both microsomal and nonmicrosomal enzymes are very low to nondetectable during the embryonic period and low to detectable during fetal and early neonatal life (Bend et al., 1975; Neims et al., 1976; Waddell and Marlowe, 1976; Juchau, 1981). For example, various studies (Galloway et al., 1980; Filler and Lew, 1981; Legraverend et al., 1984) have demonstrated that P450-dependent biotransformation reactions can occur during very early embryogenesis and prenatal life in rodents, but rates of such reactions appear to be orders of magnitude less than those measured in hepatic preparations of mature animals. Since these rates are so low, the question of biological significance has been raised.

Surprisingly, studies using human and primate embryonic and early fetal tissues showed comparatively high rates of metabolism (Pelkonen and Karki, 1973; Pelkonen et al., 1975). A variety of P450-dependent systems (P450 NF/P450-5{P450IIIA3};P450 MP/P450-8{P450IIC9}; P450-9; P450 HFLa) were detected in human livers and adrenal glands, with relatively high specific activities during approximately the second half of the first trimester (i.e., weeks 6 through 12). Human fetal tissues were also reported to have relatively high activities for various conjugation reactions, including glutathione, sulfation, acetylation, and reductive and epoxide hydrolase reactions (Juchau et al., 1980). Glucuronyl transferase activity, another conjugation pathway, was measured only at extremely low levels in human fetal tissue (Juchau, 1981).

Research in rodents has shown that although such biotransformation pathways appear to be very low in early rodent development, inducers can elicit the precocious development of both monooxygenase and conjugative enzymes (Dutton, 1978; Filler and Lew, 1981; Juchau, 1981). Giachelli and Omiecinski have used two specific oligonucleotides to confirm previous general observations that phenobarbital (PB) can induce P450b and e (P450IIB1 and P450IIB2) mRNAs in the rat fetus by day 22 in gestation (Cresteil et al., 1982; Giachelli and Omiecinski, 1986). The levels of these mRNAs increased approximately two-fold from gestational day 21 to day 22 in PB-induced liver (Giachelli and Omiecinski, 1987). Using a "multiprobe approach," Yang et al. (1988) have suggested the presence of three constitutive P450 isozymes and one inducible form in various tissues of the rat conceptus as early as day 11 of gestation.

Studies by Nebert's group (Shum et al., 1979; Legraverend et al., 1984) and others (Juchau et al., 1985; Faustman-Watts et al., 1986) have demonstrated that the manifestation of developmental toxicity in rodent embryos is correlated with their capacity to respond to inducers. 3-Methylcholanthrene pretreatment of rat embryos in vivo in early organogenesis was shown to enhance the in vitro developmental toxicity of aromatic amines. This enhanced developmental toxicity was correlated with increased embryo metabolism of the amine to ring hydroxylated metabolites (Juchau et al., 1985; Faustman-Watts et al., 1986). Carbon monoxide inhibition studies suggested a P450-dependent pathway for this metabolism (Faustman-Watts et al., 1986).

The ontogeny of epoxide-metabolizing enzymes, such as epoxide hydrolase (EH) and glutathione S-transferases (GSTs), is also important in predicting toxicity. Utilizing cloned cDNA probes for human microsomal EH, significant levels of EH mRNA have been detected in human fetal lung, kidney, adrenal gland, and liver as early as gestation day 54 (C. Omiecinski, personal communication). Phenobarbital has been shown to induce GST within 5 days postpartum, but no induction was detected in day-22 rat fetuses (Hales and Neims, 1976). Homogenates of day-10 rat embryos and yolk sacs have been shown to have measurable GST activity toward chlorodinitrobenzene, benzo[a]pyrene-oxide, p-nitrostyrene-7,8-oxide, and aflatoxin-8,9-oxide. The embryonic/adult activity ratios varied for each substrate (Faustman et al., 1988). Human fetal liver GSTs have been shown to be active toward methyl parathion, and this activity was substantially greater than that reported for purified isozymes of rat liver GST (Radulovic et al., 1987).

Both inter- and intra-species differences in metabolism appear to be extremely important in developmental toxicity. Studies examining the human fetal hydantoin syndrome have shown that lymphocytes prepared from affected subjects (children with the syndrome) had higher rates of arene oxide detoxification than did those from unaffected children (Spielberg, 1987). These studies suggest that pharmacokinetic differences in drug metabolism can play a role in defining sensitivity to developmental toxicity. Future studies should focus on such genetic differences in metabolism and their possible role in determining sensitivity to teratogens.

c. Placental

The human placenta has been examined for biotransforming capabilities. The majority of these investigations have shown that, compared to hepatic tissues, the xenobiotic metabolizing capability of the placenta is almost negligible quantitatively unless the mother was exposed to inducing agents of the 3-methylcholanthrene (MC) type during pregnancy (Pelkonen et al., 1979; Juchau, 1980). However, Kulkarni and his colleagues have been investigating rodent and human placental tissues for alternative (non-P450-dependent) pathways of xenobiotic oxidation. They have reported activities of flavin-containing monooxygenases (Osimitz and Kulkarni, 1982), indanol dehydrogenase (Kulkarni et al., 1985), peroxidase (Nelson and Kulkarni, 1986), NADPH-Fe^{2+}-dependent lipid peroxidation (Kulkarni and Kenel, 1987), and GST (Radulovic et al., 1986).

Placentas from women who smoke exhibit aryl hydrocarbon hydroxylase (AHH) activities that are similar to those of adult rat livers (Juchau, 1976; Juchau, 1980). Substrates that are more rapidly biotransformed in vitro by such induced placental tissues include a variety of carcinogens, mutagens, and teratogens. Induction of placental enzymes by MC-type inducers has been observed to favor activational rather than inactivational pathways, but a study examining the offspring of smoking women has observed that placentas from normal infants had high levels of AHH activity in comparison with placentas from abnormal infants (Manchester and Jacoby, 1984).

In a series of pharmacokinetic studies, Slikker and his colleagues have also demonstrated the importance of placental metabolism in defining potential developmental toxicity (Slikker et al., 1982; Slikker, 1987). Their results indicate that it is the relative lack of fetal and placental metabolism of synthetic estrogens (e.g., diethylstilbestrol) and glucocorticoids (e.g., triamcinolone acetonide) as compared to the naturally occurring congeners that is at least partially responsible for their greater developmental toxicity (Slikker, 1987). Thus, the contribution of placental metabolism to teratogen activation is a topic meriting further delineation.

4. Elimination

a. Renal

The diminished plasma albumin levels and binding ability observed during pregnancy could elevate the levels of free compound, and this might result in increased excretion. Increases in renal plasma flow and glomerular filtration rate would also favor additional elimination. Renal plasma flow changes do occur during early pregnancy (Dunlop, 1981). Average renal plasma flow in nonpregnant women was determined to be 480 mL/min. Increases to as much as 840 mL/min were observed in the first 20 weeks of pregnancy. A mean flow rate of 891 mL/min has been determined at 20 to 30 weeks and 771 mL/min at 30 to 40 weeks (Dunlop, 1981). Elevation of glomerular filtration rates results in an increased filtration fraction that is proportionately more elevated than renal plasma flow. Both of these changes would function to accelerate renal excretion. Drugs such as ampicillin, digoxin, and lithium, which have predominantly renal elimination and low levels of protein binding, show increases in total clearance during pregnancy that are consistent with pregnancy-induced changes in renal pharmacokinetics (Krauer, 1987).

b. Extra-Renal

Changes in extra-renal methods of elimination have also been identified. A decrease in biliary elimination of bromosulphthalein has been observed. Pulmonary excretion of gases and volatile compounds would also be expected to be increased due to increased respiratory rate, tidal volume, and minute volume. Fecal excretion would be expected to be decreased as a result of decreased gastrointestinal motility.

c. Compensatory Mechanisms/Repair

Compensatory mechanisms and repair could be considered elimination processes or reactions on the cellular or tissue level. Cellular necrosis is a normal event during morphogenesis and plays a critical role in tissue diferentiation, organ shaping, and metamorphic processes (Menkes et al., 1970). However, when cellular necrosis occurs outside the context of normal development, as a consequence of teratogen exposure, dysmorphogenesis may result.

A common observation in teratological studies has been that localized chemically or physically induced tissue necrosis in the developing embryo may result in the malformation of the affected structures (Scott, 1977). However, this correlation between necrosis and dysmorphogenesis does not always apply to cytotoxic teratogens (Scott, 1977). A chemical may produce cell death and terata at high doses but only cell death at low doses. A second exception lies with a subset of cytotoxic agents that produce initial necrosis in exposed embryonic tissues, but no abnormality is exhibited in the same tissues at birth. These exceptions suggest the existence of a compensatory mechanism in the developing embryo that can maintain the normal developmental program in a particular tissue in the presence of some types of tissue damage (Scott, 1977).

An extreme case of such a regenerative capacity was illustrated in mouse blastocysts exposed to mitomycin C (Snow and Tam, 1979). The embryo was reduced to 10 percent of its normal size by exposure just prior to organogenesis, and within 48 hours the embryo had once again approached normal size. Pedersen (1987) cited a number of studies that provide additional evidence for the ability of the early embryo to recover from extensive tissue damage. The ability of an affected tissue to exhibit such capabilities may depend upon a number of different factors, including extent of proliferation, embryonic stage of development, individual regenerative capacity, and tissue interactions. Additional studies by Snow and colleagues with mitomycin C suggest that this compensatory hyperplasia may be induced in dysmorphogenesis as well (Snow, 1987). Tissue interactions may be a critical factor in tissue repair during morphogenetic differentiation, because the affected tissue must restore the lost cells within a narrow window of time in order to maintain structural integrity and prevent malformation

(Ritter, 1977; Neubert et al., 1980). Such a disruption in the normal schedule of developmental events could lead to a wide range of possible abnormalities. Examples of such critical windows would be neural tube closure, palatal shelf fusion, and digit formation.

A special instance of this compensatory mechanism may be DNA repair processes, especially in regard to the subset of cytotoxic teratogens that may produce their effects through the generation of critical DNA lesions (Manson, 1981; Bochert et al., 1987). Two excellent reviews of DNA repair mechanisms are available elsewhere (Hanawalt et al., 1979; Friedberg, 1985). If cells have the specific ability to remove the cytotoxic macromolecular lesion, they could eliminate the sequence of events leading to necrosis and possibly malformation. This process could also explain the increased sensitivity to cytotoxic agents by rapidly proliferating tissues, in that they do not have sufficient time to repair such damage. Very little work has been done in the evaluation of DNA repair in teratogenesis; however, embryonic rodent tissues have been shown to remove a variety of DNA adducts, including dibenzo[a,e]fluoranthene (Perin-Roussel et al., 1985), O^6-alkylguanines (Bochert et al., 1978; Muller and Rajewsky, 1983), and N^3-alkyladenine (Bochert et al., 1978). Human fetal tissues have also been shown to contain O^6-methylguanine methyltransferases, and a preliminary report suggests that this activity is inducible by certain xenobiotics (Krokan et al., 1983; D'-Ambrosio et al., 1987). Investigators have suggested that DNA modifications are a primary cause of embryotoxic effects (Bochert et al., 1987).

Unscheduled DNA synthesis was observed in ultraviolet- (UV) exposed murine oocytes (Masui and Pedersen, 1975) and blastocysts (Pedersen and Cleaver, 1975) by use of autoradiographic techniques. Additional studies have shown that oocytes are also capable of the postfertilization repair of DNA damage in spermatozoa exposed to UV and alkylating agents (Pedersen and Mangia, 1978; Generoso et al., 1979; Dean, 1983). These findings are especially significant in light of the demonstrated inability of the mature spermatozoan to repair its own DNA (Masui and Pedersen, 1975; Dixon and Lee, 1980). These findings suggested that these cells have the ability to excise UV-induced DNA changes and by analogy may be capable of "long patch" nucleotide excision repair. Other studies with UV-exposed embryos suggest that the ability to perform postreplication DNA repair may vary with developmental age (Eibs and Spielmann, 1977). Additional studies are required to determine how DNA repair capacity varies with embryonic development. Such studies should contribute to our understanding of differential sensitivity between tissues, developmental stages, and species.

PHARMACOKINETIC MODELING APPLIED TO DEVELOPMENTAL TOXICOLOGY

1. Development of Pharmacokinetic Models

The development of models for pharmacokinetics consists of two parts: choice of body regions and compartments, and formulation of the mathematical relationships to represent chemical transport, clearance, and so forth. A basic question that occurs in the initial stages of model development is how much detail is required for model generation. In practice, many body areas can be lumped together as "body regions," and many processes are simplified. Figure 13-2 shows examples of pharmacokinetic models. The number of compartments should be based on physiochemical properties of the compounds under analysis. For example, if a compound is not lipid-soluble, then a consideration of adipose tissue is less important (Bischoff, 1987). Most commonly, due to a lack of specific information on membrane transport, an assumption is made of flow limitation or perfusion limitation. This means that the amount of chemical transported across membranes is dependent on the amount of chemical delivered to the tissue or organ, hence the names "flow-limited" or "perfusion-limited" models. Previous sections have highlighted the lack of information for developmental conditions.

The time scale of PK reactions under consideration is also important for model building. This is particularly important when examining potential developmental toxicants. Are only events occurring during the first pass of blood through the body or during the first 24 hours (60 circulations/hour) of interest, or are consequences of repeated or chronic dosing of interest? In particular, information on routes of exposure is important in these considerations. Frequently, a two-compartment model can be used to discuss a semilog plot of concentration in blood versus time. The first phase observed is dominated by distribution of compound between body parts and the second phase by compound elimination (Bischoff, 1987).

Figure 13-2 shows the development of classical pharmacokinetic compartment models. Early evaluations by Jusko (1972) extended such pharmacodynamic principles to examine teratogenic outcomes. In particular, the information presented here has been adapted from an excellent discussion/review article by Young (1983), which presents pharmacokinetic modeling for teratologists. The simplest model, the one-compartment open model, is shown first (Fig. 13-2, section A.1). In this example, the compound of interest was not metabolized and was eliminated through the renal system. Thus, the concentration of this agent in the blood over time could be described with a slope equal to $-k_{BU}$, the elimination constant. To arrive at this simplification, two assumptions were made: (1) volume of distribu-

A. Single-Compartment Models
   1. One-Compartment Open Model

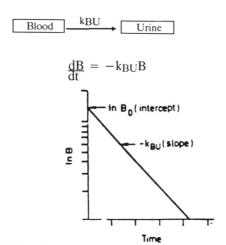

$$\frac{dB}{dt} = -k_{BU}B$$

   2. One-Compartment Model with Parallel Elimination

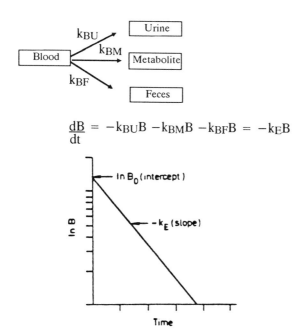

$$\frac{dB}{dt} = -k_{BU}B - k_{BM}B - k_{BF}B = -k_{E}B$$

Figure 13-2. Examples of pharmacokinetic models.
Source: Adapted from Young, 1983.

3. One-Compartment Absorption Model

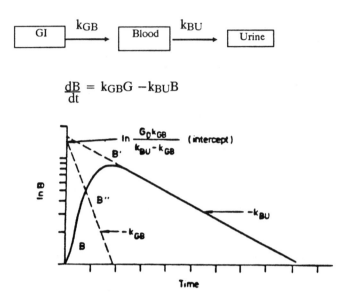

$$\frac{dB}{dt} = k_{GB}G - k_{BU}B$$

Note: Assumes rapid absorption

B. Multi-Compartment Models
1. Two-Compartment Model

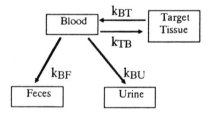

Figure 13-2 (continued).

B. Multi-Compartment Models
1. Two-Compartment Model (continued)

$$\frac{dB}{dt} = -k_{BT}B + k_{TB}T - k_{BU}B - k_{BF}B \cong -k_E B$$

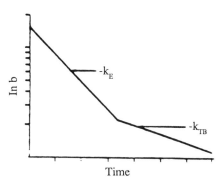

Note: $k_E = \dfrac{k_{BU} + k_{BF}}{1 + \dfrac{k_{BT}}{k_{TB}}}$, biphasic-compatible with deep compartment, $k_{TB} < < k_E$

Key:

K_{ij} = rate constant for movement from compartment i to compartment j.
Subscript = B refers to the Blood compartment
U refers to the Renal compartment (urine)
M refers to the Metabolism
F refers to the Fecal compartment
T refers to the Target Tissue compartment
G refers to the Gastrointestinal Tract
k_E = rate constant for elimination

(For a more detailed explanation, please refer to Young, 1983.)

Figure 13-2 (continued).

tion was constant throughout elimination, and (2) elimination was a first-order process. Other physiological functions, such as blood flow, pH, and renal clearance were assumed to be constant and thus not incorporated into the model. Solving the differential equations, the area under the blood concentration versus time curve can be obtained. If only urine data were available, mathematical manipulation of the equation would still allow for the determination of k_{BU}.

Figure 13-2, section A.2, shows a slightly more complex model where metabolism and fecal elimination are incorporated as parallel elimination routes. A similar approach to that described above was used to derive a differential equation, but in this example, the elimination constant (k_E) is a function of all three specified elimination routes. When a chemical follows this type of kinetics, only the disappearance of the compound from the blood (or appearance of metabolites) plus the final amounts of each elimination product would be needed to calculate all of the kinetic parameters (Young, 1983). As in the example described above, several assumptions would need to be made for this model to be appropriate. In this example, an assumption of instantaneous excretion of the metabolite (no accumulation) was made. Whenever a new situation is modeled, each of these assumptions must be carefully examined to determine if they are true. The third model, described in Figure 13-2, section A.3, shows a one-compartment absorption model and describes absorption of the compound from the gastrointestinal tract and elimination by the renal route. In this case, no metabolic pathway is considered. The log blood concentration versus time curve shown in this section makes the assumption that absorption is complete. Using several similar assumptions as described above, an estimate for the absorption constant ($-k_{GB}$) and area under the curve can be calculated. If absorption is less than 100 percent, the curve would extend above the dashed line at B', and the estimates for $-k_{GB}$ would be invalid (Young, 1983).

Multi-compartment models can also be described. Figure 13-2, section B.1, shows a simple two-compartment model. In this situation, both blood and the target tissue are modeled as compartments, and both fecal and urinary elimination are considered. The double arrows, representing rates between the blood and tissue compartments, describe an equilibrium and define the nature of the peripheral compartment (target tissue). If an equilibrium is achieved rapidly, then the peripheral compartment is referred to as a "shallow compartment" with limited capacity; if an equilibrium is never reached, or is reached very slowly, then the compartment is known as a "deep compartment." The "depth" of peripheral compartments is related to the ratio of k_{BT} and the sum of the elimination constants, k_{BF} and k_{BU}. If the rate at which the compound enters the peripheral compartment is 10 times the rate of elimination and the volume of distribution is limited, then it is a shallow compartment. Likewise, if the rate k_{BT} is less than 10 times the elimination rate and the volume of distribution in the tissue compartment is relatively large, then it is a deep compartment (Young, 1983). The graph shown in Figure 13-2, section B.1, is biphasic and compatible with a deep compartment.

Garrett (1987) discusses the embryonic/fetal compartment as a deep compartment and suggests that such a consideration can demonstrate why a substance that is harmless to the pregnant woman can be toxic to the conceptus. Upon chronic administration, such a substance would persist in the embryo/fetal compartment and would accumulate. The presence of a deep compartment would be confirmed by evidence of a very slow, constant terminal rate of elimination or metabolism and would be monitored as the rate at which the toxicant (or metabolite) would appear in the urine or feces.

An example of the application of a two-compartment model where the fetus is acting as a rapidly equilibrating, shallow compartment is the analysis of the developmental toxicity of salicylate by Kimmel and Young (1983). These investigators defined a two-compartment model with both fecal and renal routes of elimination and the formation of two metabolites, hydroxyhippuric acid and gentisic acid. Their model's predictions for teratogenic outcomes were accurate for 74 percent of the litters in the 95 percent confidence interval when they used a combination of either the k_{TB} or the 24-hour maternal blood concentration with the 45-minute maternal blood concentration.

Studies on caffeine have used a similar two-compartment model with parallel first-order elimination, but the central and peripheral compartments were not combined to fit blood concentration data points (Young, 1987). Paths of elimination included urine, feces, and the metabolites theobromine and the sum of theophylline and paraxanthine. Since only 30 percent of the administered dose of caffeine could be accounted for in urine and feces as the tri- and dimethylxanthines, an additional compartment X was used for mass balance fit. The results of pharmacokinetic analysis revealed that the teratogenic end points of number and percentage per litter of fetuses with gross malformations, specific malformations (caudal or lumbar cartilage abnormalities) or combined total malformations, or total affected per litter correlated with half-life for return from the peripheral compartment, total biological half-life, area under the blood concentration-time curve (AUC), and several specific time point concentration values (Young, 1987).

2. Physiologically Based Pharmacokinetic Modeling

Models that are developed to define the interactions between chemicals and biological tissues can range dramatically in complexity. Their complexity is dependent on the number of sites of action, parent compound versus (possibly multiple) metabolites, routes of exposure(s), paths of activation, inactivation, etc. The basic ideal of physiological pharmacokinetics (PPK) is to extend pharmacokinetic modeling so that quantitative aspects of other biological areas could be incorporated, such as known physiological differences and similarities among species, membrane biophysics, and biochemical kinetics (Bischoff, 1987). Certain similarities exist between this approach and the traditional compartmental modeling methods of mathematical biology, which are referred to as classical pharmacokinetics and are primarily oriented to the prediction of blood levels following various dosage schedules (Fig. 13-3) (Gibaldi and Perrier, 1982).

Frequently, compartments used in classical PK are based only on abstract mathematical constructs whose qualities are derived from curve-fitting experimental blood sample data. These models provide useful information on quantitative "operation of the body" but usually neglect specific organ levels. PPK models evaluate organ, tissue, and sometimes even intra- and extra-cellular concentrations. Utilization of known anatomical and physiological functions was proposed by Teorell as the basis for PK models in 1937 but was not pursued until computers were advanced enough to solve the type of

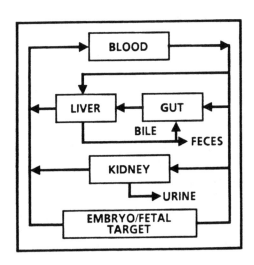

Figure 13-3. Physiological pharmacokinetic model
for gestational considerations.

differential equations formulated by Bischoff and Brown (1966). Dedrick (1973) was the first to use the term "physiological pharmacokinetics." Figure 13-4 shows the extension of PPK models to more complex PK models (Lutz and Dedrick, 1987). In this diagram, a relatively simple compartmental model for the pregnant women is presented. In addition, an expansion of the embryo/fetal target is shown, describing the interactions of parent compound or reactive metabolites with cellular/intracellular targets. Repair and elimination processes within the developing organism are also included. This figure proposes that it is the C* or biologically effective dose (critical target dose) of the developmental toxicant that needs to be quantified for accurate risk assessment.

3. Biological Basis for Physiological Pharmacokinetics

One of the applications of such physiologically based PK models (Lutz and Dedrick, 1987) has been to understand species differences. Large species differences are known to exist in sensitivity to teratogenesis and response to a number of specific teratogens, such as thalidomide, methotrexate, warfarin, glucocorticoids, valproic acid, and retinoids (Nau, 1986a). These species differences have been postulated to be due to two factors: differences in the intrinsic sensitivities of the developing tissues, and differences in the embryonic exposure during sensitive periods (Nau, 1986a). Differences in the embryonic exposures are probably due to pharmacokinetic differences in absorption, distribution, metabolism, or elimination.

Investigators have attempted to identify an orderly variation of anatomic and physiological properties that change with body weight and thus begin to account for some species differences (Bischoff, 1987). Allometry, the study of disproportionate changes in size (or function) that occur when specific features of animals are compared across species, has been used to provide the basis for such interspecies comparisons (Lindstedt, 1987). Such investigations have shown that the variation of physiological processes as the 0.7-0.8 power of body weight and other anatomic variables shows an almost first-degree dependence on body weight. Thus, investigators have devised scaling factors to account for these differences and to allow for extrapolation (Nau, 1986a; Bischoff, 1987). Purely physiochemical interactions of exogenous chemicals with biological tissues are fairly constant. For example, knowing partition coefficients can allow for prediction of tissue and blood levels across species. Qualitative differences, such as the lack of a gall bladder in some species, and dramatic differences in placental absorption can be exceptions to these generalizations. In the earlier sections of this chapter, we have highlighted some of these differences. It is hoped that more research will be done to define physiological changes during pregnancy and to

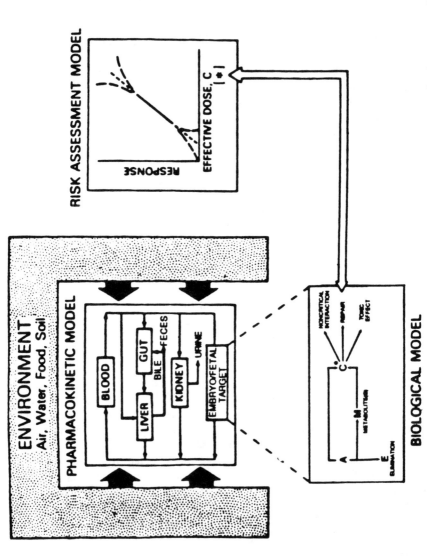

Figure 13-4. Physiological pharmacokinetic model with an expansion of the embryo/fetal target and quantitation of the critical target dose (C*) for risk assessment. Source: Adapted from Lutz and

apply this information in pharmacokinetic models in order to develop better means of risk assessment.

4. Identifying Mechanisms

The ability to correlate pharmacokinetic events with developmental toxicity end points would be a powerful tool in extrapolating adverse outcomes to other species. Relating the toxicologic effect (incidence/magnitude) to measurable pharmacokinetic parameter(s), such as maximum concentration, average concentration, minimum concentration, or total dose, would enable the investigator to begin to understand the mechanisms of toxicity and to improve both intra- and interspecies comparisons. The toxicologic response should most closely relate to the maximum concentration of the unbound biologically active form(s) when (Gillette, 1987):

- The response occurs almost instantaneously after active forms interact reversibly with receptor sites

- The response is a result of irreversible interaction of a substance (or enzyme) that turns over rapidly in the body

- Biologically active forms cause physiological or biochemical changes that exceed the capacity of homeostatic mechanisms to adjust, thus leading to irreversible damage

The toxicologic response should relate to the average concentration of unbound biologically active forms when the response is due to certain irreversible mechanisms that come into play when rates of replacement or repair of the sites of action are slow. The adverse developmental response should most closely relate to the minimum concentration of unbound active forms when the response is caused by noncompetitive, but reversible, inhibition of an enzyme that alters the concentration of a vitally important endogenous substance, or in the case of certain kinds of irreversible mechanisms (Gillette, 1987). The total dose of the biologically active forms most closely relates to the toxicologic response when that response is due to an irreversible accumulation of toxic products in the body. This response has been used to refer to transformed cells (viewed as accumulation of toxic products) that serve as clones for tumors (Gillette, 1987).

An example of a teratogen whose response has been shown to be related to the area under the concentration versus time curve is cyclophosphamide (CP) (Reiners et al., 1987). In these studies, the embryotoxicity of CP was strongly dependent on pharmacokinetic parameters. A very low, steady-state concentration of CP, maintained for a 24-hour period of infusion, was shown to be as teratogenic as a 100-times-higher peak concentration produced by injection. It has been postulated that the effects of CP are due to effects on DNA, and the pharmacokinetic observations are consistent with the hypothesis that repair of CP-induced DNA lesions are slow in comparison with processes leading to a teratogenic effect (Mirkes et al., 1983; Mirkes, 1985; Reiners et al., 1987).

Pharmacokinetic studies on valproic acid by Nau and his colleagues have shown that the total drug exposure (AUC or administered dose) did not correlate with valproic acid-induced exencephaly in the mouse (Nau, 1986b). A threshold concentration had to be reached, either by a series of short-lived drug concentration peaks or by steady-state concentrations, to produce developmental toxicity (Nau, 1986b). These pharmacokinetic studies are now being extended in primates (Mast et al., 1987).

5. In Vitro Studies: Pharmacokinetic Considerations

A variety of in vitro models have been proposed for assessing developmental toxicity (Faustman, 1988). Reasons for the development of such models include screening for potential developmental toxicants as well as establishing "simple" systems to examine mechanisms of developmental toxicity. Pharmacokinetics considerations have been incorporated into the design of such in vitro systems (Sadler et al., 1988).

Incorporation of metabolizing capacity into in vitro systems is one example. The inclusion of monooxygenase systems (Fantel et al., 1979; Kitchin et al., 1981; Faustman-Watts et al., 1983; Shepard et al., 1983) or coculture of hepatocytes in whole rodent postimplantation culture systems (Oglesby et al., 1986) are examples of such considerations. In particular, use of liver from pregnant female rodents as a source of hepatocytes is an excellent illustration of developing in vitro systems to more closely model the pharmacokinetics occurring in vivo (Oglesby et al., 1987). Others have used serum from treated humans as a source of culture medium (Chatot et al., 1980) to test the effects of "true" human metabolites. These are just a few examples of how metabolizing systems are being incorporated into in vitro systems to more closely model pharmacokinetic changes and their relationship to developmental toxicity. Other in vitro approaches to examining pharmacokinetics have taken advantage of available human tissues. Placental transport has been assessed in vitro using human term placentas; however, because of the time-specific changes occurring in placental tissue, term placentas are probably not truly representative of changes occurring during embryonic development (Schneider et al., 1972; Miller and Berndt, 1975; Miller et al., 1976).

Other in vitro approaches have included tissue dosimetry measurements in in vitro systems and comparisons to in vivo effects. Examples of this approach include recent embryo dosimetry studies with substituted phenols in vivo and in the postimplantation embryo culture system (Copeland et al., 1988) and coordinated in vivo and in vitro limb studies with alkylating agents by Bochert and his colleagues (Bochert et al., 1981). Tissue dosimetry studies where actual reactive intermediates are monitored indirectly as covalently bound reactants rather than using only administered dose levels should validate our in vitro approaches and provide better estimates of the risk for other organisms.

CONCLUDING STATEMENTS

The preceding pages have highlighted the importance of pharmacokinetic considerations in defining differences in species susceptibility to developmental toxicants. In order for us to effectively use in vivo and in vitro animal models for developmental toxicity and to extrapolate these findings to predicting human risk, pharmacokinetic considerations must be extended to the cellular and molecular levels. As illustrated by the recent number of reviews and volumes on this topic (Nau, 1986a; Mattison and Jelovsek, 1987; Nau and Scott, 1987; Young, 1987), investigators are attempting to incorporate this type of information in their explanations of differential sensitivity to developmental toxicity. It is important that such efforts not only be incorporated into in vitro studies but that they also be extended to biochemical epidemiology studies. Molecular dosimetry studies may provide the missing link in these cross-comparison studies. It is hoped that this review will stimulate and encourage researchers working in these fields to continue their important efforts in this area and that it will encourage efforts for cross-laboratory collaboration and funding.

14.
FETAL PHARMACOKINETIC AND PHYSIOLOGICAL MODELS

Donald R. Mattison

Models of many types are used in all phases of biological research (National Academy of Sciences, 1985). They are simplified rules or systems used to organize our view of structure and function. In both an experimental and theoretical sense, models are used to define responses of complex organisms or organ systems to external forces or factors. In this discussion, mathematical models that can be used to predict human risk for adverse reproductive outcome following xenobiotic exposure will be explored. Depending on their formulation, predictive models fall into one of two broad categories: qualitative or quantitative.

QUALITATIVE MODELS

Qualitative models define the system of interest in verbal or pictorial terms. For example, the illustrations in an embryology or gross anatomy text represent qualitative models. The first step in the construction of a quantitative model is frequently the establishment of a qualitative model, and in subsequent discussions we will define qualitative models of the mother, fetus, and placenta. One of the interesting developments that has occurred over the past decade, with the development of super computers and rapid techniques for parallel processing and matrix manipulations, is the ability to develop visual or graphic representations of qualitative models from complex quantitative models. These techniques have blurred the distinction between qualitative and quantitative models, and they appear to have potential in reproductive and developmental toxicology.

QUANTITATIVE MODELS

Quantitative models both require and provide numerical information. Although these models have generally been felt to be more rigorous than qualitative models, the computer methods described above have removed that distinction. The development of quantitative models that can be used to formulate qualitative models will not be described in this discussion; rather, the focus will be on two approaches to risk assessment based on quantitative models of the mother, fetus, and placenta. The two approaches explored will be classical, compartmental pharmacokinetic models and physiological-pharmacokinetic models. Also note that statistical models of the type that may have no biological basis but simply fit data to curves will not be discussed.

1. Pharmacokinetic Models

Classical pharmacokinetic models often begin with compartmental descriptions of the structure of interest. Although they are of enormous value in therapy or in situations where total body processing of a xenobiotic is of interest, these models may be limited in defining the target tissue dose of a compound. As such, these compartment models represent static images of the system at a particular time or stage of development. This should not be interpreted as suggesting that these models are of little value; on the contrary, classical pharmacokinetic models can be and have been used to provide insight into the effects of hormonal alterations, placental function, and physiological changes during pregnancy, development, and growth on xenobiotic processing and toxicity.

2. Physiological Models

Physiological models represent a useful approach to the formulation of a quantitative model of a biological process. This approach is appealing to many biologists because the models retain biological, physiological, and anatomical information as discrete entities or parameters that can be modified over time. The ability to modify the model over time is especially desirable for biologists exploring reproductive or developmental processes with changing vulnerability. Physiological models are also attractive to toxicologists because they allow a direct approach for the evaluation of target tissue toxicity and metabolic interplay between organs (e.g., maternal liver-placenta-fetal liver). Physiological models that may be of use in reproductive and developmental biology will be described, but detailed examples will not be provided.

MODELS OF THE MOTHER, FETUS, AND PLACENTA

Complex alterations in pulmonary, cardiovascular, renal, gastrointestinal, and hepatic function occur during pregnancy (Hytten and Leitch, 1971; Hytten and Chamberlain, 1980). These physiological changes during pregnancy may alter the uptake, distribution, metabolism, and clearance of xenobiotics by the pregnant woman, placenta, and fetus. Physiological alterations during pregnancy may also alter maternal response to environmental toxicants. This discussion will review physiological changes occurring during pregnancy that may alter pharmacokinetics. The effect of these changes will also be explored using classical one- and two-compartment pharmacokinetic models. The formal structure of physiological models for maternal, fetal, and placental compartments will be described but not solved.

1. Maternal Organism: One-Compartment Models

A one-compartment model will be used to describe the effect of physiological adaptations to pregnancy on xenobiotic pharmacokinetics in the mother (Fig. 14-1). In a one-compartment model, pharmacokinetic

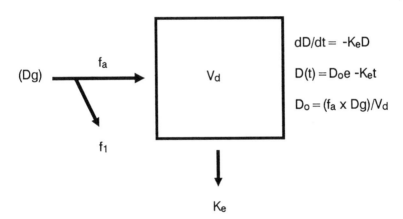

Figure 14-1. One-compartment pharmacokinetic model, assuming exposure by intravenous ad ministration. The dose given is D_g, the fraction of the dose absorbed is f_a, and the fraction lost is f_1. The volume of distribution is V_d, and the elimination rate constant is K_e. In this model, the xenobiotic is immediately absorbed and distributed throughout the designated volume of distribution, The initial concentration of the xenobiotic in the maternal compartment is D_o. The changing concentration of the xenobiotic in the maternal compartment $D(t)$. Source: Mattison, 1986.

parameters, which can change during pregnancy, include the amount of xenobiotic absorbed, volume of distribution, and rate of elimination (Wagner, 1979).

a. Uptake

During pregnancy, physiological changes occur in several systems that can alter the rate and amount of a xenobiotic that will be absorbed. Intestinal motility is decreased and gastric emptying time is increased during pregnancy (Hytten, 1980a). This means that xenobiotics will spend a longer time in both the stomach and the small intestine. If the xenobiotic is absorbed through the small intestine, increased residence time in the stomach will act to delay the time to peak concentration in the maternal compartment. In addition, the xenobiotic may be metabolized in the stomach so that increased residence time will decrease the amount of parent compound available for absorption. If absorption is via the stomach, however, added residence time will increase the fraction absorbed. If the ingested xenobiotic passes through the stomach unaltered, the longer time in the small intestine will increase the fraction absorbed.

Pulmonary function also changes significantly during pregnancy. Although the respiratory rate (breaths per minute) is unchanged (deSwiet, 1980b), the tidal volume (the volume of air exchanged per breath) is increased from 487 to 678 mL, a 39 percent increase (Table 14-1).

This means that the amount of inhaled xenobiotics is significantly increased during pregnancy. For example, if the work environment contains arsenic at a concentration of 0.2 mg/m^3, a nonpregnant woman will inhale 0.72 mg in an 8-hour working day. During pregnancy, that same woman will inhale 1.01 mg arsenic in the course of an 8-hour day (Table 14-2). Similar increases in pulmonary dose of benzene and ethylene oxide will occur during pregnancy.

TABLE 14-1. PULMONARY FUNCTION CHANGES DURING HUMAN PREGNANCY

Function	Nonpregnant	Pregnant	Change (%)
Respiratory rate	15	16	—
Tidal volume (mL)	487	678	+ 39
Minute ventilation (mL)	7,270	10,340	+ 42
Minute O₂ uptake	201	266	+ 32
Vital capacity (mL)	3,260	3,310	+ 1

Source: Data from deSwiet, 1980a.

TABLE 14-2. PULMONARY DOSE OF SELECTED XENOBIOTICS DURING
PREGNANCY

Xenobiotic	Nonpregnant (mg)	Pregnant (mg)
Arsenic (0.2 mg/m^3)	0.72	1.01
Benzene (31 mg/m^3)	111.60	156.35
Ethylene Oxide (90 mg/m^3)	324.00	454.00

Source: Mattison, 1986.

It is not known if this change in pulmonary dose during pregnancy is responsible for increased maternal toxicity. However, a recent study (Gerhardsson and Ahlmark, 1985) suggests that women are more vulnerable to silicosis than men, a difference that may have been influenced by pregnancy. The mean duration of exposure to diagnosis was significantly ($p < 0.001$) shorter for women (20.5 ± 8.6 years) than men (28.1 ± 10.1 years). The authors do not comment on the number of pregnancies or duration of work exposure during pregnancy. However, if these women worked during pregnancy, they would be inhaling substantially greater doses of dust. Interestingly, this phenomenon of shorter latency to onset of pulmonary disease in women has also been observed in the German fire clay industry (Gerhardsson and Ahlmark, 1985).

There are also substantial changes in blood flow to different regions of the body during pregnancy. Blood flow to the hand has been said to increase approximately sixfold during pregnancy, from 3 to 18 mL/min/100 mL tissue (de Swiet, 1980a). Blood flow to the foot doubles during gestation, increasing from 2.5 to 5 mL/min/100 mL tissue. Over this same period of gestation there are only small increases in blood flow to the forearm and leg. Increased blood flow to the hand could have a significant impact on amount of xenobiotic absorbed; this will be explored using a two-compartment model.

b. Distribution

During pregnancy there are changes in body weight, total body water, plasma proteins, body fat, and cardiac output that can alter the distribution of xenobiotics (Hytten and Leitch, 1971; Hytten and Chamberlain, 1980): Maternal cardiac output increases approximately 40 percent to 50 percent by the middle of the second trimester and remains elevated throughout gestation; maternal weight increases from approximately 50 kg at the start of pregnancy to approximately 63 kg at 40 weeks; total body water increases from 25 L at the start of pregnancy to 33 L at term; maternal extracellular fluid volume increases from 11 L to 15 L over the course of pregnancy; plasma volume increases from 2.5 L to 3.8 L over the 40 weeks of gestation. Maternal body fat also increases about 25 percent during gestation (Hytten, 1980b). At the beginning of pregnancy, the maternal body contains approximately 16.5 kg adipose tissue. At 20 weeks of gestation, maternal body fat has increased to 18.5 kg and by 30 weeks to 20 kg. There may be a slight decrease in body fat over the last 10 weeks of gestation. This increase in body fat during pregnancy will increase the body burden of lipid-soluble xenobiotics during pregnancy, and may have an impact on the delivery of xenobiotics to the infant through lactation.

The increase in plasma volume and total body water during pregnancy will decrease the concentration of many xenobiotics in the maternal organism. If the volume of distribution in the nonpregnant woman is 5 L, and if 50 percent of a xenobiotic (100 mg) is absorbed, the initial concentration could be as high as 10 mg/L. Suppose that during pregnancy the volume of distribution increases to 6, 7, and 8 L at 20, 30, and 40 weeks, respectively; this increase in volume of distribution will proportionately decrease the concentration of the absorbed xenobiotic (e.g., to 8.3, 7.1, and 6.3 mg/L).

c. Metabolism

The altered hormonal milieu of pregnancy is associated with changes in hepatic and extrahepatic metabolism of xenobiotics (Lewis, 1980, 1983). In addition, metabolism by the fetus and placenta during late gestation may slightly alter maternal levels of the parent xenobiotic or its metabolites. Placental and fetal metabolism may also influence fetal or placental toxicity produced by a xenobiotic.

Using classical pharmacokinetics, Gillette (1977) has evaluated the impact of fetal metabolism on maternal and fetal levels of hypothetical xenobiotics. He suggests that fetal metabolism has only a small effect on the maternal concentration of a lipid-soluble xenobiotic that is rapidly transported into the fetal compartment. The effect of fetal metabolism may lower the fetal concentration by half. If the xenobiotic is slowly transported to the fetus, metabolism in fetal tissues may have an even greater impact on fetal concentration. With a slower rate of transport to the fetus, metabolism may reduce fetal concentrations significantly in comparison to the concentration that would be obtained if fetal metabolism does not occur. Placental metabolism may also play a similar role in altering maternal and fetal concentration of some xenobiotics.

d. Elimination

During gestation, alterations in renal blood flow, glomerular filtration rate, hepatic blood flow, bile flow, and pulmonary function may alter maternal xenobiotic elimination. Maternal renal plasma flow increases from 500 mL/min/1.73 M^2 body surface area to approximately 700 mL/min/1.73 M^2. The glomerular filtration rate also increases during pregnancy. At the beginning of gestation, the glomerular filtration rate is approximately 100 mL/min/1.73 M^2 body surface area. By mid-gestation (20 weeks) the glomerular filtration rate has increased to approximately 150 mL/min/1.73 M^2.

Both increased renal plasma flow and glomerular filtration rate will increase the elimination rate constant for xenobiotics cleared by the kidney. If the rate constant for elimination is 0.5 at the beginning of gestation and increases to 0.7 at mid-gestation and 0.9 at term, the xenobiotic will be cleared more rapidly during pregnancy. Note that use of physiological models will directly account for this change in elimination by increased renal blood flow (Finster et al., 1984a,b), while it is accounted for in pharmacokinetic models by increases in the rate constant.

Consider, for example, a xenobiotic whose volume of distribution increases in proportion to maternal weight during pregnancy, and whose rate of elimination also increases from 0.10 to 0.15 during the first trimester. As pregnancy advances, the increased volume of distribution decreases the concentration of the xenobiotic in maternal plasma. The increase in the elimination rate constant increases the rate at which the xenobiotic is cleared from the body (i.e., the slope of the log concentration vs. time is more negative). This suggests that for some xenobiotics, maternal tolerance may actually increase during pregnancy. However, increased renal clearance during pregnancy may increase toxicity to the maternal bladder epithelium by increasing the amount of xenobiotic delivered to the bladder.

2. Fetal and Maternal Organisms: Two-Compartment Models

Following the above exploration of some effects of physiological adaptation to pregnancy on pharmacokinetics in the maternal organism, it may be instructive to consider the effects of these alterations on the amount of xenobiotic reaching the fetal compartment (Fig. 14-2). The two-compartment model used is composed of maternal and fetal tissues (Wagner, 1979). Xenobiotic elimination is only through the maternal compartment. Exchange between maternal and fetal compartments occurs across the placenta.

The parameters used in defining this model are illustrated in Table 14-3. Absorption will be defined by blood flow to the hand or pulmonary function. Volume of distribution in the maternal and fetal compartments will be defined by maternal and fetal weights, respectively. The rate of elimination from the maternal compartment will be determined by renal plasma flow.

TABLE 14-3. PARAMETERS USED IN THE TWO-COMPARTMENT
PHARMACOKINETIC MODEL OF PREGNANCY

	Absorption		Distribution			Elimination
Gestation (weeks)	Hand blood flow (mL/min per 100 mL tissue)	Pulmonary function (minute volume in mL)	Maternal weight (kg)	Placental weight (g)	Fetal weight (g)	Renal plasma flow (mL/min per 1.73 M[2a])
0	3	7,270	50	-	-	500
10	4.5	7,997	51	25	8	760
20	6	8,724	54	160	310	760
30	12	9,451	59	275	1,350	680
40	18	10,340	63	380	3,500	720

[a]Body surface area.
Source: Mattison and Jelovsek, 1987.

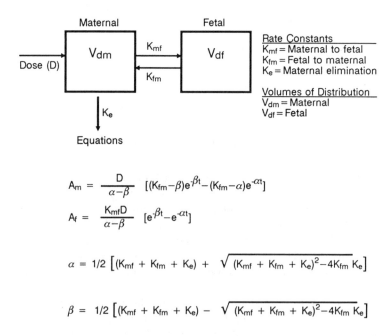

$$A_m = \frac{D}{\alpha - \beta} \left[(K_{fm} - \beta) e^{-\beta t} - (K_{fm} - \alpha) e^{-\alpha t} \right]$$

$$A_f = \frac{K_{mf} D}{\alpha - \beta} \left[e^{-\beta t} - e^{-\alpha t} \right]$$

$$\alpha = 1/2 \left[(K_{mf} + K_{fm} + K_e) + \sqrt{(K_{mf} + K_{fm} + K_e)^2 - 4 K_{fm} K_e} \right]$$

$$\beta = 1/2 \left[(K_{mf} + K_{fm} + K_e) - \sqrt{(K_{mf} + K_{fm} + K_e)^2 - 4 K_{fm} K_e} \right]$$

Figure 14-2. Two-compartment pharmacokinetic model during pregnancy.

The rate of transfer of xenobiotics between the maternal and the fetal compartment will be determined by placental weight.

a. Xenobiotic Absorbed through the Hand

During pregnancy, blood flow to the hand increases approximately sixfold. If the hand is the major site of xenobiotic absorption, there could be as much as a sixfold increase in maternal dose (Table 14-4). According to the chosen parameters, the dose absorbed through the hand could increase from 100 mg in the nonpregnant state to 600 mg at 40 weeks gestation. Over the same period, the maternal volume of distribution (V_{dm}) would increase from 5.0 L to 6.3 L, proportional to the increase in maternal blood volume. The fetal volume of distribution (V_{df}) would change from 0.0008 L at 10 weeks to 0.35 L at 40 weeks. The rate constant for elimination from the maternal compartment (K_{mo}) would increase from 5.0 to 7.2 over the 40 weeks of gestation. In this model, we will assume that transfer from the maternal to the fetal compartment occurs 10 times faster than transfer from the fetal to the maternal compartment (K_{fm}), and the rate of transfer is proportional to the placental weight. The parameters for the two-compartment model of pregnancy are summarized in Table 14-4, and the results of the calculations are summarized in Table 14-5.

TABLE 14-4. XENOBIOTIC ABSORBED THROUGH THE HAND

Gestation (weeks)	Dose absorbed (mg)	V_{dm} (L)	V_{df} (L)	K_{mf}[a] (m^{-1})	K_{fm}[a] (m^{-1})	K_{mo} (m^{-1})
0	100	5.0	-	-	-	5.0
10	150	5.1	0.0008	0.25	0.025	7.6
20	200	5.4	0.031	1.6	0.16	7.6
30	400	5.9	0.135	2.8	0.28	6.8
40	600	6.3	0.350	3.8	0.38	7.2

[a]K_{mf} is proportional to placental weight and K_{fm} is assumed to occur at a rate that is 1/10 the rate of K_{mf}.

TABLE 14-5. EFFECT OF INCREASED ABSORPTION THROUGH THE HAND[a]

Gestation (weeks)	Xenobiotic absorbed (mg)		Maximum blood concentration (mg/L) Maternal		Fetal		Maximum amount (mg) Fetal	
	+	-	+	-	+	-	+	-
0	100	100	20.0	20.0	-	-	-	-
10	150	100	29.4	19.6	5,860	3,910	4.69	3.13
20	200	100	37.0	18.5	1,050	526	32.60	16.30
30	400	100	67.8	16.9	790	198	106.00	26.70
40	600	100	95.2	15.9	537	90	188.00	31.30

[a]In the columns marked " +," maternal dose through the hand is increasing during pregnancy. In the columns marked "-," maternal dose through the hand does not change during pregnancy.

These calculations were done in two different ways. In the first series of calculations, the dose absorbed through the hand increases sixfold over the course of gestation, along with the previously defined changes in the maternal and fetal volumes of distribution, the maternal elimination rate constants, and placental transfer rates (Tables 14-3 through 14-5). In the second set of calculations, the dose absorbed is constant throughout pregnancy (100 mg), but the volume of distribution, rate of transfer, and rate of elimination are changing (Table 14-5). The maximum concentrations shown are predicted by the model, but insufficient data are available on transdermal absorption to indicate if they are realistic. Because of the increase in the dose of xenobiotic absorbed through the hand, there is an increase in concentration in the maternal and fetal compartment in comparison with that seen in the simulation where maternal dose does not increase.

With both simulations there is a distinct difference between the maternal and fetal compartments with regard to the time during gestation of peak xenobiotic concentration. Maximum concentration in the fetal compartment occurs at 10 weeks in both cases. Peak maternal concentration occurs at 0 weeks in the simulation without increasing dose, while in the simulation with increasing maternal dose, peak concentration occurs at 40 weeks.

If environmental exposure to a xenobiotic is via transdermal absorption on the hand, increasing absorption will increase the dose delivered to the fetus throughout gestation. Interestingly, this two-compartment model predicts that the maximum fetal concentration will occur early in gestation. Maternal dose, however, will continue to increase with increasing absorption through the hand, so that maximum maternal concentration will occur late in gestation at the time of maximum absorption through the hand.

b. Xenobiotic Absorption through the Lung

The two-compartment pharmacokinetic model can also be used to explore the effect of increased pulmonary dose during gestation on xenobiotic in the maternal and fetal compartments (Tables 14-3 and 14-6). In this simulation, the xenobiotic absorbed through the lung is distributed rapidly to both maternal (V_{dm}) and fetal (V_{df}) compartments. The volume of distribution in maternal and fetal compartments is proportional to maternal and fetal weights, respectively (Table 14-3). The rate of elimination from the maternal compartment (K_{mo}) is proportional to the maternal renal blood flow. Transfer between maternal and fetal compartments (K_{mf} and K_{fm}) is proportional to the placental weight. Since the xenobiotic absorbed is rapidly distributed, the rate constant for transfer between maternal and fetal compartments is assumed to be equal in both directions, but increasing with gestation.

TABLE 14-6. XENOBIOTIC ABSORBED THROUGH THE LUNGS

Gestation (weeks)	Dose absorbed (mg)	V_{dm} (L)	V_{df} (L)	K_{mf}	K_{fm}	K_{mo}
0	100	5.0	–	–	–	5.0
10	110	5.1	0.0008	0.25	0.025	7.6
20	120	5.4	0.031	0.016	0.016	7.6
30	130	5.9	0.031	0.16	0.16	6.8
40	140	6.3	0.350	0.38	0.38	7.2

In this simulation, as in the previous two-compartment pharmacokinetic simulation for absorption through the hand, there is a difference in the time during gestation at which maximum maternal and fetal concentrations are reached (Table 14-7). Maximum fetal concentrations occur early in gestation — at 10 weeks. Over the rest of gestation, fetal concentrations decrease. As expected, however, the fetal concentrations are higher in the simulation with increased pulmonary absorption.

In the maternal compartment, maximum xenobiotic concentration occurs at 0 weeks in the simulation in which increased pulmonary absorption does not occur. If pulmonary absorption increases during gestation, maximum maternal concentrations are achieved at 20 weeks and maintained at 30 and 40 weeks of gestation.

3. Placenta

In the two-compartment model defined in the previous section, the placenta was represented simply by two rate constants, one for maternal to fetal transfer and the other for fetal to maternal transfer. Although this results in algorithms that can be solved, it neglects the complex nature of the placenta as well as the role of the placenta in controlling pregnancy.

Following implantation in humans, the placenta begins to exert control on the maternal organism and becomes a dominant organ controlling growth and development of the fetus. The first signal sent by the placenta, human

TABLE 14-7. EFFECT OF INCREASED ABSORPTION THROUGH THE LUNGS[a]

Gestation (weeks)	Xenobiotic absorbed (mg)	Maximum blood concentration (mg/L)		Maximum amount (mg) Fetal	
		Maternal	Fetal		
	+	-	+	-	+	-	+	-
0	100	100	20.0	20.0	-	-	-	-
10	110	100	21.6	19.6	442	402	0.35	0.32
20	120	100	22.2	18.5	74	61	2.28	1.90
30	130	100	22.0	16.9	33	26	4.51	3.47
40	140	100	22.2	15.9	17	12	6.02	4.30

[a]In the columns marked " + ," maternal dose through the lungs is increasing during pregnancy. In the columns marked "-," maternal dose through the lungs does not change during pregnancy.

chorionic gonadotropin (hCG), stimulates continued ovarian production of progesterone. In the absence of hCG production, or in the face of ovarian inability to respond to hCG, miscarriage will occur. During implantation, the success of the pregnancy depends on interactions between the ovary and placenta. Following its establishment, the placenta will determine the success of the pregnancy, just as the dominant follicle determined the success of the menstrual cycle it controlled.

Initially during implantation, the placenta invades the endometrium, the lining of the uterus that formed under the hormonal control of the ovary. During the process of implantation, both maternal and fetal placental circulatory systems are created. The maternal portions of the placental circulation—the lobules—are poorly defined regions separated by incomplete septa in primates. The fetal portion of the placental circulation forms within cotyledons. There are generally several cotyledons within each lobule. Exchange of proteins, amino acids, carbohydrates, fats, gases, and other chemicals, including xenobiotics, occurs across the placenta (Table 14-8).

The rate constants for transfer between the maternal and fetal circulatory systems are simply measures of the rate of exchange of a chemical across the placenta and as such do not consider species differences in placental type or

TABLE 14-8. TISSUE LAYERS SEPARATING MATERNAL AND FETAL CIRCULATIONS

Placental type	Maternal Tissue			Fetal Tissue		
	Epithelium	Connective tissue	Endothelium	Trophoblast	Connective tissue	Endothelium
Epitheliochorial Pig Horse Donkey Cow	***	***	***	***	***	***
Syndesmochorial Sheep Goat	***	***	***	***	***	***
Endotheliochorial Cat Dog Ferret			***	***	***	***
Hemochorial Man Monkey				***	***	***
Hemoendothelial Guinea Pig Rabbit Rat						***

Source: Mossman, 1987.

structure. They also do not consider differences in placental structure during pregnancy or differences in fetal or maternal blood flow rates through their respective circulatory units in the placenta. These considerations limit the usefulness of purely pharmacokinetic models, but they can be addressed by physiological models.

Defining the effect of any chemical on the fetus, either directly or indirectly, requires elucidation of placental metabolism and transfer. At the present time, research using human fetal tissues from first or second trimester pregnancies is quite difficult for legal, ethical, and procedural reasons. Because of this, most research has been restricted to defining placental transfer and metabolism using the term human placenta. It is hoped that these restrictions will eventually be eased. With greater experience in defining placental function through use of the term placenta, we might then be able to better characterize placental function—transport and metabolism—in the first and second trimester human placenta.

By the third trimester, much of the structure of the fetus has been defined. During this period, however, many of the functional characteristics of the fetus are being developed. For example, cellular communication, (e.g., neuronal contact) is being developed, as is cell number in many organ systems. In addition, the fetus remains vulnerable to cytotoxic or disruptive processes during the third trimester. Finally, during the third trimester, issues of fetal effects from environmental exposure remain a substantial concern.

Existing evidence suggests that placental transfer from the maternal to the fetal circulatory system occurs for most compounds tested (Cummings, 1983; Krauer and Krauer, 1977; Philipson, 1979). Placental metabolism is less common, although it has been demonstrated for selected compounds (Pelkonen, 1980; Juchau and Faustman-Watts, 1983). Nevertheless, when placental metabolism occurs, it can have significant impact on fetal or placental toxicity. In addition to mediation of placental/fetal toxicity by altering transference of parent compound or metabolites into the fetal circulatory system, placental toxicity involving destruction of placental cells or alteration of placental functions may have similar disruptive effects on the fetus. For example, in experimental animals, prenatal exposure to cadmium produces fetal death (Clarkson et al., 1983). This effect appears not to be the result of direct fetal toxicity but is thought to be the result of placental toxicity. For that reason, xenobiotic uptake and effect on placental function may, in some cases, be as important as placental transport of the parent xenobiotic or metabolism and transport of metabolites to the fetus.

PHYSIOLOGICAL MODELS

Physiological models appear to offer significant opportunity for cross-species extrapolation to determine the effects of physiological changes during pregnancy on maternal or fetal toxicity. In addition, physiological models may allow appropriate extrapolation between species, because comparable stages of pregnancy as well as placental and fetal development can be compared in the risk assessment process. Another attraction of physiological models for risk assessment in developmental toxicology is that similar approaches are being developed for risk assessment in carcinogenesis. This means that all risk assessment procedures that use physiologically based models could be linked by the common denominator of biological structure and function.

1. Physiological Models of the Maternal Compartment

At the outset, a physiological model of the maternal compartment begins with a detailed qualitative model of the maternal organism (Fig. 14-3). The

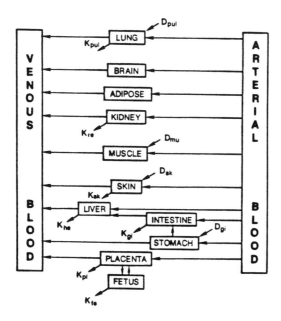

Figure 14-3. Physiological model of the maternal compartment during pregnancy. Routes of exposure or dosing may include the lung, muscle, skin, and gastrointestinal system. Routes of elimination include lung, kidney, skin, liver, gastrointestinal system, placenta, and fetus. Metabolism or uptake may occur in any organ.

model will include all major organs and systems. Environmental exposure may occur through the lungs (D_{pul}), skin (D_{sk}), muscle (D_{mu}), or gastrointestinal system (D_{gi}). Elimination may occur through the lung (K_{pul}), kidney (K_{re}), skin (K_{sk}), liver (K_{he}), intestine (K_{gi}), placenta (K_{pl}), or fetus (K_{fe}). Metabolism or uptake of a xenobiotic of interest may occur in any organ or tissue in the maternal compartment and will be reflected by an arterial to venous gradient across that organ.

Characterization of this physiological model for a developmental toxicant in experimental animals, followed by definition of the uptake, distribution, and metabolism in organs in the human maternal compartment, should form one of the first steps in human risk assessment. Another step in this process will be to define animal and human distribution in the fetal compartment of the physiological model.

2. Physiological Models of the Fetal Compartment

Like the physiological models of the maternal compartment, the physiological models of the fetal compartment are much more detailed and complex than the two-compartment model reflects (Fig. 14-4). Disregarding the unusual situation of exposure through the amniotic fluid, the major route of fetal exposure will be through the placenta. Reabsorption of parent xenobiotic or metabolites, however, may occur through the amniotic fluid. Potential reabsorption routes include stomach and skin. Although true elimination can only take place across the placenta into the maternal compartment, metabolism can occur in any fetal organ.

3. Physiological Models of the Placenta

As suggested by Table 14-8, the human placenta is relatively simple anatomically in comparison to the placentas of other species. Physiological models of the placenta will also vary in complexity across species. Much of the research effort defining physiological models of the placenta comes from a literature devoted to fetal and placental physiology that is more than a decade old (Bartels, 1970; Longo and Bartels, 1973). Most of this research used sheep models of pregnancy and reflects the impact of Barron and Dawes on fetal and placental physiology. More recently, efforts of researchers using term human placenta for isolated dual perfusion of cotyledons and lobules offer the greatest potential for defining physiological models of placental function.

For the sake of definition and completeness, one physiological model for the human placenta will be illustrated (Fig. 14-5).

In the two-compartment pharmacokinetic model, transfer between maternal and fetal circulations was characterized by two rate constants. In the

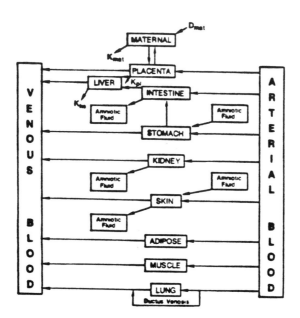

Figure 14-4. Physiological model of the fetal compartment. Xenobiotics gain access to the fetal compartment across the placenta. Elimination may occur in the placenta, fetal gastrointestinal system, kidney, or skin. Xenobiotics eliminated into the amniotic fluid are available for reabsorption through the skin and gastrointestinal system and through the lungs during fetal breathing movements.

more complex physiological model, transfer between maternal and fetal circulations depends on several parameters (Table 14-9).

Note that this physiological model of the placenta is specifically for the term placenta. An accurate physiological-flow model for the preterm placenta will require an additional cellular layer between the maternal and fetal circulations—the cytotrophoblast. This additional layer will obviously require additional rate constants. It is apparent that physiological models are relatively complex; however, characterization of the effect of these parameters on placental transport functions, coupled with sensitivity analysis to identify critical parameters, may make appropriate simplification possible.

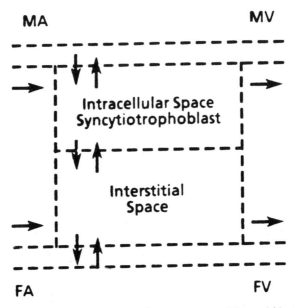

MA   **MV**

Intracellular Space
Syncytiotrophoblast

Interstitial
Space

FA   **FV**

Figure 14-5. Physiological model of the term human placenta. Maternal blood flowing into the intervillous space through the maternal artery (MA) encounters the epithelium of the syncytiotrophoblast. Maternal blood percolates across the villi and then leaves the intervillous space through maternal veins (MV). Fetal blood enters the cotyledon through the fetal artery (FA), passes through a capillary network in the terminal villi, and then leaves the placenta through the fetal veins (FV).

TABLE 14-9. PARAMETERS INFLUENCING TRANSPLACENTAL TRANSFER

Flow Parameters
  Maternal artery (MA)
  Maternal vein (MV)
  Fetal artery (FA)
  Fetal vein (FV)

Transfer Parameters—Rate Constants
  MA to intracellular space
  Intracellular space to MV
  Intracellular space to interstitial space
  Interstitial space to intracellular space
  Interstitial space to FV
  FA to interstitial space

15.
TESTS FOR DEVELOPMENTAL TOXICITY

Ronald D. Hood

A great deal has been written about tests for developmental toxicity. Although by no means all-inclusive, a list of pertinent articles might include: Tuchmann-Duplessis (1972), Palmer (1974, 1976, 1978, 1980, 1981), Committee (1975), Schardein (1976a,b), Wilson (1977b,c, 1978), U.S. Environmental Protection Agency (EPA) (1978), Staples (1979), Bass and Neubert (1980), Wendler (1980), Interagency Regulatory Liaison Group (IRLG) (1981), Kimmel (1981a), Organization for Economic Cooperation and Development (OECD) (1981), Barlow and Sullivan (1982), Johnson (1983a), Nisbet and Karch (1983), Schardein (1983), U.S. EPA (1984), World Health Organization (WHO) (1984), Baeder et al. (1985), Chitlik et al. (1985), Ross (1985), Saxen (1985), Schardein (1985), Schardein et al. (1985), U.S. EPA (1986b), Kimmel et al. (1986), Hardin (1987), Neubert et al. (1987). A few selected issues related to the topic of developmental toxicity tests are discussed below.

ADEQUACY OF CURRENT STANDARD TESTS

1. In Terms of Experimental Design

a. Numbers of Animals: Fixed Guidelines vs. Estimating the Numbers Required Based on the Desired Degree of Precision and the Estimated Variability Expected in the Data

Federal guidelines for developmental toxicity tests specify minimum numbers of animals per dosage group, but such numbers typically do not assure adequate power to detect small treatment-related effects (Palmer, 1985). Changes in continuous variables, such as fetal weight, are considerably more easily detected than are those in discrete variables, such as prenatal death.

The appropriate numbers of animals per test group that would allow detection of a difference of a specified magnitude can be calculated a priori, based on the expected variance (calculated from historical or preliminary data) (e.g., Healey, 1987). When Nelson and Holson (1978) made such an estimate for A/J mice, they found that 22 litters might allow detection of a

10 percent fetal weight reduction. For various strains, it was estimated that from 12 to 16 litters of rats or from 22 to 50 mouse litters would be needed to allow detection of a 10 percent decrease in mean fetal weight. Finding a 10 percent decrease in survival of the conceptus would require from 235 to 324 litters for mice and 216 to 248 for rats.

Since only 20 rodents or 12 rabbits per dosage group are required by EPA guidelines regarding tests for developmental toxicity ("teratogenicity"), it can easily be seen that these minimal numbers do not allow for a very sensitive test in terms of many of the parameters measured. As Palmer (1974, 1985) reminds us, such test group sizes allow detection of only the most potent developmental toxicants. On the other hand, it must be realized that such tests are quite expensive and that expense rises as numbers of test animals are increased. This fact must not become such an overriding consideration, however, that tests that are so insensitive as to be useless are routinely employed.

Indeed, it has been stated that the use of smaller numbers of rabbits than rats is based entirely on economics. Strictly scientific reasoning would require more rabbits than rats, due to the inherently greater variability of data derived from the former. In the case of primates, the number of individuals per treatment group should be even higher, as they typically have only one offspring per dam and tend to yield "all or none" responses (Environmental Health Criteria 30, 1984).

One possible way to help overcome this problem would be to employ species and strains of test animals that are sufficiently uniform as to give the best possible sensitivity with small numbers of litters. Nevertheless, it must also be realized that considerable genetic variation would be useful in order to allow manifestation of the broadest possible range of responses. This may more closely approximate the situation in humans, where sensitive subpopulations in terms of toxic effects often exist. Such an approach has been advocated by Kocher (1977b) and Kalter (1978), who suggested use of crosses of inbred strains in developmental toxicity tests, but the issue has received relatively little attention. It is also uncertain whether the best use of such F_1 hybrids would be as the test offspring or as the female parents (Palmer, 1969). More recently, Kalter (1981) suggested the concurrent use of several inbred mouse strains in order to achieve a wider range of possible responses.

b. Species of Test Animals

For a discussion of the relative merits of different mammalian species, see Chapter 17 (Animal Models of Effects of Prenatal Insult).

c. End Points Measured

In developmental toxicity testing, measures of maternal toxicity are observed in order to allow determination of the relative health status of the dam. The commonly used end points for maternal toxicity are shown in Table 15-1 taken from U.S. EPA (1986b), wherein they are discussed in some detail. Most of the end points listed are routinely measured because they are easily observed. In general, however, these measures are relatively crude indicators of toxicity, and in cases such as maternal body weight change in the rabbit, they may at times be of little value. Some of the possible end points listed, such as enzyme markers and clinical chemistries, are infrequently used and may be difficult to interpret as measures of toxicity (U.S. EPA, 1986b). Although gross manifestation of maternal toxicity is generally easily determined, more subtle effects may pass unnoticed because of the nature of the end points observed, making determination of maternal no-observed-effect levels (NOELs) and lowest-observed-effect levels (LOELs) uncertain.

TABLE 15-1. END POINTS OF MATERNAL TOXICITY

Mortality
Fertility Index (no. with seminal plugs or sperm/no. mated)
Gestation Index (no. with implants/no. with seminal plugs or sperm)
Gestation Length (when allowed to deliver pups)
Body Weight
  Treatment days (at least first, middle, and last treatment days)
  Sacrifice day
Body Weight Change
  Throughout gestation
  During treatment (including increments of time within treatment period)
  Posttreatment to sacrifice
  Corrected maternal (body weight change throughout gestation minus gravid uterine
    weight or litter weight at sacrifice)
Organ Weights (in cases of suspected specific organ toxicity)
  Absolute
  Relative to body weight
Food and Water Consumption (where relevant)
Clinical Evaluations (on days of treatment and at sacrifice)
  Types and incidence of clinical signs
  Enzyme markers
  Clinical chemistries
Gross Necropsy and Histopathology

Source : U.S. EPA, 1986b.

End points for assessment of developmental toxicity are shown in Table 15-2, also taken from U.S. EPA (1986b), wherein they are discussed in detail in terms of their utility and interpretation. Further discussion of both mater-

TABLE 15-2. END POINTS OF DEVELOPMENTAL TOXICITY

Litters with implants
    No. implantation sites/dam
    No. corpora lutea (CL)/dam[a]
    Percent preimplantation loss [(CL - implantations) x 100]/CL[a]
    No. and percent live offspring/litter
    No. and percent resorptions/litter
    No. and percent litters with resorptions
    No. and percent late fetal deaths/litter
    No. and percent nonlive (late fetal deaths + resorptions) implants/litter
    No. and percent litters with nonlive implants
    No. and percent affected (nonlive + malformed) implants/litter
    No. and percent litters with affected implants
    No. and percent litters with total resorptions
    No. and percent stillbirths/litter
Litters with live offspring[b]
    No. and percent litters with live offspring
    No. and percent live offspring/litter
    Viability of offspring[c]
    Sex ratio/litter
    Mean offspring body weight/litter[c]
    Mean male body weight/litter[c]
    Mean female body weight/litter[c]
    No. and percent externally malformed offspring/litter
    No. and percent viscerally malformed offspring/litter
    No. and percent skeletally malformed offspring/litter
    No. and percent malformed offspring/litter
    No. and percent litters with malformed offspring
    No. and percent malformed males/litter
    No. and percent malformed females/litter
    No. and percent offspring with variations/litter
    No. and percent litters having offspring with variations
    Types and incidence of individual malformations
    Types and incidence of individual variations
    Individual offspring and their malformations and variations (grouped according to litter
      and dose)
    Clinical signs[c]
    Gross necropsy and histopathology

---

[a]Important when treatment begins prior to implantation. May be difficult in mice.
[b]Offspring refers both to fetuses observed prior to term or to pups following birth. The end points examined depend on the protocol used for each study.
[c]Measured at selected intervals until termination of the study.
Source : U.S. EPA, 1986b.

nal and developmental toxicity end points may be found in Chitlik et al. (1985) and in Rands et al. (1982a,b). It appears that most of the readily observable prenatal end points for developmental toxicity, at least survival, growth, and morphology, are currently being used. Little attention is paid in the United States, however, to measures of functional or biochemical effects. This is true in terms of both research (U.S. EPA, 1986a) and required testing, although in some cases postnatal testing has been required when reversibility of effects was in question (U.S. EPA, 1986b).

It must be remembered that the end points observed in laboratory animals are not necessarily the same as those seen in humans for any given agent (Kimmel et al., 1986). Also, developmental toxicity end points are quite diverse, a wide range of end points may be produced by a single chemical, and the comparability of end points among test species is also uncertain with our present state of knowledge (Kimmel et al., 1984).

d. Timing of Treatment

Treatment timing has been somewhat controversial in that the currently used protocol requiring treatment throughout organogenesis is considered to be somewhat inefficient in revealing the potential of a test agent to induce malformations. As Johnson and Christian (1984) state, the Segment II type study (U.S. Department of Health, Education and Welfare, 1966; Food and Drug Administration [FDA], 1982), although called a "teratology study," is not really designed for the production of malformations ("terata"). They give detailed evidence to support the contention that the Segment II type protocol is more efficient for production of death of the conceptus or toxicity to the dam than for induction of structural abnormalities in the surviving offspring.

Wilson (1973) contended that use of a series of three-day treatment periods spanning organogenesis would prove superior for production of terata and would have the added benefit of preventing effects on dose-response due to enzyme induction and the resultant increase in metabolism of the test compound. It has also been proposed that both short- and long-term treatments be used for each agent tested (Committee, 1975).

There has often been a tendency to be more alarmed in the case of chemicals that cause malformations than in the case of those that produce other manifestations of developmental toxicity. As pointed out by Palmer (1980), however, "it may not be necessary to make fine distinctions between teratogenicity, embryotoxicity or growth retardation, since none would be considered acceptable in the human case." When it is considered that species differences in reaction to a given test agent may result in prenatal mortality in one species versus severe malformation in another (e.g., the case of the effect of thalidomide in the rat versus its effect in humans), this distinction becomes even less relevant. When the additional consideration of the inefficiency of chronic dosing of the conceptus is taken into account, the distinction between "teratogenic" and embryo/fetotoxic becomes even less relevant. Thus, as concluded by the IRLG Workgroup (Kimmel et al., 1986), "both are valid indicators of developmental toxicity," a point of view echoed by Johnson and Christian (1984).

If the point of view is taken that other measures of toxicity to the conceptus, in addition to terata, are also valid (e.g., Palmer, 1976, 1980; Schardein, 1983; U.S. EPA, 1986a), the Segment II type test protocol can be seen to be relatively useful. Although it may not be the most efficient protocol for discovering the potential of a chemical for inducing malformations, it is nevertheless a relatively efficient means for displaying potential for developmental toxicity (Palmer, 1980; Johnson and Christian, 1984). This is true because it severely tests the ability of the conceptus to withstand both direct and maternally mediated adverse effects (including possible cumulative effects or buildup of metabolites) during a major part of gestation. The standard test protocol avoids the necessity for the additional treatment groups that would be needed if several short-term treatment segments were employed, each at a series of dose levels. It also more closely mimics human exposure, which is more commonly chronic than acute (Palmer, 1980).

As has been recently suggested (Palmer, 1976; Brown and Fabro, 1983; Johnson and Christian, 1984; U.S. EPA, 1986a), what is needed may be sounder scientific interpretation of the data, rather than a revised test protocol in terms of timing of treatment and dose levels employed. It has also been proposed that if no other testing is to be done during the preimplantation period, treatment initiation prior to implantation would be useful, since coverage of all periods of development is of more significance than timing of initiation of a given study (U.S. EPA, 1986a).

A test of the effects of peri- and postnatal exposure to possible toxicants can be obtained by use of the so-called Segment III type study, where pregnant females are dosed during the fetal period and through parturition, lactation, and weaning of their offspring. Such a study can yield information on effects on parturition and early offspring development and survival. Treatment during this period allows observation of outcomes that might be diminished by maternal tolerance due to enzyme induction or the like when longer treatment periods are used. Cross-fostering can be done if needed to determine if observed effects are due to maternal toxicity or direct effects on the young (Palmer, 1981).

e. Timing of Assessment

Current protocols for Segment II type tests for developmental toxicity require evaluation prior to the expected time of parturition. For the purpose of detecting strictly prenatally manifested effects, this is the appropriate choice. It allows manifestation of the full range of possible visible effects on the conceptus without risk of potential loss of data associated with birth of the offspring.

There are, however, drawbacks to the current timing of evaluation if only Segment II type tests are done. For example, effects that are only manifested postnatally cannot be observed (Schardein, 1983). Examples include pup stunting and mortality (e.g., Snow and Tam, 1979) and a variety of functional deficits such as those discussed in the current document. It has therefore been suggested that tests of developmental toxicity should be designed to include evaluation of postnatally manifested effects caused by prenatal or early postnatal insult (Simmons et al., 1984; Kimmel et al., 1986). Exactly how this is to be done is still a matter for debate, but such data could prove valuable for risk assessment.

One further suggested shortcoming of the current timing of assessment is the inability to distinguish early deaths due to severe malformation of offspring from those due to other toxicity end points. For the purpose of risk assessment, however, as was pointed out above, death of the offspring should be considered equally undesirable an outcome as malformation (Johnson and Christian, 1984).

2. In Terms of Coverage

a. Which End Points Are the Most Sensitive Indicators of Developmental Toxicity?

There does not appear to be a clear-cut agreement on which end point or combination of end points is superior for assessment of developmental toxicity (White et al., 1981). Various studies have attempted to use end points ranging from specific malformations to combinations of malformations or variations, weight reduction, and/or death to indicate developmental toxicity. Biochemical (Andrew, 1976) and functional (Butcher et al., 1972) parameters have also been suggested as sensitive indicators as well.

Use of certain end points, such as skeletal variation, is said to have the advantage of allowing true quantitation of events that are frequent enough to allow for greater sensitivity (Palmer, 1977). These may be useful if one considers that any manifestation of effect on the conceptus is of biological relevance. Khera has suggested that such effects are of little relevance because they are commonly encountered in the presence of maternal toxicity and their significance is unclear (Khera, 1981). Whether or not the effect is maternally mediated, however, it is nevertheless an effect on the offspring and can be regarded as an appropriate end point in attempts to delineate a developmental toxicity NOEL. According to Palmer (1977, 1980), events such as appearances of extra ribs often occur at lower doses of test agents than do true malformations and are thus more sensitive end points of developmental toxicity.

Fetal or pup weights are also a sensitive measure of effects on the off-spring, but a decrease may merely reflect general undernutrition of the dam rather than toxicity to the offspring. It has been suggested, however, that in postnatal tests changes in pup weights were a better measure of developmental delay or acceleration than was measurement of delays in developmental landmarks, e.g., surface or air righting, pinna unfolding, eye opening (Lochry et al., 1985)

The sensitivity of fetal weights as an end point may be affected by the tendency of weight to be influenced by relative position in the uterine horns, according to studies such as those of McLaren and Michie (1959, 1960), Barr et al. (1969), Norman and Bruce (1979), Stuckhardt et al. (1981), Chahoud et al. (1984), and Domarus et al. (1986), and some investigators found no such effects (Fasel and Schowing, 1980). Unfortunately, however, the differences reported were not uniform across species or even among studies in the same species. Nevertheless, it might be possible to adjust fetal weights for intrauterine location, at least within a given study, in order to increase the ability of data analysis to detect treatment-related differences. Also, use of a short mating period can decrease variability in fetal weights (e.g., Endo and Watanabe, 1988). Nevertheless, it should be kept in mind that sensitivity of fetal weight is already relatively high—for example, one can often detect differences of less than 10 percent. Even for apparent changes of this magnitude, there is sometimes a question of biological relevance.

b. How Are the Various End Points Interrelated?

The various end points measured in tests for developmental toxicity are often analyzed and used in interpretation of results as though they were all independent and unrelated. This is not always appropriate, however, as some parameters such as malformation and death of the conceptus are at times related.

The above mentioned example was discussed at length by Kalter (1980). He proposed that in some cases, the lethal and malforming characteristics of a teratogen were unrelated, and the frequencies of these two events would increase independently with increasing dose. In the alternative situation, the agent would primarily cause malformation at low doses. As dose increased, an inverse relationship would then be seen between malformation and prenatal mortality. This would occur as the severity of the induced defects increased to the point of causing deaths among the offspring. In at least some cases, these two scenarios might be confounded and not clearly separable. Additionally, Kalter (1980) suggests that a given agent may cause nonspecific fetal death under certain experimental conditions and kill by first lethally malforming the offspring under other conditions.

Another situation where developmental toxicity end points may be related is the common association of decreased fetal weight, diminished crown-rump length, and retarded ossification (Hart et al., 1988). These effects are probably related, in that they are all manifestations of developmental retardation. They may be due to direct factors, such as general toxicity to the conceptus or to the placenta, or to indirect effects of maternal toxicity or undernutrition. Thus, instead of a possible cause and effect relationship, as might at times be seen for malformation (or functional deficit) and death, here the relationship among end points is more likely merely a shared etiology.

Litter size and fetal weight have also been said to be interrelated, with fetal weight tending to decrease as litter size increased (U.S. EPA, 1986b). This may not be a universal occurrence, however, as Norman and Bruce (1979) and Chahoud et al. (1984) failed to find such a relationship in litters of Wistar rats or Han/NMRI mice. Fetal weight is also influenced by the sex of the fetus, with males tending to weigh more than females (U.S. EPA, 1986b).

It has also been suggested that maternal toxicity is related to various developmental toxicity end points. This has been discussed previously in Chapter 7 (Maternal vs. Developmental Toxicity).

c. Should We Use Additional Tests or Measure Additional Parameters?

Several additions to the standard test protocols for developmental toxicity have been proposed, but none have as yet reached widespread use. This lack of innovation is probably due at least in part to cost considerations as well as to inertia on the part of those involved in testing as well as those regulating test protocols. If a new test or measurement of an additional end point added significantly to the sensitivity or reliability of a test, however, it would likely be adopted eventually.

Zeindl and Sperling (1977) suggested cytogenetic analysis under the assumption that chromosomal breakage may be associated with developmental toxicity. The authors agreed, however, that the effects seen on the conceptus were probably not caused by the clastogenic effects of the treatments used in their study.

Although fetal organ weights are not often measured in developmental toxicity tests, Mosier et al. (1982) found that specific organ weights in rat fetuses were differentially affected. This effect was seen both in absolute terms and relative to body weight following maternal treatment with various glucocorticoids.

Biochemical techniques have also been recommended. Andrew (1976) suggested assessment of developmental enzyme patterns as a likely technique for evaluating adverse effects on development. Such an approach was indeed used by Karp et al. (1985), but they found that while mercuric acetate could affect maternal activities of glucose-6-phosphate dehydrogenase and glycogen phosphorylase (but not cytochrome c oxidase) in the kidneys of pregnant hamsters, activities of these enzymes in their developing offspring were not altered. It was possible that these negative results may have been due to lack of sufficient mercury reaching the conceptus, however, and tests involving effects on enzyme activities probably deserve more attention in the future.

An additional biochemically based assay was reported by Klose et al. (1977), who used isoelectric focusing and electrophoresis to examine the pattern of proteins produced by mouse embryos. It was proposed that this protein mapping technique might be used to look for changes induced by developmental toxicants. None of these methods has been studied thoroughly to determine if it would add to our ability to efficiently detect developmental toxicants. Such tests would require considerable effort to validate their usefulness, and the funds required have not been abundantly available. While such assays have considerable appeal from a theoretical point of view, their practicality is in question. Although they may give additional answers to some of the questions asked in testing for developmental toxicity, tests that measure broader arrays of end points appear more likely to detect a variety of developmental toxicants. To achieve a similar result, an extensive battery of single or narrow end point tests might be required, thus decreasing any possible advantages of speed, simplicity, and low cost.

d. Should Testing Be More (or Less) Rigidly Standardized?

• *In terms of the specific tests to be done.* There are arguments both for and against standardization of the particular tests to be performed for evaluation of potential developmental toxicants. In general, however, requiring the same general types of tests seems desirable. It allows comparability of results across a wide variety of test chemicals and thereby facilitates the regulatory process. Both the reviewers and the individuals generating the data can become more familiar with the range of likely results. This greatly aids not only in interpretation of the data generated but also in terms of consistency of test conduct and data handling.

It can be argued that in specific cases, the low likelihood of significant human exposure makes a full range of testing unnecessary. Nevertheless, for those chemicals requiring a full battery of tests, the merits of a relatively standardized test selection outweigh any obvious drawbacks.

• *In terms of how the tests are to be conducted.* There are also some advantages in a considerable degree of standardization of the conduct of the required tests. This has typically been suggested by regulators (e.g., IRLG, 1981; U.S. EPA, 1984), but some degree of flexibility has always been allowed as long as the minimum standards of test conduct have been met or exceeded. Test standardization is not only of use within the United States but also allows for greater international uniformity of testing and regulation as well (Walker, 1984).

There have been reasonable pleas for retaining at least some flexibility in test protocols, allowing the researcher some latitude in modifying a given test to fit a specific chemical (e.g., Palmer, 1978). An example of such a modification was published by Perraud et al. (1984). In their study of piroxicam, a nonsteroidal anti-inflammatory drug, treatment of pregnant rats was discontinued a few days prior to parturition. This allowed assessment of the agent's potential for postnatal effects on the offspring without interference due to the drug's ability to delay parturition. Delayed parturition is a common effect of nonsteroidal anti-inflammatory agents, and such an effect had been confirmed for piroxicam in initial trials.

Other possibly useful departures from standard protocols might include dosing more or less often or performing two or three studies with shorter dosing periods that together spanned the entire period of interest (Palmer, 1980). Such possible modifications would be based on the unique properties of a compound or its cumulative toxicity or ability to induce enzymes.

'IN VITRO' TESTS AND OTHER 'PRESCREENS': UTILITY AND VALIDATION

1. Need for Prescreens

An amazing variety of biological models have been proposed as possibly useful in screening for developmental toxicity (Goss and Sabourin, 1985). These have included use of organisms as diverse as viruses and embryonic chicks; this diversity can be appreciated upon examination of Table 15-3, which lists many of the suggested test species. Although most of the proposed short-term "prescreens" for developmental toxicity do not employ pregnant mammals, there has been considerable interest in the approach of Chernoff and Kavlock (1982), which uses the pregnant mouse.

According to the Second Task Force for Research Training in Environmental Health Science (1977), the development of rapid, relatively inexpensive methods for screening potential teratogens is an important goal. This view has been echoed in numerous other statements in the literature, including those of Neubert and Barrach (1977a), Wilson (1978), and Johnson (1981). It has also been the subject of conferences and workshops, such as

TABLE 15-3. PROPOSED SHORT-TERM SCREENING
SYSTEMS FOR DEVELOPMENTAL TOXICITY

Test Species	Test System	References
Brine Shrimp (*Artemia salina*)	developing nauplii	Sleet & Brendell (1983, 1985), Kerster & Schaeffer (1983)
Chicken	embryos in ovo cell cultures	Jelinek (1977, 1982), Marhan & Jelinek (1979), Jelinek et al. (1985), Greenberg (1983)
Cricket (*Acheta domesticus*)	eggs developing to first instar nymphs	Walton (1981, 1983)
Drosophila *melanogaster*	embryonic cell cultures whole embryos reared to adults	Bournias-Vardiabasis & Teplitz (1982), Bournias-Vardiabasis & Flores (1983), Bournias-Vardiabasis et al. (1983), Buzin & Bournias-Vardiabasis (1984), Ranganathan et al. (1987), Schuler et al. (1982), Hood & Davis (1984), Kundomal & Baden (1985), Schuler et al. (1985)
Fishes (e.g., Medaka, salmon, zebra fish)	embryos in ovo reared to hatching	Laale (1981), Birge et al. (1983), Baumann & Sander (1984), Cameron et al. (1985)
Frogs (*Xenopus laevis* and various others)	embryos in ovo or reared to tadpole stage	Birge et al. (1983), Dumpert & Zietz (1984), Dawson et al. (1985) Fulton & Chambers (1985), Sabourin et al. (1985)
Hydra (*Hydra attenuata*)	artificial "embryos" differentiating from groups of reaggregating cells	Johnson (1980a), Johnson & Gabel (1982, 1983), Johnson et al. (1982), Johnson (1984), Sabourin et al. (1985)
Mammals (rats or mice)	cell cultures cultured whole embryos	Braun et al. (1982a, b), Hassel & Horigan (1982), Clayton & Zehir (1982), Pratt et al. (1982), Braun & Horowicz (1983), Kistler (1985), Pratt & Willis (1985), Sharma et al. (1985), Kochhar (1981), Fantel (1982), Sadler et al. (1982), Klein & Pierro (1983), Warner et al. (1983), Kitchin & Ebron (1984), Sadler & Warner (1984), Beck et al. (1985), Katayama & Matsumoto (1985), Klug et al. (1985), Sadler (1985), Steele (1985), Kitchin et al. (1986), Oglesby et al. (1986)

TABLE 15-3. PROPOSED SHORT-TERM SCREENING SYSTEMS FOR
DEVELOPMENTAL TOXICITY (CONTINUED)

Test Species	Test System	References
Mammals (continued)	organ cultures	Neubert & Barrach (1977b), Manson & Simons (1979), Kochhar (1981, 1983), Kwasigroch & Skalko (1983), Saxen (1979),
	pregnant dams allowed to litter and their pups reared to various ages	Chernoff & Kavlock (1982), Gray et al. (1983), Gray & Kavlock (1984), Schuler et al. (1984), Plasterer et al. (1985), Seidenberg et al. (1986), Hardin (1987), Hardin et al. (1987b), Kavlock et al. (1987), Seidenberg & Becker (1987), Wickramaratne (1987), Wier et al. (1987)
Planarians *(Dugesia sp.)*	regenerating fragments and growing intact individuals	Best & Morita (1982), Sabourin et al. (1985)
Sea urchins *(Strongylocentrotus purpuratus)*	developing embryos	Hose (1985)
Viruses (vaccinia WR)	virions in cultured monkey kidney cells	Keller & Smith (1982)

the Consensus Workshop on In Vitro Teratogenesis Testing, sponsored by the EPA and FDA in 1981.

New chemicals are produced more rapidly than they can be tested for developmental toxicity (Wilson, 1977b; Johnson, 1981; Hill, 1983). This fact substantiates the urgency of developing more efficient screening systems. Such tests would be useful at the lowest level of a "tier system" for screening (Johnson, 1980a; Neubert, 1981). Tests in successive tiers would be increasingly more complex and costly but would be expected to be more accurate predictors of relative hazard. By eliminating the more obviously harmful agents, a successfully validated, appropriate new test could allow the screening of significantly greater numbers of chemicals at lower cost.

The potential importance of useful prescreens for developmental toxicity is reflected in the increasing number of reviews on the topic. These include: Kochhar (1975), Staples, (1975), Neubert and Barrach (1977a, 1979), Wilson (1977b, 1978), Saxen (1979), Barrach and Neubert (1980), Pratt et al. (1980), Flint (1981), Johnson (1981), Neubert (1981, 1985), Beck (1982b), Brown and Fabro (1982), Freese (1982), Kimmel et al. (1982), Hill (1983), Shepard et al. (1983), Snell (1983), Environmental Health Criteria 30 (1984), Ornoy (1984), Braun (1985), Goss and Sabourin (1985), Kimmel (1985), Saxen (1985), Brown et al. (1986), U.S. EPA (1986b), Brown (1987), Collins (1987), Flynn (1987), Friedman (1987), Johnson et al. (1987), Kimmel (1987), Schmid (1987), Welsh (1987), Whitby (1987), and Welsch (1988). Some reviews, however, reflect a relatively negative view of the potential of in vitro prescreens except in limited roles (e.g., Neubert and Barrach, 1979; Neubert et al., 1985).

2. Characteristics of Prescreens

What then are the essential characteristics of a screen for developmental toxicity? Obviously it must be capable of displaying end points of toxicity that are highly correlated with adverse significant effects in developing mammals in general and in humans in particular. Also, according to Johnson (1981), a basic attribute of any adequate test system is that "it must differentially detect agents to which the conceptus is uniquely susceptible." As proposed by Karnofsky (1965), virtually any chemical may interfere with development if given in a high enough dose at the right time to a susceptible organism. Thus, the task at hand is not to merely determine if a test chemical has an adverse effect on the conceptus, but to assess the magnitude of any difference in effect between the offspring and its mother. If this differential is slight, maternal toxicity may be an overriding concern. If it is large, developmental effects become increasingly important. In addition, a useful test must be able to consistently show dose-response relationships.

Johnson (1981) proposed that a teratogenesis screen must be able to detect disruption of any of the basic developmental effects that are essential for normal embryogenesis. Further features of an in vitro test system have been proposed by Wilson (1977c). He stated that it is essential that the system: (a) "use biological subjects available in large numbers," (b) "involve progressive development," (c) "be relevant to mechanisms of teratogenesis," and (d) "be easily performed, yielding interpretable results." It is desirable that the system: (a) "use an intact organism capable of absorbing, circulating and excreting chemicals," (b) "give few false negatives (compared with mammals)," and (c) "react to varied types of agents."

A useful screen must be amenable to validation. Chemical agents that give a positive response in mammals, especially humans, must consistently give a positive response in the test system. Similarly, presumptive non-teratogens should give negative responses. A moderate percentage of false positives would be acceptable, as these could be further investigated if warranted by the potential usefulness of the test agent (Shepard et al., 1983). Ideally, the percentage of false negatives should be minimal, as substances passing the initial screen might not be tested further (Wilson, 1977c; Johnson, 1981).

3. Types of Proposed Prescreens and Their Utility

Although the need for more efficient tests has been frequently acknowledged, such a system remains to be perfected. In fact, the majority of screening systems tested appear to have a variety of shortcomings. Nevertheless, at least some appear to hold promise, and most if not all are yet in need of adequate validation.

In order for a prescreen to be useful, Neubert (1981) believes that it must provide answers to two definitive questions: (1) If the results of a test are negative, has the test provided enough information for us to judge that no further testing is necessary? If so, we could eliminate much of the currently needed testing. (2) If the test results are positive, is this truly indicative of a hazard for humans? Again, if such a relationship could be firmly established, little or no further testing might be required.

Of course, establishing the above for any single prescreen or battery of prescreens will be exceedingly difficult, as such relationships remain controversial even for the standard in vivo tests.

With regard to the potential utility of in vitro methodologies, Neubert and Barrach (1983) contend that although such tests may often detect chemicals that have a general capacity to interfere with developmental events, they may fail to reveal agents that require "special pharmacokinetic parameters" in order to have an adverse effect. They further state that highly specific teratogens (those that interfere with only a specific developmental event) may also go undetected. They contend that the main use of in vitro testing will be for evaluating series of derivatives of already well-defined developmental toxicants, and that they are likely to be of little use in screening for new environmental agents.

Such negative views notwithstanding, research with potential prescreens is proceeding in a number of laboratories and has met with considerable interest (e.g., Kimmel et al., 1982). Nevertheless, it will be difficult in the short term to evaluate the true merit of any prescreens that may come into wide use. This is because the only currently available basis for such a judgment lies in whether or not it allows potent human developmental toxicants to escape detection (Shepard et al., 1983). Furthermore, it has repeatedly been pointed out that prescreens are currently not intended as substitutes for traditional testing in pregnant mammals when the need for a more thorough test is indicated (U.S. EPA, 1986a).

a. In Vitro Tests

According to Wilson (1977b), any screening systems that do not employ a pregnant mammal have been referred to as "in vitro" systems. Among the alternative in vitro screening methods that have been proposed are those that rely on the culture of rodent embryos (e.g., Fantel, 1982; Sadler et al., 1982; Klein and Pierro, 1983; Beck et al, 1985; Sadler, 1985; Oglesby et al., 1986). Such techniques are useful in experimental approaches to the mechanisms of teratogenesis. As prescreens, they appear to offer little advantage over traditional methods involving pregnant rodents, however, in that both are expensive and time-consuming, and cultured embryos are apparently somewhat hypoxic as well (Netzloff et al., 1968; New, 1970). Moreover, conditions for any culture system must be precisely controlled in order to give consistent results (Palmer, 1985).

More esoteric versions using cultured embryonic organs or tissues have also proven to be highly useful experimental tools (e.g., Manson and Simons, 1979; Kochhar, 1981, 1983; Kwasigroch and Skalko, 1983; Saxen, 1979), but may lack utility as the basis for a truly practical screen. In some cases, teratogenicity has been seen in vitro when it was not observed in vivo (Kwasigroch and Skalko, 1985), but it has not been established whether such an occurrence should be considered an artifact or merely an increase in test sensitivity.

According to Barrach and Neubert (1980) for example, such tests: (1) cannot predict embryolethal potential, growth retardation, or the production of functional deficits, (2) are apt to give false negatives with other than "general" (i.e., nonspecific) teratogens, (3) are sensitive to slight variations in culture conditions, (4) do not allow for more than partial control of variables due to metabolic effects, and (5) some components of the culture medium may interact with the test agents. In addition, Neubert (1981) and

Neubert et al. (1985) pointed out that culture systems may not allow adequate testing of compounds that are poorly water soluble, the serum often used in culture media may vary in composition over time, and concentrations of the test chemical used may be unrealistic. Such techniques also may be expensive, and they require high expertise — obviously undesirable characteristics for a practical test system.

Since mammalian embryos do not possess the adult repertoire of xenobiotic metabolizing capabilities, some systems have employed adult liver fractions to add this capability (e.g., Kitchin and Ebron, 1984). Care must be taken, however, that the enzyme system not harm the embryos, and under some circumstances it might produce metabolites that would never reach the embryo under in vivo conditions. According to Kitchin and Ebron (1984), the problem of water solubility may be solved by use of corn oil or low concentrations of certain other solvents (at least for culture of whole rat embryos). Much more needs to be learned of such possibilities as well as effects of such factors as constant contact with the test chemical and solvent in culture systems.

Similar and more cogent arguments could be used against the reliability and utility of tests using cells, tissues, or organs from nonmammalian species. In addition, although the techniques of molecular biology offer fascinating insights into both normal and abnormal development, the level of our knowledge at this time does not allow the use of such methods as accurate predictive toxicologic tools (Johnson, 1981; Neubert, 1981).

Although the avian embryo has frequently been used in testing, it also has acknowledged drawbacks. Foremost of these is that, except for exchange of respiratory gases, the bird embryo in its shell is a closed system. It is sensitive to mechanical, osmotic, and pH effects, and to buildup of metabolites. Also, the great amounts of yolk present may interact with test agents. A World Health Organization Study Group (WHO, 1967) concluded that the chick embryo ". . . is too sensitive to a wide range of agents. . . ." and that as a teratogenicity screen ". . . its use is not recommended," a view reiterated by Kimmel and coauthors (1982).

Embryos of certain fishes, such as the Medaka (Cameron et al., 1985) and the zebra fish (Baumann and Sander, 1984), have also been recommended for screens and may have some promise. No such test involving fishes has been validated, and the costs and skill involved are not insignificant. Amphibian embryos may be less useful than those of fishes, because they are surrounded by a jelly coat that might interfere with permeability (Wilson, 1977b). They have been tried, however, especially *Xenopus laevis,* and may have some value (Birge et al., 1983; Dumpert and Zietz, 1984; Dawson et al., 1985).

Invertebrates have been suggested as test organisms. Among these is *Hydra attenuata,* whose dissociated cells can be packed into pellets by centrifugation (Johnson, 1980a). Such pellets are said to act as artificial "embryos" which react to a number of test agents (Johnson and Gabel, 1983). Such "embryos" possess a modest range of tissues and few complex structures, with a limited repertoire of responses compared with those of higher organisms. Thus, they may not always respond in a manner similar to mammalian embryos when challenged with developmentally toxic insults. In addition, they live in an aqueous medium, and may be difficult to treat with chemicals that are relatively insoluble in water. The same arguments can be made against the utility of planarians, which have been proposed for use in screens (Sabourin et al., 1985). Nevertheless, at least in the case of the hydra assay, good concurrence between the prescreen results and those in mammals has been reported for a number of compounds (cf., Johnson and Gabel, 1983).

Another invertebrate, *Drosophila melanogaster*, has also received a degree of attention as an organism on which to base a prescreen (e.g., Hood and Davis, 1984; Kundomal and Baden, 1985; Schuler et al., 1985). Some of the objections to aquatic organisms (such as problems with non-water-soluble chemicals) may be overcome with this organism; it can metabolize xenobiotics, and much is known of its biology, but results of validation studies are encouraging.

In vitro tests have been proposed relying on organisms phylogenetically remote from humans, such as slime molds, bacteria, and viruses (cf., Keller and Smith, 1982). In addition to the drawbacks discussed above, these systems suffer from the disadvantage of being even more metabolically, physiologically, and physically unlike humans (Wilson, 1977c).

b. Tests Employing Pregnant Mammals

Considerable interest has recently been generated by a test first proposed by Chernoff and Kavlock (1982) in an attempt to overcome some of the shortcomings of previously proposed assays. Currently referred to as the Chernoff/Kavlock Assay or CKA (Gray and Kavlock, 1984), the method involves treatment of pregnant mice for 5 consecutive days, or on single days, during gestation days 8 through 12. The test dams are given a "minimally toxic dose" as determined in an initial toxicity test. The dams are allowed to litter, and their pups are counted and weighed on the day after parturition and again 2 days later. Any dead pups are examined for abnormalities and dams that have not delivered by 3 days after the expected delivery date are killed and inspected for implantations.

Because of promising early results (Chernoff and Kavlock, 1982), the CKA has been further evaluated and altered during follow-up studies to see if it can correctly identify putative "teratogens" (Chernoff and Kavlock, 1983; Gray et al., 1983; Gray and Kavlock, 1984; Seidenberg et al., 1986; Hardin, 1987; Hardin et al., 1987b; Kavlock et al., 1987; Seidenberg and Becker,

1987; Wickramaratne, 1987; Wier et al., 1987). In general, the results of the several published permutations of the CKA have been favorable in terms of their agreement with the outcomes of more traditional developmental toxicity evaluations. Averaged over a number of these studies, the apparent false positive rate was around 12 percent (Hardin et al., 1987a). Such a rate may be acceptable, considering the need to minimize false negatives, and the possibility that there were false negative results in the original literature upon which the conclusion was based must also be considered. The apparent false negative rate of the actual CKA data (8.6 percent) was likely due at least in part to the use of insufficiently high doses in several cases (Hardin et al., 1987a).

The CKA has some advantages, in that (1) it allows for interaction between the mother and conceptus and for biotransformation of the test compound, (2) no complex culture methodologies are needed, and (3) water-insoluble agents may be tested. As pointed out by Hardin et al. (1987a), the level of expertise required to conduct the test is less than that needed for a standard teratology screen, and it also provides data on the neonate. It is relatively rapid and inexpensive, and allows for the wide range of responses inherent in the mammalian repertoire, but it may yet be subject to further refinement.

A number of suggestions have been made for variations and possible improvements to the original CKA. These have included, for example, the use of alternative animal species, initial determination of maternal toxic dose in pregnant (rather than nonpregnant) dams, extension of the treatment period, use of additional dose levels or dose-setting criteria, extension of the period of postnatal observation, and evaluation of further pup-related parameters (Francis and Farland, 1987; Hardin, 1987; Kavlock et al., 1987; Seidenberg et al., 1986; Wickramaratne, 1987; Wier et al., 1987). There have also been requests to make the design of CKA-derived assays more flexible (Hardin et al., 1987a; Palmer, 1987). Some of the suggested changes (e.g., use of either rat or mouse, a longer dosing period, use of two dose levels) have already been incorporated in testing guidelines published by the EPA's Office of Toxic Substances (OTS) (U.S. EPA, 1984) and also published in the Federal Register (50 FR 39428). According to Francis and Farland (1987), the CKA as defined by the OTS has been referred to as the "preliminary developmental toxicity screen."

A modified CKA appears particularly useful in certain situations, such as comparison of structurally related compounds and prioritization of chemicals with regard to possible further developmental toxicity testing (Hardin et al., 1987a; Wickramaratne, 1987). The CKA has not met with unqualified acceptance, however, and it has been little used by industry (Francis and Farland, 1987).

Criticisms from industry scientists have included concerns that use of maternally toxic doses would result in too many false positives, but results of the validation tests mentioned above do not bear out the likelihood of such an outcome. Perhaps a more important criticism is that a CKA assay costs nearly as much as a standard developmental toxicity test when conducted by contract laboratories under Good Laboratory Practices (GLP) guidelines (48 FR 53922) that require use of separate animal rooms for each individual chemical tested. If the GLP guidelines could be modified to allow several compounds to be tested simultaneously with a single control group in the same room, the costs could be greatly decreased (Francis and Farland, 1987).

Christian et al. (1987) question the use of the CKA on the grounds that it is not an efficient use of testing resources in comparison with other possible screening procedures, such as the type of pilot study often used as a dosage range-finding assay prior to a standard developmental toxicity test. They suggest that the pilot study would assess many of the same maternal and developmental end points at modest expense and that if a full developmental toxicity study were later required, the range-finder's results would already be at hand. Their points seem well taken, but they do not mention one useful aspect of the CKA that is not duplicated in the range-finder: the assessment of effects that are only detectable postnatally (cf., Gray and Kavlock, 1984). Thus, the CKA as a stand-alone test is somewhat more comprehensive in its coverage.

4. Test Validation

For a developmental toxicity prescreen to be accepted as useful, it must pass extensive and rigorous validation testing (Kimmel et al., 1982; Kimmel, 1985), but it must be realized that most prescreens are unable to provide information on all developmental processes of interest. Factors related to maternal metabolism or toxicity, possible maternally mediated effects, fetal death due to delayed parturition, and postnatal functional deficits would be difficult or impossible to screen for in a system that does not involve a relationship between a mammalian mother and offspring (Neubert, 1981; Neubert and Barrach, 1983). Unless a Chernoff/Kavlock type assay can be perfected, no prescreen can be expected to test for anything more than unique susceptibility of a developing offspring to the direct effect of a toxic agent (or in some cases, its metabolites). Accordingly, validation should consider whether the prescreen can successfully differentiate between unique hazards to the conceptus and what Johnson et al. (1982) refer to as "coeffective teratogens," those that exhibit developmental toxicity only at doses that are also toxic to adults.

Johnson et al. (1982) proposed a set of premises on which validation of prescreens for developmental toxicity might be based. Many of these same considerations have been mentioned by others as well (e.g., Shepard et al., 1983). Briefly, these premises are as follows:

• The test system must concur with the best data from mammals, including man.

• Uniform protocols for both testing and dose selection must be employed without any modifications based on facts already known about a given test chemical.

• The test must yield uniform end point assessments.

• The test results must be capable of being used to rank chemicals based on their relative hazard potentials so that they may be prioritized in terms of the need for further testing.

• Dose-response relationships must be revealed by the test results.

• Ideally, the system should provide for metabolism of test compounds.

• The system must be capable of assaying both unknown chemicals and mixtures of uncertain composition.

In order to allow validation, a prescreen must use defined, specific end points that are readily quantifiable and can be analyzed statistically (Kimmel, 1985). Kimmel also points out that the type of statistical analysis used must be reported along with the data so that the results can be critically evaluated. He further states that the techniques used to expose the system to the test agents must be spelled out in detail. The rationale for dose selection and exposure timing, including their relationship to in vivo exposure, were also said to be important.

We must also be aware that agents that are merely cytotoxic may appear to be selective developmental toxicants even though they are not (Neubert, 1985; Neubert et al., 1985). The choice of test systems and interpretation of results is critical to weeding out such agents and eliminating prescreening systems that cannot identify them.

In order to permit greater comparability and standardization of prescreens, it has been suggested that a list of test chemicals be made up and such compounds be made available for validation studies (Kimmel et al., 1982; Kimmel, 1985). Such a list has been made available (Smith et al., 1983), and a test chemical repository has been established.

Another approach has been proposed by Neubert et al. (1985). They state that use of known developmental toxicants for validation is a biased method, and that concurrently testing unknowns in vitro and in vivo is a superior method.

16.
MALFORMATIONS vs. VARIATIONS AND 'MINOR DEFECTS'

Ronald D. Hood

DETECTION AND IDENTIFICATION

A "malformation" may be defined as "a permanent structural change that may adversely affect survival, development, or function" (U.S. EPA, 1986b). The same document classifies a variation as "a divergence beyond the usual range of structural constitution that may not adversely affect survival or health" and correctly points out the difficulty in distinguishing between malformations and variations, due to their existence on a continuum ranging from the normal to the abnormal.

Variants and anomalies have been defined in a variety of ways. For example, Palmer (1977) considers "variants" to be "structural changes occurring in more than 5 percent of the populations," while he describes "minor skeletal anomalies" as "slight, relatively rare structural changes not obviously detrimental." Palmer thus classifies manifestations of delayed development as either variants or minor anomalies, depending on their incidence, blurring possible distinctions between delays and structural changes. Also, in some cases, it cannot be determined merely by observation at necropsy if an alteration is a permanent variation or whether it is a transient effect caused by retarded development of the structure relative to the norm or relative to other tissues of the same individual. Whether an alteration would be classified as a variant or as a minor anomaly can even vary by species and by strains within species.

His definitions are somewhat arbitrary, but according to Palmer (1977), they were based on the concept that "the more frequently an anomaly arises, the less detrimental it will be," as it would otherwise be more heavily selected against in natural populations. As a matter of practicality, Palmer's (1977) categorization often results in situations where variants are frequently common enough to allow statistical analysis of their incidence; "minor anomalies" could not be so analyzed unless a toxic insult greatly increased their incidence. When the presence of frank malformations is clearly related to treatment, variants provide little additional relevant evidence, but when the data are equivocal, analysis of the incidence of variants may allow resolution of the ambiguity.

Another confounding factor is the lack of uniformity in recognizing and in categorizing variations and malformations (U.S. EPA, 1986b). For example, some investigators classify any visible, additional ossified structure lateral to the spine as an "extra rib," while others count only those at least one-half or one-third as long as the preceding rib, and some ignore such structures altogether (Palmer, 1977). In addition, there are sometimes differences of opinion as to whether a given structural change should be viewed as harmful to the individual possessing it (and thus considered a "malformation") or benign (and therefore classified as merely an anomaly). Because of the strain and species differences in incidences of background levels of variants and minor anomalies, as well as malformations, any developmental toxicity data must be analyzed in the context of historical results from the same laboratory if possible. Thus, it is incumbent upon the investigator to collect such control data and use them to temper judgment of the significance of test results. Unfortunately, this is not always done, and such data are often not available in published accounts of research, even when it had been relied upon in the evaluation by the author. Background incidence data from the literature can also be used as a supplement to in-house historical data (e.g., Cozens, 1965; Palmer, 1968; Perraud, 1976; Crary and Fox, 1980; Stadler et al., 1983).

STANDARDIZATION ACROSS LABORATORIES

Until recently, there appears to have been little organized effort to standardize either the terminology or the criteria used in categorizing malformations, variations, or developmental delays (Black and Marks, 1986; U.S. EPA, 1985, 1986b), or to categorize them specifically in published guidelines. The hazard evaluation guidelines published by the EPA's Office of Pesticide Programs (U.S. EPA, 1985), do contain a partial listing of malformations and variations, but only as examples, with no attempt to be comprehensive. As a result of the current state of affairs, there is only a limited degree of interlaboratory standardization, and the evaluation of developmental toxicity data for regulatory purposes is thus made more difficult.

RELATIVE SIGNIFICANCE OF DELAYED DEVELOPMENT AND SKELETAL VARIATION

There is considerable controversy among developmental toxicologists regarding the significance of the developmental delays and skeletal variations frequently seen in test offspring. Both are manifestations of developmental perturbation but may have the same or different etiologies.

Delayed development is most commonly manifested as small, immature-appearing fetuses or reduction of skeletal ossification and could be caused by direct effects on the fetus or placenta (Goldman, 1977). Such outcomes have recently been suggested to be secondary results of maternal toxicity (Khera, 1984b, 1985), but according to Kavlock et al. (1985), only supernumerary ribs were relatively consistently related to maternal toxicity in mice. Supernumerary ribs following maternal stress in mice (but not in rats) were also reported by Beyer and Chernoff (1986).

There has been a tendency to consider delayed development as of minor consequence, unless it is especially severe, and to view it as a separate matter from teratogenicity or prenatal mortality (Johnson, 1983b). Indeed, it is widely believed that offspring surviving insults that resulted in mild developmental delays are likely to fully recover, and there is evidence in the experimental literature supporting that view (Palmer, 1977). Nevertheless, infants small for gestational age (SGA) are a major problem in humans, and it has been well documented that their morbidity and mortality rates are higher than those of individuals closer to the norm (Dubowitz, 1974; Neubert and Barrach, 1983).

Decreased weight is not invariably a sign of developmental retardation. Small fetuses may appear to be fully developed in terms of the maturity of their anatomical components. Conversely, fetuses of normal weight may exhibit retarded skeletal development (Aliverti et al., 1979). With few exceptions, the causes of SGA individuals are not well established (Chez et al., 1976), but toxic insults could well be a contributing factor (Neubert and Barrach, 1979), and such maternal stressors as cigarette smoking are among the known causal elements (Tuchmann-Duplessis, 1979).

When assessing data on variants, minor anomalies, and retarded development, a particularly important factor is whether or not the data appear to be dose-related (Johnson, 1983b). Although such increases in variants, retardation, and so forth, more commonly appear at doses that are maternally toxic, this does not mean they can be ignored. In fact, Waddell and Marlowe (1976) and Khera (1984b) suggest that causes of frank malformations may be maternally mediated, although malformations may be more commonly caused by direct effects on the conceptus (Neubert and Barrach, 1983). Due to species differences, the result of maternal toxicity during gestation may at times be more (or less) serious for the human conceptus than for the offspring of test species (Johnson, 1983b).

Palmer (1977) has suggested the following as specific changes that may be of particular significance in assessing whether retarded development is due to toxic effects:

• Retarded general ossification relative to fetal weight and size
• Precocious general ossification relative to fetal weight and size

- Specific retardation of ossification at one locus relative to the occurrence of more obvious malformation at the same locus

It is often assumed that an agent that only causes an increase in minor anomalies or variants has a lower probability of being significantly hazardous to humans than would a chemical that results in malformations or prenatal death. It has also been said that developmental delays may be less serious than malformations or mortality, and their relative significance should be weighted accordingly (Marks et al., 1982). Additionally, the teratogenicity of a given agent may result from different mechanisms of action than those causing prenatal death (Neubert and Barrach, 1983). Nevertheless, any significant dose-related alteration in the offspring may be an indication of hazard (Johnson, 1983b) and must be considered. Such alterations provide additional end points for assaying effects on the conceptus and may provide evidence of the potential for more serious effects in humans (Palmer, 1985, 1988). Thalidomide, which produces only minor effects on the skeletal development of rats but severe malformations in humans, is a case in point (Palmer, 1974). As we are reminded by Neubert and Barrach (1983), syndromes of minor abnormalities should be considered a significant risk in terms of undesirable human outcomes, and the SGA baby has an increased risk of mortality. Further, Mehes (1985) and Holmes et al. (1985) state that the presence of certain minor anomalies and major malformations in human neonates is highly correlated, and according to Hoyme (1987), patterns of "minor anomalies" constitute important features defining malformation syndromes.

PERMANENCE OF EFFECT

Defects categorized as malformations should, by definition, be limited to developmental alterations that are essentially permanent. This has apparently not always been the case with developmental delays or even variations. In 1981, Khera recognized that such findings may be transitory, that even some conditions often referred to as malformations may in fact be self-correcting, and that follow-up studies were needed to determine the true significance of observations such as delayed ossification and "wavy ribs." Indeed, more recent studies have found that wavy ribs may become increasingly normal in appearance postpartum and be hardly distinguishable at weaning (Nishimura et al., 1982; Wickramaratne, 1988). Certain skeletal variations have been found, moreover, to persist into adulthood and to serve as markers for prenatal teratogen exposure (Beck, 1983).

Delayed ossification may also be temporary in nature (Collins et al., 1987). A considerable degree of variation in ossification can be seen even in untreated rodent and rabbit fetuses, with the variability decreasing at later examination times (Fritz, 1975; Aliverti et al., 1979). Additionally, skeletal ossification has been found to increase at different rates dependent upon which specific bones were assessed (Ariyuki et al., 1980, 1982).

Other anomalies, such as hydronephrosis in the rat, have also been said to be potentially temporary in nature and subject to considerable developmental variability in the timing of their disappearances (Woo and Hoar, 1972). At least some strains of both rats and mice appear to exhibit a considerable spontaneous incidence of hydronephrosis even when examined as adults (Burton et al., 1979; Goto et al., 1985).

HOW SIGNIFICANT ARE TRANSIENT EFFECTS?

1. Are They Useful Indicators of Potential for Other Types of Developmental Toxicity?

The general utility of transient effects as warning signs of an agent's potential to cause more lasting and harmful effects in other species, such as humans, is not well documented. Currently, the tendency is to be concerned about any dose-related changes in the conceptus even though their true significance is as yet undefined (Johnson, 1983b; Palmer, 1985; U.S. EPA, 1986b).

2. Are Offspring More Vulnerable to a Second Insult (by the Same or Different Agents) during a Transient Effect?

This question has been posed (Kimmel et al., 1986), but it has rarely been addressed in the literature. It seems likely that the answer would be positive, however, at least in specific cases. This is because any deviation from the normal developmental timing or pathways is likely to lower the threshold for more significant and longer-lasting effects. As discussed by Palmer (1985), malformations probably occur only when a developing system is in an unstable state. Once such a state has been induced by toxic insult, it would seem likely that further insult could more easily push the system toward disorganization and death.

One possible example can be seen in the work of Tabacova et al. (1983), who treated pregnant rats and two subsequent generations of dams with carbon disulfide by inhalation. They reported that the treated F_2 offspring of F_1 dams that had themselves been exposed while in utero were significantly more sensitive to the chemical's developmental toxicity than their parental generation had been. Not only were higher incidences of defective fetuses seen in the F_2 fetuses, but also the types of effects were altered.

Additionally, the F_1 dams appeared to be more sensitive to carbon disulfide than their (F_0) dams had been. Thus it appeared that past exposure to a developmental toxicant had a sensitizing effect not only on the F_1 generation but also on their offspring.

17.
ANIMAL MODELS OF EFFECTS OF PRENATAL INSULT

Ronald D. Hood

The problem of the adequacy and proper use of animal models in the assessment of developmental toxicity has been addressed on a number of occasions (Tuchmann-Duplessis, 1972, 1977; Schardein, 1976b, 1983, 1985; Palmer, 1980; Wilson, 1977b; Fraser, 1980; Kimmel et al., 1986; Brown and Fabro, 1983; Hendrickx et al., 1983; Nisbet and Karch, 1983; Khera, 1984a; Kimmel et al., 1984; Ross, 1985). Among the most useful and provocative of these reviews are those of Palmer (1978, 1985) and Schardein et al. (1985).

HOW GOOD ARE OUR CURRENT ANIMAL MODELS AS PREDICTORS OF HUMAN EFFECTS?

Several authors have reviewed the developmental toxicity literature in attempts to assess the utility of laboratory animals as predictors of response in humans. Although this is a difficult undertaking because of the lack of sound, comparable data, the authors have tended to come to certain conclusions. It was pointed out that with the apparent exception of coumarin anticoagulants (which are particularly toxic to rodents), all reasonably established human teratogens have caused malformations in at least one commonly used species of laboratory animal. Use of more than one species of animal to test each compound was recommended, because different species often differ in their responses to a given agent, and no one species was obviously a superior predictor of the human response (Schardein et al., 1985). Furthermore, the responses of humans and test animals were often not identical, although they have been very similar in some cases (Brown and Fabro, 1983; Khera, 1984a). This supports the belief that end points other than malformations should be considered in evaluating teratogenicity potential, as well as general developmental toxicity (Hemminki and Vineis, 1985; Kimmel et al., 1984; Schardein et al., 1985).

It has been stated that human teratogens have generally been identified through case reports (or in some cases, epidemiologic studies), and such findings are only supported by animal data (Schardein et al., 1985). Kimmel et al. (1984), however, contend that this has not actually been the case. According to these authors, most human teratogens were actually predicted by animal studies, but the data were typically ignored.

Although use of high doses in developmental toxicity assays has at times been deplored, it has been shown that humans are significantly more sensitive than laboratory animals to known teratogens (Brown and Fabro, 1983; Schardein, 1983; Khera, 1984a). Such evidence appears to support the use of reasonably high test doses in animal studies, although the basis for the apparent human sensitivity may merely be that the only confirmed human developmental toxicants are those to which humans are especially sensitive.

Unfortunately, although much has been made of the need for using animal models whose pharmacokinetic profile and biotransformation pathways for the chemicals tested are similar to those of humans (e.g., World Health Organization, 1967; Schardein, 1976b; Spielberg, 1984), there is said to be little evidence in the literature to show that this leads to improved concordance with human developmental outcomes (Khera, 1984a). Also, the needed data on pharmacokinetics are often lacking (Tuchmann Duplessis, 1972). Even similarities of blood levels and metabolites produced do not guarantee identical outcomes following exposure to a developmental toxicant, such as thalidomide (Hendrickx et al., 1983).

Animal tests have often been criticized for yielding numerous "false positive" results. This is because many agents have been shown to cause malformations in laboratory animals but that have not been shown to be developmental hazards in humans. Such a simplistic assessment is unfair, in that human data exist for only a few chemicals, and even in these cases exposure levels have generally been low, unknown, or confounded with other agents. Group sizes have almost invariably been small and confounding factors numerous. The power of most such studies to detect events that are likely to be relatively rare, such as malformations, is quite low. It is thus unsurprising that most human studies would yield negative results, and the so-called false positive results in animals may appear false largely because definitive human data are unavailable (Brown and Fabro, 1983).

WHAT FACTORS ARE INVOLVED IN MAKING A SUPERIOR ANIMAL MODEL?

There has been much discussion of the presumptive attributes of desirable animal models for developmental toxicity hazard assessment, but such speculation has had little, if any, impact on the choice of test species, breeds, or strains. In practice, such selection seems to be dominated by factors based on practicality. Animal models are selected on the basis of how many criteria they possess, such as: ready availability, low cost, ease of handling, high fertility, ease of breeding, large litters, short gestation length, ease of mating time determination, low rates of spontaneous deaths and developmental abnormalities, ease with which their fetuses can be examined, and the amount of information available on their reproduction, development, and response to developmental toxicants (Tuchmann-Duplessis, 1972; Palmer, 1977, 1980). The rationale for using such criteria is that none of the animal models tested is an obvious counterpart of humans in response to developmental toxicants. This leaves issues of practicality foremost in the selection process.

Although each of the numerous proposed test species has desirable characteristics, most also have overriding liabilities. Also, it is widely accepted that although submammalian species may eventually be shown to have utility in prescreens or for testing low priority chemicals, only an intact mammal has the numerous characteristics needed to mimic the human situation when more definitive answers are required (Brown and Fabro, 1983).

Nonhuman primates, especially those that appear closest phylogenetically to humans, have been assumed to be good models of the human response, but this belief is somewhat controversial. It has been said that while monkeys, such as the rhesus, have generally responded with positive results to known human teratogens, there is some discordance (e.g., Wilson, 1973, 1977c; Schardein et al., 1985).

Recently, Hendrickx et al. (1983) stated that the concordance between nonhuman primate and human data was actually quite good and supported the use of such models when definitive data are essential. The use of monkeys in efforts to obtain more reliable data on the likely human response has also been suggested by Palmer (1985), but he further pointed out the impracticality of using such species for initial safety evaluations. This is due to well-known drawbacks, such as cost and time constraints, associated with use of adequate numbers of primates per test. In fact, as mentioned by Brown and Fabro (1983), most if not all apparent "false negative" results obtained with monkeys are probably due to lack of adequate numbers of test animals. Use of primates has also been supported by Korte et al. (1987) based on extensive experience with rhesus and (to a greater extent) cynomolgus monkeys.

Since it is impractical to use nonhuman primates for most safety evaluation studies, investigators have turned to the rat and, to a lesser extent, the mouse, with the rabbit being the most used when a nonrodent species is required. These models are employed because they, to a greater extent than currently known alternatives, embody the desirable elements of the criteria listed above (Tuchmann-Duplessis, 1977). Although neither these nor other species are ideal models, we can make reasonably intelligent use of them because we have so much background information to aid in interpretation of experimental outcomes (Palmer, 1980). Even so, we cannot accurately predict, a priori, whether one of these or an alternative species would be the best to use in a given situation (Palmer, 1985). Indeed, support for or criticism of a particular animal on the basis that it either does or does not respond in a manner identical to that of humans is often based on an unfortunate emphasis on malformations, and at times on specific defects. If developmental toxicity is seen in a broader context, even the rat provides a warning of problems with thalidomide (Palmer, 1985).

ARE THERE ONE OR A FEW 'BEST MODELS,' OR CAN THE CHOICE OF MODEL BE TAILORED TO THE SPECIFIC AGENT TO BE EVALUATED?

Although use of the rabbit has been encouraged because it is sensitive to the teratogenic effects of thalidomide, this is not evidence that it would react like humans when tested with an agent with a different mechanism of action (Palmer, 1980).

Even the rat and rabbit can have unique drawbacks in certain situations. For example, the rabbit is dependent on gut organisms for proper digestion of its diet and cannot be used to test antibiotics that might interfere with this process (Schardein et al., 1985). Chemicals that alter gut motility, such as beta-adrenergic blocking agents, can also cause species-specific adverse effects in rabbits (Palmer, 1980). Rats, on the other hand, sequester arsenicals in their erythrocytes, and both adult and conceptus are uniquely sensitive to such compounds (Hood, 1985).

It has been suggested that use of pharmacokinetic data would allow selection of the best alternative among competing animal models. In fact, such data have been shown to provide suggestive evidence regarding reasons for differences in susceptibility to developmental toxicants among strains or species (Kimmel, 1981a; Brown and Fabro, 1983). The problem lies in applying such selection criteria to chemicals prior to their initial developmental toxicity testing. Knowledge of the pharmacokinetics, and especially the biotransformation, of a test agent in both human beings and prospective test animal species would be needed before an informed decision could be made. Since such information is rarely at hand even for prospective drugs or food additives and virtually never available for environmental or industrial chemicals, such an approach looks better in theory than in practice. It seems that such selection criteria are more likely to be employed to resolve conflicts in animal data once the primary developmental toxicity testing has already been done. It is possible that data interpretation may be improved and a superior animal model for further testing may be chosen more intelligently based on pharmacokinetic evaluation, but it appears unlikely that such data will be widely used in selection of models for initial testing.

Another point often brought up in discussions of animal models is the possibility of an influence on test outcomes due to differences among species in placental type and presumptive differences in placental function. The most common inference is that animals dependent upon an inverted yolk sac during embryogenesis may respond differently to teratogens than would humans (Palmer, 1978). Yet with the possible exception of rare agents, such as trypan blue, which may act by inhibiting histiotrophic nutrition, a specific placental structure has not been shown to affect teratogenesis. Indeed, humans also depend on histiotrophic nutrition but switch over to hemotrophic nutrition earlier in development in comparison with rodents, rabbits, and ferrets (Beck, 1982a). Molecules that are capable of traversing the placenta, particularly those that are small and/or lipophilic, are likely to do so regardless of placental type or developmental stage (Brown and Fabro, 1983).

Since susceptibility to developmental toxicants is presumed to be based in part on genetic factors associated with both offspring and mother, better animal models might be created by appropriate selective breeding or crossing. Possible use of the offspring of crosses between inbred mouse strains to provide a superior model possessing a combination of genetic uniformity with heterozygosity (Kocher, 1977b; Kalter, 1978) has been mentioned previously in this document. Whether this is a practical or useful approach has not been well evaluated, and it does suffer from the necessity of maintaining inbred and thus less fertile stocks from which to derive the desired F_1s. This method would be restricted to use with mice because of the need for highly inbred parental strains. Also, according to Kalter (1978), even such strain crosses do not approximate the heterogeneity of human populations.

Evidence from the literature indicates that mice can be selected for susceptibility to specific developmental toxicants (Kalter, 1978). Such an approach to developing superior test animals appears problematic, however, in that enhanced susceptibility to one teratogen may not ensure greater susceptibility to others. Also, susceptible strains are likely to be more developmentally unstable and thus exhibit a higher frequency of spontaneous defects. Such a characteristic would make such strains less useful as test animals.

HOW COMPARABLE ARE END POINTS ACROSS SPECIES?

As previously mentioned, end points of developmental toxicity may vary considerably in frequency of response among species exposed to the same developmental toxicant. Certain end points, such as prenatal death and reduced weight gain, are often seen across species treated with teratogens, even if malformations are not observed in all cases (Palmer, 1978). Maternally mediated effects may also occur and could confuse interpretation of end points. At present, there does not seem to be agreement as to the comparability of end points among test species and particularly between animals and humans.

18.

USE OF HUMAN DATA

Maureen C. Hatch

Researching the risks to developing humans from toxic exposures is a difficult enterprise. There are so-called critical periods for toxicity; effects can be expressed either morphologically or functionally; the outcomes are relatively rare and may be subtle (e.g., depressed mental performance or disordered behavior), yet are highly significant; effects may be detectable at or soon after birth, or not until later in life; in the case of the brain, the final stages of development occur long after the main period of organogenesis, so that both postnatal and prenatal exposures may be influential; and, particularly for intrauterine exposures, it is hard to estimate the delivered dose to developing tissues. In spite of the difficulties, epidemiologic approaches must play a role in developmental research — even more so as the focus expands to include effects on behavior, cognition, and social functioning, as well as structural defects.

At present, there are some 30 known human teratogens (cf., Schardein, 1985), most of them pharmacologic agents. Many additional chemicals test positive in laboratory animals, but data are currently lacking to evaluate their developmental effects in humans. The following discussion reviews the approaches that have been, or can be, used to identify new teratogens and other developmental toxicants, and suggests the kinds of studies that are needed.

PAST APPROACHES

1. Registries

A number of population- or hospital-based birth defects registries exist both in the United States and abroad for purposes of ongoing monitoring and further epidemiologic studies. The monitoring systems are intended to detect significant change in the incidence of congenital defects, while the epidemiologic component — sometimes referred to as "case-control surveillance" (Oakley, 1985) — aims to elucidate etiology. The monitoring function of registries is exemplified by the Eurocat Project, which involves 17 regional registries in 10 countries of the European Economic Community (Weatherall et al., 1984), and the Birth Defects Monitoring Program, which covers a third of all U.S. births (Edmonds et al., 1981). Such systems have identified important secular change in incidence of specific malformations but have rarely been able to identify or even suggest a responsible agent. Certainly it is difficult to pursue temporal or spatial clusters of events if no plausible theory about cause presents itself. In such cases, follow-up may focus on exposure to known risk factors, to rule out obvious explanations. In spite of the difficulties, it is clearly essential to continue to document trends in birth defects frequency. Also, such registries are a source of cases for specially mounted studies to test hypotheses about new hazards.

Two examples of registries designed for epidemiologic studies are Finland's matched-pair register of selected indicator malformations (Saxen, 1983), a supplement to its national Register of Congenital Malformations, and the Metropolitan Atlanta Congenital Defects Program (MACDP) (Edmonds et al., 1981). The MACDP protocol includes interviews conducted with mothers of children born with certain major malformations, concerning a broad spectrum of potentially relevant exposures. Tests of hypothesized associations are carried out by comparing the exposure histories of mothers in the case group of interest with the histories of mothers of children with other birth defects; this strategy assumes that a given exposure relates to only one, or at most a few, group(s) of malformations. The Finnish program uses a more conventional case-control strategy; each new case is matched to a normal birth, and standardized interviews are carried out with both case and control mothers. These two systems have made use of already collected data to test new hypotheses concerning such agents as spermicides (Cordero and Layde, 1983) and video display terminals (Kurppa et al., 1985).

There are at least two ways in which registries could be strengthened for purposes of developmental research. First, a great deal more effort should be directed to means of acquiring detailed exposure data, either by interview or by linkage with other data sources. Second, registration should be extended to end points other than birth defects, such as low birthweight, fetal loss, and developmental disabilities. This has been suggested previously (e.g., Kline et al., 1977; Oakley, 1985) and is strongly recommended in a recent report of a World Health Organization meeting (El Batawi et al., 1987).

2. Case Reports/Clusters

Case series of developmental effects have produced important etiologic clues. It has frequently been remarked that most known hazards to humans were in fact identified through clusters of illness for which clinicians and patients sought an explanation in some common exposure. The developmental effects of polychlorinated biphenyls (PCBs), methylmercury, and hexachlorobenzene began as clinical hunches that were confirmed in follow-up research studies. Associations that are not sufficiently striking to be noticed by clinicians or the public are less likely to be detected. Some means should be found for institutionalizing the "astute clinician." An example of such an approach is the Food and Drug Administration's teratogen information system, which solicits case reports from health professionals in addition to compiling information on suspected associations from many other data sources (Morgan et al., 1988). Another approach might involve establishing a coordinated surveillance network.

3. Record Linkage

Existing data systems also have potential for use in developmental research, providing a means can be found to associate exposure information with outcome. One possibility is to use exposure data contained in the record of outcome itself. The 1989 revision of the fetal death certificate will add items concerning the parents' occupation and industry in the year prior to the loss (Freedman et al., 1988), and it can be hoped that medical records will increasingly include a standard occupational and environmental history. Another option is to link records of outcome to geographically based environmental data, as in an ecologic study. One example of this approach is the study of low birthweight among babies born to mothers residing in more and less highly exposed areas of Love Canal (Vianna and Polan, 1984).

Ideally, one wants to link outcome to exposure at the individual level. The Nordic countries have used record linkage based on unique personal identifiers as a way of examining associations between registered data on exposure (e.g., union or employer registers) and reproductive outcomes (Selevan et al., 1986; Lindbohm and Hemminki, 1988). Although not without some limitations, the use of available records is economical and can mitigate potential biases in interview-based studies. At present, this strategy is unavailable to American researchers, but a recent Federal task force on human health and the environment recommended that the United States adopt a unique health record numbering system to facilitate such linkage (Dixon et al., 1986). The Social Security number has sometimes been used as an identifier but is not ideal in the best of circumstances and certainly is problematic if one wants to link prenatal or early postnatal exposures to reproductive or developmental outcomes. The National Health and Nutrition Examination Survey (National Center for Health Statistics, 1981) includes biological measurements of environmental toxicants, such as metals and pesticides, and could be an important source of exposure data for record linkage studies if identifying information were available. The exposure files to be established by the newly created Agency for Toxic Substances and Disease Registry are another potential resource.

4. Special Epidemiologic Studies

Epidemiologic studies of exposures suspected as hazardous on the basis of toxicologic research or anecdotal reports have also been productive in evaluating developmental hazards. Such studies have used mainly cross-sectional and case-control designs. For example, a case-control study, based on the MACDP register described above, was initiated by the Centers for Disease Control to examine the question of father's service in Vietnam and risk of birth defects in the offspring (Erickson et al., 1984). A cross-sectional study in Scotland examined current blood lead concentrations in relation to cognitive ability and school performance in children six to nine years old (Fulton et al., 1987). Particularly for such neurobehavioral outcomes, the emphasis now is on prospective studies and, more recently, longitudinal cohort studies. The longitudinal approach involves a costly and demanding protocol but will support the most secure inferences. Because repeated measures of exposure and outcome are available, such studies can distinguish effects of exposure during critical periods from effects of cumulative exposures. They also can differentiate developmental delay from long-term deficits (e.g., McMichael et al., 1988).

NEW DIRECTIONS THAT MAY CONTRIBUTE TO RISK ASSESSMENT

While striking associations or strong relationships are bound to come to attention in time, associations involving smaller increases in risk and less obvious health effects will not be detected without careful regard for minimizing sources of error.

Better measures of exposure are needed, particularly in studying agents for which self-reports or environmental exposure data poorly approximate individual dose because of vagaries in uptake and pharmacokinetics. There is a real risk of underestimating or missing causal associations if individuals whose delivered dose is trivial are included among the "exposed." Biological dosimeters may be needed to make a proper assessment of risk. It was not, for instance, until the advent of work measuring lead in primary dentition that an association between moderate lead exposure in childhood and cognitive/behavioral functioning could be adequately evaluated. For developmental research, samples of placental and fetal tissue, amniotic fluid, cord blood, and breast milk may also be useful for evaluating certain exposures.

With respect to measurement of outcome, precision is again important in order to identify etiologically similar subgroups of cases for purposes of causal research. Understanding of mechanism is also enhanced when more precise descriptions of outcome are used. Mechanistic data would ultimately improve the ability to extrapolate findings from species to species, as well as from compound to compound. In addition to measures that refine diagnosis of clinical outcomes, biological measures of early response or subclinical effects can also contribute insight into process. If observations are extended along a continuum, dose-response relationships can be more rigorously tested. Thus, consideration should be given in general to development of clinical and preclinical end points.

In terms of end points for investigation, emerging data suggest the possibility that head circumference may be a sensitive parameter of central nervous system (CNS) effects. Reassessment of Japanese atomic bomb survivors irradiated in utero shows effects on head size even at low doses (Miller and Blott, 1972); in many cases, small head size was accompanied by frank mental retardation (Otake and Schull, 1984). In addition, preliminary results from further studies of this cohort indicate a radiation dose-dependent decrement in school grades and IQ scores (Brown and Scialli, 1986). For infants exposed prenatally to PCBs, Fein and colleagues (1984) observed reductions in head size over and above effects on birthweight and gestation. Finally, evaluation of data from the Woman and Infant Children program found that the main benefit from maternal food supplementation in pregnancy is a small but significant increase in infant head circumference (David Rush, personal communication). It has also been proposed that minor physical anomalies—particularly multiple minor anomalies—are a sensitive indicator of teratogenicity (Holmes et al., 1985), and perhaps especially of neurodevelopmental toxicity (Firestone and Prabhu, 1983). In addition, there is much current interest in end points relating to cognition, behavior (including sexual behavior), and social functioning (for example, recent follow-up studies of children exposed to PCBs, e.g., Rogan et al., 1988).

Finally, the case of diethylstilbesterol (Steinberger and Lloyd, 1985) makes clear the need for long-term follow-up of cohorts exposed prenatally to compounds that may affect reproductive capacity in the male or female offspring. Of particular concern are agents that could alter fetal gametogenesis, fetal sex hormone production, or the structure and function of the reproductive tract.

19.
STRUCTURE-ACTIVITY RELATIONSHIPS

Roman Osman

INTRODUCTION TO STRUCTURE-ACTIVITY RELATIONSHIPS

The purpose of formulating a Structure-Activity Relationship (SAR) is to express in a coherent way the relationship between chemical structure and biological activity induced by a series of compounds. The underlying assumption is that a causal relationship exists between the observed biological activity and the structure of the molecules responsible for the biological activity. The logical link in such a relationship is demonstrated in the following diagram:

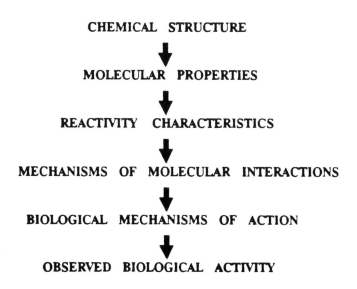

The biological activity at the bottom of the diagram is linked logically to the chemical structure through a set of well-defined steps. Thus, the observed biological activity is caused by a combination of biological mechanisms of action (e.g., stimulation or inhibition of enzymatic activity, transport, ion conduction, cell division). These biological mechanisms are in turn caused by specific molecular interactions (e.g., substrates or inhibitors with enzymes, drugs with receptors, ions with channels), that are controlled by the reactivity characteristics of the interacting molecular components. The molecular properties, which are determined by chemical structure, are responsible for the reactivity characteristics, thus establishing the logical causal relationship between chemical structure and biological activity.

The SAR diagram presented above serves as a branching point for two different approaches to the elucidation of SARs and to their applicability. One approach is concerned with the formulation of the causal relationships in the above sequence. Its main thrust is therefore mechanistic, and its applicability is to the understanding of the basic mechanisms of biological activity. The other approach, quantitative structure-activity relationship (QSAR), is concerned with the formulation of quantitative relationships between the measured biological activity and a set of parameters that represent structure. Its main thrust is to formulate a mathematical equation that will have predictive strength with respect to the biological activities of new compounds that have not been included in the initial set from which this relationship was constructed.

In spite of the predictive power that these formulations may have, their ability to suggest mechanisms is limited. The main reasons for this limitation lie in the restricted meaning of the structural and molecular parameters used in the correlation and in the purely statistical (usually linear) nature of the quantitative formulation of the SAR.

The field of developmental toxicology can benefit from both approaches to SARs. The first approach, being investigative in character, will help establish the spectrum of well-defined biological activities that contribute to the complicated processes in teratogenesis. It will help to determine which molecular properties encoded in the chemical structure are responsible for the molecular reactivities. These lead to specific interactions that, in turn, modulate the biological activity. The second approach, being statistical in nature, can be used to screen drugs and other chemicals for their potential toxicity in a rapid and fairly reliable way. While the first approach is a long-range commitment, it is a necessary foundation for the formulation of the meaning of the parameters and the quantitative relationships in the QSAR.

The two approaches complement each other, and efforts should be devoted to the refinement of the QSAR approach by introducing into it parameters that have a mechanistic basis. The QSAR approach will then become a powerful quantitative tool for the prediction and explanation of toxicity based on sound causal relationships.

PREVIOUS ATTEMPTS AT APPLYING SARs DEVELOPMENTAL TOXICOLOGY

The recent literature on SARs in developmental toxicology can be divided into three main categories. One category is represented by the rather limited efforts to apply QSAR to this field. For example, this is represented by work such as that of Enslein (Enslein et al., 1983; Enslein, 1984; and references cited therein), which draws heavily on the standard techniques of QSAR. This is a purely statistical approach based on a large number of chemicals with varying degrees of developmental toxicity.

The strength of Enslein's approach is the impartial representation of chemicals according to their structural parameters. The problems associated with this approach have to do, to some extent, with the apparent strength. That is, the impartial method of describing the molecule in the form of structural parameters cannot produce a mechanistic hypothesis which could be followed by other techniques to refine the SAR. Furthermore, this model deals with a heterogeneous data set not only with respect to the chemicals included in the correlation, but more importantly, with respect to their biological activity. Even classifications such as "teratogenic" and "nonteratogenic" are both subjective and limited in predictive power.

As discussed below, developmental toxicity (and even teratogenesis) cannot be considered as a uniform biological end point. Therefore, the predictive power of such statistical approaches may be accidental. Nevertheless, the usefulness of these approaches for rapid screening is obvious if they can be shown to work in suitable studies. It is important to mention in this respect the need of extensive data bases for the construction of the statistical QSAR; the resources available for this purpose have been discussed by Wassom (1985).

THE SEARCH FOR RELEVANT STRUCTURAL FEATURES OF DEVELOPMENTAL TOXICANTS

The second category of SAR literature that deals with developmental toxicity encompasses attempts to define the chemical variability in the structure of related compounds that is relevant to the biological end point. The quality of work varies from the simple and limited to the more extensive and sophisticated. Examples of the former are characterized by a simple classifying approach in which a series of drugs is declared as teratogenic based on very limited data (Lloyd et al., 1965) or classified into two structural groups without a significant relationship to teratogenic activity (Teramoto et al., 1981). Alternatively, a rank order is established (Korhonen et al., 1982) or a non-dose-related classification is suggested (Keller et al., 1984).

Better SAR studies concentrate on the elucidation of the correlation between certain types of structure and toxicity, but they rarely yield a formulation of the molecular mechanism that may be responsible for the biological action. For example, an increase in the chain length of alkoxy acids lowers their embryotoxicity, but from the paper it is not clear why (Rawlings et al., 1985). Similarly, benzo[a]pyrene is an active carcinogen in the mouse fetus, while its K-region metabolite, benzo[a]pyrene-4,5-oxide, is not. The ultimate metabolite, BPDE, which is not a K-region metabolite, shows even higher activity as a carcinogen (Rossi et al., 1983). The puzzle, although interesting in itself, is not resolved. It nevertheless prompts the authors to come to the conclusion that K-region metabolism is not activating the compounds to become carcinogenic, while the ultimate metabolism has a major contribution to this property.

The review by Woo (1983) is a vast compilation of data on derivatives of carbamates but leads only to the conclusion that some ordering ideas are important for the SAR of these compounds. An important observation of this author is that small structural changes may have profound effects on the carcinogenic, mutagenic, and teratogenic activities of these compounds. No suggestions as to possible mechanisms for such extreme sensitivity to molecular alterations are offered.

Opposite conclusions are reached concerning the structural requirements of retinoids for induction of terata (Willhite et al., 1984; Willhite, 1986). The identification of the molecular properties is carefully delineated, but the molecular link is missing. Similar approaches appear in the analysis of the stereochemistry of steroidal amine teratogens (Gaffield and Keeler, 1984) or the redox potential of nitroheterocyclics (Greenaway et al., 1986).

A series of papers on steroid teratogens (Brown and Keeler, 1978a-c) carefully analyzes their SARs and suggests that their activity comes about from the inhibition of hormone action. This proposed mechanism is not, however, supported by studies that would demonstrate that such competition is indeed operational.

These SAR studies illustrate the need to define relationships in molecular mechanistic terms that will eventually lead to the formulation of the causal relationship between structure and biological activity.

IDENTIFICATION OF MECHANISMS OF DEVELOPMENTAL TOXICITY

The third class of SAR literature is concerned with the identification of the biological mechanisms responsible for teratogenicity or other developmental toxicity. An unsuccessful attempt to relate the protective properties of nicotinic acid against organophosphate-induced teratogenesis to mechanisms involving altered rates of metabolism (Roger et al., 1969) is a good example of the approach to the characterization of the biological spectrum of teratogenic activity. A thorough discussion of the need of metabolism for the activation of chemicals to their toxic form is presented by Druckrey (1973), but the SAR components in this presentation are not clear. A somewhat different approach is the attempt to define teratogenicity as the consequence of enzyme induction (Poland and Glover, 1973, 1980; Lucier and McDaniel, 1979).

Thalidomide is one of the most widely studied developmental toxicants, but the mechanism by which this chemical induces teratogenesis is still not clear. Some suggestions relate its activity to induction of metabolizing enzymes (Neubert and Krowke, 1983). However, in a series of publications by Jonsson and coworkers (Jonsson, 1972a,b; Jonsson et al., 1972), the extreme selectivity of thalidomide out of 17 structurally related compounds was not explained. Extending the chemically related series of molecules and expanding the investigation into probing which of the two rings is responsible for the activity also left the mechanism unresolved. Nevertheless, the authors produced an interesting speculation about the interaction of thalidomide with nucleic acids, represented as a molecular interaction. This led to the hypothesis that this interaction is involved with some factors that regulate skeletal tissue formation (Jonsson, 1972b).

The complexity of teratogenicity is illustrated by the teratogenic and anti-teratogenic effects of compounds that are structurally very similar (Uyeki et al., 1982). A careful study of cyclophosphamide (Nau et al., 1982) identified, through the use of isotopic substitution, the crucial step in the conversion of cyclophosphamide to the toxic phosphoramide mustard. In a different approach, the biological spectrum of adenosine analogues has been identified, and all these activities have been linked to the inhibition of SAH-hydrolase. This inhibition supposedly disturbs transmethylation in rapidly proliferating systems (Holy, 1982).

In two other publications (Abramovici and Rachmut-Roizman, 1983; Johnson et al., 1984) important concepts of embryotoxicity are described, and the distinction between teratogenicity and lethality is clearly stated. Finally, a very extensive review of the agents that may affect the male reproductive system (Bernstein, 1984) makes an important point about using the SAR as an alerting tool for the prediction of potential toxicity of certain structures.

It should be quite clear from these publications that an attempt to define developmental toxicity as a product of a single biological event would not produce the correct representation. Developmental toxicity is probably the consequence of the combination of many biological processes that are influenced by the various toxic agents. Thus, in order to be able to define the relationships between chemical properties and developmental effects, the biological spectrum involved should be more clearly defined. Subsequently, the biological processes responsible for the ultimate activity could be cast in molecular terms that will eventually lead to elucidation of the causal relationship between structure and biological activity.

20.
STATISTICAL ANALYSIS OF DEVELOPMENTAL TOXICITY DATA

Vernon M. Chinchilli

A number of difficulties arise in the statistical analysis of data from developmental toxicity studies. First, the sheer volume of data and the diverse types of end points can be overwhelming. A typical study might include a wide variety of end points measuring fertility, maternal toxicity, teratogenesis, and fetal developmental toxicity. Some of these end points are measured directly on the parental animal, while the majority are measured on the fetus or pup. End points can be expressed on a continuous scale (such as weight, crown-to-rump distance, etc.) or a discrete scale (presence/absence of an effect, severity of an effect on a four-point scale, etc.). If a dichotomous end point is to be expressed in terms of the litter rather than the fetus, the result is a proportional response (proportion of fetuses with a certain effect). This latter situation leads to the question of whether the fetus or the litter is the experimental unit.

EXPERIMENTAL UNIT

From a statistical viewpoint, it is reasonable to assume that the litter (and not the fetus) is the experimental unit (Palmer, 1974; Haseman and Hogan, 1975). This is because the parental animal is randomized to treatment, the parental animal receives the treatment directly, and fetuses/pups within a litter usually exhibit a litter effect, in that they do not respond independently of one another. Regardless of whether the response of interest is measured on a continuous or dichotomous scale, ignoring the litter effect when it actually exists leads to invalid statistical tests. In this situation, the statistical test would be too liberal in the sense that the Type I error rate is inflated (the null hypothesis is rejected more often than it should be). On the other hand, employing a statistical test that incorporates a litter effect when no such effect exists usually results in a conservative test (the null hypothesis is not rejected as often as it should be).

The best approach to resolve this issue within a particular study is to use a more general statistical model that incorporates a litter effect. Under a set of parametric assumptions, the model without a litter effect is a special case of the more general model. Then it is possible to conduct a preliminary test to determine whether the litter effect is significant. If it is, the more general model is retained; otherwise, the simpler model, without a litter effect, is invoked. Unfortunately, this approach is not applicable in a nonparametric setting (e.g., with rank statistics) because a model without litter effects cannot be expressed as a special case of a model with litter effects.

ANALYSIS OF A CONTINUOUS RESPONSE VARIABLE

Usually an analysis of variance (ANOVA) model provides a reasonable setting for analyzing a continuous response variable from a developmental toxicity study. In particular, a nested ANOVA model is an appropriate choice for incorporating litter effects:

$$Y_{ijk} = \mu + \tau_i + \beta_{ij} + \varepsilon_{ijk} \qquad [20\text{-}1]$$

where μ represents the overall mean, τ_i the fixed effect due to the ith treatment $(1 \leq i \leq t_i)$, β_{ij} the random effect due to the jth litter nested within the ith treatment group $(1 \leq j \leq m_i)$, and ε_{ijk} the random effect due to the kth fetus nested within the litter of the ith treatment $(1 \leq k \leq n_{ij})$. In the classical nested ANOVA model (Searle, 1971), it is assumed that the β_{ij} are independent and identically distributed as normal random variables with null mean and variance σ^2_b, the ε_{ijk} are independent and identically distributed with null mean and variance ε^2_e, and the β_{ij} and ε_{ijk} are independent.

The null hypothesis of no litter effect is equivalent to H_0: $\sigma^2_b = 0$, and an F-test is easily constructed as the ratio $MS_{L(t)}/MS_e$, where $MS_{L(t)}$ is the mean square for litter within treatment and MS_e is the mean square for error. Assuming that the litter effect is significant, an overall test of treatment differences is constructed as the F-ratio of $MS_t/MS_{t(L)}$. The latter F-test only reveals whether differences among the groups exist, and it does not indicate what those differences are. A multiple comparison procedure, such as Dunnett's test (Dunnett, 1955; Miller, 1981), can be applied to determine which treatment groups differ significantly from control. For Dunnett's procedure within the nested ANOVA model, as in the overall test of treatment differences, the denominator mean square is $MS_{L(t)}$ and not MS_e.

When the levels of the treatment groups are dose levels of some chemical agent, a linear trend (dose-response) test can be constructed as an F-test on a contrast of the treatment levels. A contrast is a linear combination of the treatment effects of the form $c_1\tau_1 + c_2\tau_2 + ... + c_t\tau_t$, where $c_1 + c_2 + ...$ $+ c_t = 0$. For a contrast of linear trend, the constants $c_1, c_2, ..., c_t$ are chosen as a function of the t dose levels. If the dose levels are evenly spaced, then $c_i = i - 1/2(t+1)$, $1 \leq i \leq t$. If the doses are not evenly spaced, then complicated formulas are needed to calculate the appropriate constants. Again, the denominator mean square of the F-test of the contrast should be $MS_{L(t)}$ and not MS_e. Most ANOVA software packages for mainframe computers, such as Statistical Analysis Software System (SAS) and Biomedical Data Processing (BMDP), and some ANOVA packages for personal computers include options for testing contrasts.

In the absence of a litter effect ($\sigma_b^2 = 0$), the model in equation 20-1 reduces to a one-way ANOVA model, and the above procedures basically remain the same, except that MS_e is the appropriate denominator mean square.

For any ANOVA model, the assumptions of normality and homogeneity of variance are critical. (Heterogeneity of variance can even invalidate a nonparametric analysis.) Therefore, prior to conducting an ANOVA, it is wise to check these assumptions. The set of residuals from an ANOVA provides a convenient tool for investigating the validity of these assumptions. Most textbooks on regression and analysis of variance discuss these issues (Draper and Smith, 1981). Sometimes heterogeneity of variance can be removed via a transformation of the original data, such as a log or square-root transformation. In the case of nonnormal data, either a transformation to approximate a normal distribution (Box and Cox, 1964, 1982; Hinkley and Runger, 1984) or nonparametric analyses (Lehmann, 1975; Hettmansperger, 1984) can be applied. Unfortunately, there does not appear to be a nonparametric version of a nested ANOVA, so that multivariate nonparametric methods must be invoked in the presence of litter effects. This could be quite cumbersome, because the number of fetuses/pups per litter is not constant.

One statistical issue that has not been discussed to this point is the fact that the number of fetuses/pups per litter itself is a random variable, even though the ANOVA model assumes that this is fixed prior to the experiment. Statisticians have yet to address this problem for the analysis of a continuous response variable from a developmental toxicity study, whereas its implications have been investigated somewhat for dichotomous variables. The probable reason for this is that statisticians have concentrated on dichotomous response variables in developmental toxicity studies because they comprise the majority of measured response variables.

ANALYSIS OF A DICHOTOMOUS RESPONSE VARIABLE

Haseman and Kupper (1979) have reviewed the various approaches to the analysis of a dichotomous response variable in developmental toxicity studies. The majority of the acceptable approaches can be categorized into four groups: (1) generalized binomial models, (2) nonparametric analyses, (3) transformations of proportions, and (4) resampling techniques. The handling of the litter effect is unique for each of the four general approaches.

The beta-binomial model, as discussed by Williams (1975) for developmental toxicity studies, is the most popular generalized binomial model. It is derived by assuming that X, the number of positive responses in a litter of size n, follows a binomial distribution with probability of success θ, $0 < \theta < 1$, and that θ itself is a random variable following a beta distribution. Then the unconditional distribution of X is the beta-binomial. Whereas the binomial is a one-parameter model (θ = the probability of a positive response for any fetus/pup) and assumes that the fetuses/pups are independent (no litter effect), the beta-binomial is a two-parameter model (θ, and ϕ = the correlation between any two fetuses/pups) and assumes a nonnegative correlation among fetuses/pups. The probability model is expressed as follows:

$$P[X = x] = \left\{ \prod_{r=0}^{x-1} \left[\theta + \frac{r\phi}{1-\phi} \right] \right\} \left\{ \prod_{r=0}^{n-x-1} \left[(1-\theta) + \frac{r\phi}{1-\phi} \right] \right\} \left\{ \prod_{r=0}^{n-1} \left[1 + \frac{r\phi}{1-\phi} \right] \right\}^{-1}$$

[20-2]

Thus, the litter effect corresponds to ϕ (> 0), and analogous to the nested ANOVA model for a continuous variable, the binomial is a special case of the beta-binomial when $\phi = 0$. This permits a test for the presence of a litter effect.

For modeling the responses of the litters of all the treatment groups, it is assumed that a litter from the [i]th treatment group follows a beta-binomial distribution with parameters θ_i, and ϕ_i, $1 \leq i \leq t$. The maximum likelihood estimates of the 2t parameters can be found via a Newton-Raphson algorithm (Williams, 1975). If a trend test is of interest, a reasonable approach is to reduce the number of parameters to $t+2$ by modeling the logit of the probability parameters as a linear function of dose, i.e., $\log\{\theta_i/(1-\theta_i)\} = \alpha + \beta d_i$, where d_i is the [i]th dose level, $1 \leq i \leq t$. This form of a trend test was discussed by Kupper et al. (1986). A further reduction in parameters is possible by assuming that the correlation parameters are homogeneous across groups, i.e., ϕ_1 ϕ_2 = ... = ϕ_t. However, simulation studies conducted by

Kupper et al. (1986) indicated that biased tests of linear trend can result when this assumption is false.

Kupper and Haseman (1978) proposed another generalized binomial model, which they called the correlated binomial. It is identical to the model proposed by Altham (1978), which she called the additive generalized binomial. Altham (1978) also introduced a multiplicative generalized binomial. These generalized binomial models are slightly more flexible than the beta-binomial, in that a negative litter effect is permissible. However, these models pose a larger degree of computational difficulty in conducting a likelihood analysis, because of data-dependent restrictions on the parameters in the former and data-dependent normalizing constants in the latter. Van Ryzin (1975) considered a generalized binomial model in which the litter size is random. Some statisticians feel that the model assumptions, in particular the independence of the probability of response and the litter size, are not feasible. Van Ryzin (1975) suggested an alternative approach to estimating model parameters in the presence of dependence. However, this model has not been included in any of the simulation studies that have appeared in the literature, so its performance is not well understood.

In a nonparametric approach, the proportional responses for the litters can be ranked and a Kruskal-Wallis test applied, which reduces to the Wilcoxon rank sum test or Mann-Whitney test when t = 2. Gaylor (1978) discussed nonparametric analyses for developmental toxicity studies in detail. The nonparametric version of the trend test is known as Jonckheere's Test. Lin and Haseman (1976) have modified it to allow for ties, a situation usually encountered with the proportional responses observed in developmental toxicity studies. These rank tests are computationally easy and avoid some of the distributional difficulties of the generalized binomial models.

The one drawback to ranking the proportions is that the ranks ignore litter size. For instance, a proportion of 1/3 receives the same rank as 4/12, even though the latter proportion provides a more accurate and reliable representation of that litter. If the litter sizes do not vary much across groups, then the nonparametric approach works very well. On the other hand, if there is a great deal of variability in litter sizes across groups, a nonparametric analysis could be biased and lead to improper interpretations.

In the transformation approach, the observed binomial proportions for the litters are transformed to approximate normal random variables, so that one-way ANOVA techniques can be applied. According to Haseman and Kupper (1979), two useful transformations are the Freeman-Tukey binomial arc-sine transformation, given by

$$y = \{\sin^{-1} [x/(n+1)]^{1/2} + \sin^{-1} [(x+1)/(n+1)]^{1/2} \} \qquad [20\text{-}3]$$

and the arc-sine transformation, given by

$$y = \begin{cases} \sin^{-1}(x/n)^{1/2} & \text{if } 0 < x < n \\ \sin^{-1}(1/4n)^{1/2} & \text{if } x = 0 \\ \sin^{-1} i - \sin^{-1}(1/4n)^{1/2} & \text{if } x = n \end{cases} \qquad [20\text{-}4]$$

Analogous to the nonparametric analysis, this transformation approach does not account for varying litter sizes, so it is subject to the same criticisms.

Gladen (1979) invoked jackknife methodology to arrive at estimators of $\theta_1, \theta_2, \ldots, \theta_t$ which are weighted according to litter sizes. Then a one-way ANOVA of the jackknifed estimators, weighted by their estimated variances, can be justified asymptotically. Analogous approaches using other resampling plans, such as the bootstrap (Efron, 1982), have been suggested, but their application to developmental toxicity studies has not appeared in the literature.

COMPARISONS OF PROCEDURES FOR A DICHOTOMOUS RANDOM VARIABLE

A number of researchers have conducted simulation studies to compare the performance of the great variety of estimators and tests that have been proposed for developmental toxicity data. Haseman and Kupper (1979) reviewed these studies and concluded that none of the above procedures seems to be superior in terms of power and attainment of the desired significance level. They warned that because the nonparametric and transformation approaches do not account for varying litter sizes, they could be biased and inefficient, although most of the simulation studies they reviewed did not reveal any great loss of statistical power.

Another cautionary note they issued is that hypothesis testing within the framework of the beta-binomial model usually causes inflation of the Type I error rate (Haseman and Kupper, 1979). They indicated that this might occur because the nonnegativity restriction on the correlation parameters $\phi_1, \phi_2, \ldots, \phi, \phi_t$ results in a breakdown of the asymptotic properties of the maximum likelihood estimators when any of these parameters are truly zero. Prentice (1986) showed that actually the lower boundary of the correlation parameter need not be zero but is given by

$$\phi \geq \max\left[-\theta/(n - \theta - 1), -(1 - \theta)/(n - 1 + \theta - 1)\right] \qquad [20\text{-}5]$$

in order for the beta-binomial to be a proper probability model. Therefore, the practice of converting the maximum likelihood estimate of ϕ to zero when it is negative could be relaxed. Although this improvement might complicate the computations in the same manner as the correlated binomial, its effects have yet to be investigated.

Shirley and Hickling (1981) found the likelihood ratio tests based on the beta-binomial model to be conservative, but their simulations consisted of data generated only from the beta-binomial distribution. They reported that T-tests (F-tests for the case of more than two groups) based on the transformed proportions (via equation 20-3) performed just as well as, if not better than, the likelihood ratio tests and the nonparametric tests. Paul (1982) examined the beta-binomial, correlated binomial, and multiplicative generalized binomial. Basing his conclusions on real data sets and simulations, he determined that the beta-binomial provides a better fit to developmental toxicity data than the other two generalized binomial models. Paul (1982) also found no real differences in performance for tests based on the jackknife procedure (Gladen, 1979) and likelihood ratio tests with the beta-binomial model.

21.
MATHEMATICAL MODELING OF TERATOGENIC EFFECTS

Todd W. Thorslund

In recent years, much attention has been focused on the use of mathematical models, instead of the well-established but ad hoc safety factor approach, to define exposure levels for which no adverse effect is expected for teratogens. Many of the mathematical models suggested for use in this regard are adaptations of those commonly employed in cancer risk assessment, such as the multistage, multihit, probit, and logit models. The validity of this approach is questionable, however, due to anticipated differences in the underlying mechanisms of action for carcinogens and teratogens.

An alternative to the use of cancer models for teratogenesis, based on pharmacokinetics and drug receptor considerations, was developed by Jusko (1972). His model predicts that the fraction of intact or normal fetuses follows an n-target single hit dose-response relationship (Elkind and Whitmore, 1967). Within the context of this model, two classes of teratogens exist: those that appear to have thresholds and those that do not. In Jusko's investigations, certain agents, such as thalidomide and cyclophosphamide, appeared to attack a single target and no threshold could be determined. Other agents affected multiple targets and demonstrated practical threshold responses.

Jusko's basic model was generalized by Rai and Van Ryzin (1985) and Van Ryzin (1985) to account for the variations introduced by litters, treating litter size as a covariate. Kupper et al. (1986) used a log logistic dose-response model and generalized it to account for litter effects, which were interpreted within the context of the model as "extra-binomial" variation. The litter effect might be explained by factors such as heterogeneous fetal exposure between mothers as well as by interlitter variation in genotype. This hypothesis could be tested by obtaining fetal tissue, blood, and whole-body exposures from individual fetuses and their mothers as part of teratogenicity experiments.

22.
APPLICATION OF EXPERIMENTAL
DATA IN RISK ASSESSMENT

Ronald D. Hood

In addition to such obvious issues as appropriate statistical analyses, identification and categorization of defects, the relative significance of direct vs. maternally mediated effects on the conceptus, ability to extrapolate from animal data to humans, and the like that are discussed elsewhere in this document, some further issues are of concern and will be taken up in this section.

A/D RATIOS AND RELATED CONCEPTS

Fabro (1985) has contended that developmental toxicity tests must answer three questions: "(1) Can the agent induce developmental defects; (2) what are the effective doses; (3) are the effective doses below adult toxic doses?" A problem related to these questions is the establishment of a means for comparing the relative risk associated with exposure to different agents.

In 1981, Johnson proposed the use of the ratio between the minimally effective toxic dose in the adult organism and the minimal developmentally toxic dose in the same species. The concept was then refined, and the ratio derived was termed the A/D (i.e., adult/developmental) ratio (Johnson et al., 1982; Johnson and Gabel, 1982, 1983; Johnson, 1984). In essence, Johnson and his colleagues contend that chemicals can be categorized on the basis of their A/D ratios. Those agents found to have A/D ratios less than 3 would be considered "coeffective teratogens," in that their developmental and adult toxicities were seen at similar doses. They would not be considered uniquely hazardous to the conceptus. Substances with A/D ratios between 3 and 5 would be considered to be of some hazard to the conceptus, but not of major concern. Chemicals with A/D ratios of between 5 and 10 would be regulated as potential developmental toxicants, and those with ratios over 10 would be considered potential unique major hazards to the conceptus.

Although Johnson developed the concept of the A/D ratio while evaluating the use of the *Hydra attenuata* system for screening for developmental toxicity (e.g., Johnson and Gabel, 1982), he proposes that it is equally applicable for use with systems such as the traditional in vivo tests in pregnant mammals (Johnson, 1984). According to Johnson (1983a, 1984), the A/D ratios for a given chemical when tested in various mammalian species are remarkably similar. This was said to be true even when different routes of administration are used, with the possible exception of substances that are metabolized by individual species in a novel manner. Nevertheless, the concept of cross-species similarity of A/D ratios has recently been challenged by Daston and coworkers (1989).

In a similar vein, Fabro et al. (1982) proposed what they termed the Relative Teratogenic Index or RTI, which they defined as the ratio of the adult LD_{01} to the fetal tD_{05}, defined as "the dose required to induce an additional 5 percent malformation rate above the background rate." The authors stated that simply using the ratio between the adult LD_{50} and the fetal tD_{50} would be improper, as the dose-response slopes for the two measures of toxicity often differed. It was also suggested that the tD_{05} was used because it could be more accurately calculated than could the tD_{01}, and that data from species other than the mouse were needed in order to ascertain whether the RTI concept was widely applicable. In practice, the RTI appears similar in concept to the A/D ratio, but it unfortunately relies only on malformation as its developmental toxicity end point.

Johnson and Gabel (1983) proposed that substances with low A/D ratios not be considered unique hazards to the conceptus, even though they may be capable of causing developmental toxicity at sufficiently high doses. They further suggested that such chemical agents be regulated on the basis of their adult toxicity, under the assumption that this would provide adequate protection to the developing offspring. Nevertheless, Johnson (1984) points out that such a concept must be tempered with the recognition that there are three situations with regard to chemical hazards to the unborn: (1) Substances that are somewhat equally toxic to adults and embryos but used at or near adult toxic levels—i.e., A/D ratio near unity. The mother may recover but the embryo may be irrevocably damaged, e.g., ethyl alcohol. (2) Substances that, though used at levels below those toxic to adults, have the ability to injure the embryo at a small fraction of the adult toxic dose, i.e., A/D ratio markedly larger than 1, e.g., vinblastine and thalidomide. (3) Substances interacting in an additive or synergistic manner.

Such considerations make it clear that one cannot blindly apply a concept such as the A/D ratio or the RTI in regulation of potential developmental toxicants (Johnson and Christian, 1984). One must consider additional factors, such as likely human exposure levels, the relative need for use of the compound (e.g., cancer chemotherapeutic agents), the possibility of concurrent exposure to other factors that might increase the potential for hazard to the conceptus, and the relative magnitude and permanence of the possible developmental toxicity vs. effects likely to occur in the adult parent. Also, as was pointed out by Chitlik et al. (1985), the utility of such index systems is limited by their being based on a modest selection of dose levels, a limited set of end points, the test species selected, the numbers of test animals used, the specific dosing routes used, and various similar considerations.

DETERMINATION OF NO-OBSERVED-EFFECT LEVELS AND LOWEST-OBSERVED-EFFECT LEVELS

Quantitative risk assessment regarding developmental toxicity is highly uncertain at best. This is true because of a number of factors. For example, although known human developmental toxicants produce effects on the offspring of laboratory animals, there are often considerable species- or strain-related differences among the effects seen and these may or may not agree with the specific effects seen in humans. Thus, although false negatives appear to be rare if appropriate tests are done, it is yet difficult to extrapolate specific findings, such as a particular malformation or behavioral deficit, from animals to humans. The extent of possible false positives obtained in animal tests is even more uncertain, in that truly reliable human data are typically nonexistent. Thus, we do not yet know which of the typically measured specific end points should be monitored most closely in order to set no-observed-effect levels (NOELs) or lowest-observed-effect levels (LOELs) for developmental effects, either within or across given test species. Nevertheless, a measure of comfort may be taken from Palmer's (1980) assertion that all teratogens tested have manifested other evidence of developmental toxicity at doses lower than those required to induce malformations.

The question also arises as to whether morphologic end points are adequate or whether functional or biochemical parameters should be included as well. The answer to such a question is difficult to obtain, especially since the most useful end point(s) may well vary among different test chemicals, depending on their effects on biological systems.

A further difficulty in assessing NOELs and LOELs is that they are typically derived from tests employing only a limited number of dose levels and relatively small numbers of animals. There is generally considerable uncertainty as to whether any NOELs or LOELs obtained from examination of such data are representative of true no- or low-effect levels. The uncertainties arising from this factor and others, such as those mentioned above, require the use of larger safety factors or margins of safety than would likely be necessary if the data and their extrapolation were more certain.

STATISTICAL vs. BIOLOGICAL SIGNIFICANCE OF VARIOUS OUTCOMES

It has often been suggested that the results of statistical analyses of developmental toxicity data cannot be followed blindly (e.g., Palmer, 1978; U.S. EPA, 1986a). There are several reasons for this. One is that a number of parameters are evaluated in each such test, and if the typical 5 percent probability level is used to define "statistical significance," one outcome in twenty is expected to appear significant even when there are no real effects. On the other hand, a low incidence of a rare event may not be deemed significant by statistical analysis, but may appear biologically relevant, especially if its incidence seems to have been dose-related (Palmer, 1978). In borderline cases, performance of a second study designed to address the points in question may be in order.

Another consideration is the appearance of a low and nonsignificant incidence of a positive finding in a low dosage group coupled with significant incidences in higher dosage groups. Here it has been suggested that confidence intervals or further experimentation may be used to attempt to resolve the issue of establishing a NOEL (U.S. EPA, 1986a).

REFERENCES

Abramovici, A., and P. Rachmut-Roizman. 1983. Molecular structure-teratogenicity relationships of some fragrance additives. *Toxicology* 29:143-156.

Adams, C. E., M. F. Hay, and C. Lutwak-Mann. 1961. The action of various agents upon the rabbit embryo. *J. Embryol. Exp. Morph.* 9:468-491.

Adams, P. M., O. Shabrawy, and M. S. Legator. 1984. Male-transmitted developmental and neuro-behavioral deficits. *Teratogenesis Carcinog. Mutagen.* 4:149-169.

Adams, J., J. Buelke-Sam, C. A. Kimmel, C. J. Nelson, L. A. Reiter, T. J. Sobotka, H. A. Tilson, and B. K. Nelson. 1985. Collaborative behavioral teratology study: Protocol design and testing procedures. *Neurobehav. Toxicol. Teratol.* 7:579-586.

Alexandrov, V. A. 1969. Uterine, vaginal, and mammary tumors induced by nitrosoureas in pregnant rats. *Nature* 222:1064-1065.

Alexandrov, V. A., V. N. Anisimov, N. M. Belous, I. A. Vasilyeva, and V. B. Mazon. 1980. The inhibition of the transplacental blastomogenic effect of nitrosomethylurea by postnatal administration of buformin to rats. *Carcinogenesis* 1:975.

Aliverti, V., L. Bonanomi, E. Giavini, V. G. Leone, and L. Mariani. 1979. The extent of fetal ossification as an index of delayed development in teratogenic studies on the rat. *Teratology* 20:237-242.

Allen, L. H., and F. J. Zeman. 1973. Kidney function in the progeny of protein-deficient rats. *J. Nutr.* 103:1467-1478.

Altham, P. M. E. 1978. Two generalizations of the binomial distribution. *Appl. Stat.* 27:162-167.

Amann, R. P. 1986. Detection of alterations in testicular and epididymal function in laboratory animals. *Environ. Health Perspect.* 70:149-158.

Anderson, L. M., and L. J. Priest. 1980. Reduction in the transplacental carcinogenic effect of methyl cholanthrene in mice by prior treatment with B-naphthoflavone. *Res. Com. Chem. Pathol. Pharmacol.* 30:431-446.

Anderson, L. M., K. Van Havere, and J. M. Budinger. 1983. Effects of polychlorinated biphenyls on lung and liver tumors initiated in suckling mice by N-nitrosodimethylamine. *J. Natl. Cancer Inst.* 71:157-163.

Anderson, L. M., P. J. Donovan, and J. M. Rice. 1985. Risk assessment for transplacental carcinogenesis. In: A. P. Li, ed. *New Approaches in Toxicity Testing and Their Application in Human Risk Assessment.* New York: Raven Press, 179-202.

Andrew, F. D. 1976. Techniques for assessment of teratogenic effects: Developmental enzyme patterns. *Environ. Health Perspect.* 18:111-116.

Andrew, F. D., and P. S. Lytz. 1981. Biochemical disturbances associated with developmental toxicity. In: C. A. Kimmel and J. Buelke-Sam, eds. *Biochemical Disturbances Associated with Developmental Toxicity.* New York: Raven Press, 145-165.

Aranda, J. V., and L. Stern. 1983. Clinical aspects of developmental pharmacology and toxicology. *Pharmacol. Ther.* 20:1-51.

Ariyuki, F., K. Higaki, and M. Yasuda. 1980. A study of fetal growth retardation in teratological tests: An examination of the relationship between body weight and ossification of coccygeal vertebrae in mouse and rat fetuses. *Teratology* 22:43-49.

Ariyuki, F., H. Ishihara, K. Higaki, and M. Yasuda. 1982. A study of fetal growth retardation in teratological tests: Relationship between body weight and ossification of the skeleton in rat fetuses. *Teratology* 26:263-267.

Auroux, M., and E. Dulioust. 1984. Cyclophosphamide in the male rat: Effect on the behavior of offspring. Teratology 30:19A.

Badr, F. M., and R. S. Badr. 1975. Induction of dominant lethal mutation in male mice by ethyl alcohol. *Nature* 253:134-136.

Baeder, C., G. A. S. Wickramaratne, H. Hummler, J. Merkle, H. Schon, and H. Tuchmann-Duplessis. 1985. Identification and assessment of the effects of chemicals on reproduction and development (reproductive toxicology). *Food Chem. Toxicol.* 23:377-388.

Barlow, S. M., and F. M. Sullivan. 1982. *Reproductive Hazards of Industrial Chemicals.* London: Academic Press.

Barlow, S. M., P. R. McElhatton, and F. M. Sullivan. 1975. The relation between maternal restraint and food deprivation, plasma corticosterone, and induction of cleft palate in the offspring of mice. *Teratology* 12:97-104.

Barlow, S. M., A. F. Knight, and F. M. Sullivan. 1978. Delay in postnatal growth and development of offspring produced by maternal restraint stress during pregnancy in the rat. *Teratology* 18:211-218.

Barlow, S. M., A. F. Knight, and F. M. Sullivan. 1979. Prevention by diazepam of adverse effects of maternal restraint stress on postnatal development and learning in the rat. *Teratology* 19:105-110.

Barlow, S. M., A. F. Knight, and F. M. Sullivan. 1980. Diazepam-induced cleft palate in the mouse: The role of endogenous maternal corticosterone. *Teratology* 21:149-155.

Barnett, J. B., L. S. F. Soderberg, and J. H. Menna. 1985. The effect of prenatal chlordane exposure on the delayed hypersensitivity response of BALB/c mice. *Toxicol. Lett.* 25:173-183.

Barr, M., R. P. Jensh, and R. L. Brent. 1969. Fetal weight and intrauterine position in rats. *Teratology* 2:241-246.

Barrach, H.-J., and D. Neubert. 1980. Significance of organ culture techniques for evaluation of prenatal toxicity. *Arch. Toxicol.* 45:161-187.

Bartels, H. 1970. *Prenatal Respiration.* New York: Wiley Interscience.

Bass, R., and D. Neubert. 1980. Testing for embryotoxicity. *Arch. Toxicol. Suppl.* 4:256-266.

Baumann, M., and K. Sander. 1984. Bipartite axiation follows incomplete epiboly in zebrafish embryos treated with chemical teratogens. *J. Exp. Zool.* 230:363-376.

Beach, R. S., M. E. Gershwin, and L. S. Hurley. 1982. Gestational zinc deprivation in mice: Persistence of immunodeficiency for three generations. *Science* 218:469-471.

Beck, F. 1979. Trypan blue-induced teratogenesis. In: T. V. N. Persaud, ed. *Advances in the Study of Birth Defects, Vol. 3.* Baltimore: University Park Press, 37-51.

Beck, F. 1981. Comparative placental morphology and function. In: C. A. Kimmel and J. Buelke-Sam, eds. *Developmental Toxicology.* New York: Raven Press, 35-54.

Beck, F. 1982a. Lessons from studies in animals for the evaluation of human risks from teratogenic agents. In: H. Yoshida, Y. Hagihara, and S. Ebashi, eds. *Advances in Pharmacology and Therapeutics. II.* New York: Pergamon Press, 17-28.

Beck, F. 1982b. Model systems in teratology research. In: K. Snell, ed. *Developmental Toxicology.* New York: Praeger, 13-29.

Beck, S. L. 1983. Assessment of adult skeletons to detect prenatal exposure to acetazolamide in mice. *Teratology* 28:45-66.

Beck, F., and J. B. Lloyd. 1977. Comparative placental transfer. In: J. G. Wilson and F. C. Fraser, eds. *Handbook of Teratology, Vol. 3.* New York: Plenum Press, 155-186.

Beck, F., A. P. Gulamhusein, and I. M. Huxham. 1985. The use of human serum for studying malformations in whole embryo cultures. In: M. Marois, ed. *Prevention of Physical and Mental Congenital Defects, Part C: Basic and Medical Science, Education and Future Strategies.* New York: Alan R. Liss, Inc., 265-270.

Beckman, D. A., and R. L. Brent. 1984. Mechanisms of teratogenesis. *Ann. Rev. Pharmacol. Toxicol.* 24:483-500.

Bell, P. S., and R. H. Glass. 1975. Development of the mouse blastocyst after actinomycin D treatment. *Fertil. Steril.* 26:449-454.

Bend, J. R., M. O. James, T. R. Devereux, and J. R. Fouts. 1975. Toxication-detoxication systems in hepatic and extrahepatic tissues in the perinatal period. In: P. L. Morselli, S. Garattini, and F. Sereni, eds. *Basic and Therapeutic Aspects of Perinatal Pharmacology.* New York: Raven Press, 229-244.

Benirschke, K. 1975. Placental causes of maldevelopment. In: C. L. Berry and D. E. Poswillo, eds. *Teratology: Trends and Applications*. New York: Springer-Verlag, 148-164.

Benirschke, K. 1983. Placentation. *J. Exp. Zool.* 228:385-389.

Bergsma, D., ed. 1975. *Morphogenesis and Malformation of Face and Brain*. New York: Alan R. Liss, Inc.

Bernfield, M. 1983. Mechanisms of congenital malformations. In: J. B. Warshaw, ed. *The Biological Basis of Reproductive and Developmental Medicine*. New York: Elsevier Biomedical, 143-154.

Bernstein, M. E., 1984. Agents affecting the male reproductive system: Effects of structure on activity. *Drug Metab. Rev.* 15:941-996.

Best, J. B., and M. Morita. 1982. Planarians as a model system for in vitro teratogenesis studies. *Teratogenesis Carcinog. Mutagen.* 2:277-291.

Beyer, P. E., and N. Chernoff. 1986. The induction of supernumerary ribs in rodents: Role of maternal stress. *Teratogenesis Carcinog. Mutagen.* 6:419-429.

Biddle, F. G. 1981. The role of genetic studies in developmental toxicology. In: C. A. Kimmel and J. Buelke-Sam, eds. *Developmental Toxicology*. New York: Raven Press, 55-82.

Biddle, F. G., and F. C. Fraser. 1977. Maternal and cytoplasmic effects in experimental teratology. In: J. G. Wilson and F. C. Fraser, eds. *Handbook of Teratology, Vol. 3*. Comparative, Maternal, and Epidemiologic Aspects. New York: Plenum Press, 3-33.

Birge, W. J., J. A. Black, A. G. Westerman, and B. A. Ramey. 1983. Fish and amphibian embryos – A model system for evaluating teratogenicity. *Fundam. Appl. Toxicol.* 3:237-242.

Birnbaum, L. S., M. W. Harris, C. P. Miller, R. M. Pratt, and J. C. Lamb. 1986. Synergistic interaction of 2,3,7,8-tetrachlorodibenzo-p-dioxin and hydrocortisone in the induction of cleft palate in mice. *Teratology* 33:29-35.

Bischoff, K. B. 1987. Physiologically based pharmacokinetic modeling. In: *Pharmacokinetics in Risk Assessment, Drinking Water and Health, Vol. 8*. Washington, DC: National Academy Press, 36-61.

Bischoff, K. B., and R. G. Brown. 1966. Drug distribution in mammals. *Chem. Eng. Prog. Symp. Series* 66:33-45.

Bixler, D., D. Daentl, and L. Pinsky. 1979. Panel Discussion: Applied developmental biology. In: M. Melnick and R. Jorgenson, eds. *Developmental Aspects of Craniofacial Dysmorphology*. New York, NY: Alan R. Liss, Inc., 99-107.

Black, D. L., and T. A. Marks. 1986. Inconsistent use of terminology in animal developmental toxicology studies. *Teratology* 33:333-338.

Blake, D. A., J. M. Collins, B. C. Mayasaki, and Cohen F. 1978. Influence of pregnancy and folic acid on phenytoin metabolism by rat liver microsomes. *Drug Metab. Dispos.* 6:246-250.

Bochert, G., U. Rahm, and B. Schnieders. 1978. Pharmacokinetics of embryotoxic direct-acting alkylating agents: Comparison of DNA alkylation of various maternal tissues and the embryo during organogenesis. In: D. Neubert, H.-J. Merker, H. Nau, J. Langman, eds. *Role of Pharmacokinetics in Prenatal and Perinatal Toxicology.* Stuttgart: George Thieme Publishers, 235-251.

Bochert, G., T. Platzek, and M. Wiessler. 1981. Comparison of effects on limb development in vivo and in vitro methyl(acetoxymethyl)nitrosamine. In: D. Neubert and H.-J. Merker, eds. *Culture Techniques: Applicability for Studies on Prenatal Differentiation and Toxicity, Fifth Symposium on Prenatal Development, May 1981.* East Berlin: Walter de Gruyter, 223-235.

Bochert, G., T. Platzek, and D. Neubert. 1987. DNA modification in murine embryos: A primary cause of embryotoxic effects. In: H. Nau and W. J. Scott, Jr., eds. *Pharmacokinetics in Teratogenesis.* Boca Raton: CRC Press, 74-82.

Bolande, R. P. 1984. Symposium: Oncodevelopmental biology: Models and concepts derived from human teratogenesis and oncogenesis in early life. *J. Histochem. Cytochem.* 32:878-884.

Bournias-Vardiabasis, N., and J. Flores. 1983. Drug metabolizing enzymes in Drosophila melanogaster: Teratogenicity of cyclophosphamide in vitro. *Teratogenesis Carcinog. Mutagen.* 3:255-262.

Bournias-Vardiabasis, N., and R. L. Teplitz. 1982. Use of Drosophila embryo cell cultures as an in vitro teratogen assay. *Teratogenesis Carcinog. Mutagen.* 2:333-341.

Bournias-Vardiabasis, N., R. L. Teplitz, G. F. Chernoff, and R. L. Seecof. 1983. Detection of teratogens in the Drosophila embryonic cell culture test: Assay of 100 chemicals. *Teratology* 28:109-122.

Box, G. E. P., and D. R. Cox. 1964. An analysis of transformations. *J. Royal Stat. Soc., Series B* 26:211-243.

Box, G. E. P., and D. R. Cox. 1982. An analysis of transformations revisited, rebutted. *J. Am. Stat. Assoc.* 77:209-210.

Boylan, E. S., and R. E. Calhoon. 1981. Prenatal exposure to diethylstilbestrol: Ovarian-independent growth of mammary tumors induced by 7,12-dimethylbenz-[a]-anthracene. *J. Natl. Cancer Inst.* 66:649-652.

Braun, A. G. 1985. New perspectives in tests for teratogenicity. In: F. Homburger, ed. *Safety Evaluation and Regulation of Chemicals 2.* Basel, Switzerland: S. Karger, 230-238.

Braun, A. G., and P. B. Horowicz. 1983. Lectin-mediated attachment assay for teratogens: Results with 32 pesticides. *J. Toxicol. Environ. Health* 11:275-286.

Braun, A. G., C. A. Buckner, D. J. Emerson, and B. B. Nichinson. 1982a. Quantitative correspondence between the in vivo and in vitro activity of teratogenic agents. *Proc. Natl. Acad. Sci.* 79:2056-2060.

Braun, A. G., B. B. Nichinson, and P. B. Horowicz. 1982b. Inhibition of tumor cell attachment to concanavalin A-coated surfaces as an assay for terato-genic agents: Approaches to validation. *Teratogenesis Carcinog. Mutagen.* 2:343-354.

Braunlich, H., C. Fleck, C. Weise, and M. Stopp. 1979. Stimulation of kidney function in rats of different ages injured by nephrotoxic agents. *Exp. Pathol.* 17:486-492.

Brent, R. L. 1983. Review of developmental toxicology. *Am. J. Dis. Child.* 137:511-512.

Brent, R. L. 1986. Is hyperthermia a direct or indirect teratogen? *Teratology* 33:373-374.

Brent, R. L., and B. T. Bolden. 1968. Indirect effect of x-irradiation on embryonic development: Utilization of high doses of maternal irradiation on the first day of gestation. *Radiat. Res.* 36:563-570.

Briese, V. V., J. Fanghanel, and H. Gasow. 1984. Untersuchungen zum einflus von reintonbeschallung und vibration auf die keimesentwicklung der maus. *Ztol. Gynakol.* 106:379-388.

Brock, N., and T. von Kreybig. 1964. Experimenteller beitrag zur prufing teratogener wirkungen von argneimitteln an der laboratoriumsratte. *Naunyn-Schmiedeberg's Arch. Exp. Path. Pharmak.* 249:117-145.

Brown, N. A., 1985. Are offspring at risk from their father's exposure to toxins? *Nature* 316:110.

Brown, N. A., 1987. Teratogenicity testing in vitro: Status of validation studies. *Arch. Toxicol. Suppl.* 11:105-114.

Brown, N. A., and S. E. Fabro. 1982. The in vitro approach to teratogenicity testing. In: K. Snell, ed. *Developmental Toxicology.* New York: Praeger, 33-57.

Brown, N. A., and S. Fabro. 1983. The value of animal teratogenicity testing for predicting human risk. *Clin. Obstet. Gynecol.* 26:467-477.

Brown, D., and R. F. Keeler. 1978a. Structure-activity relation of steroid teratogens. 1. Jervine ring system. *J. Agric. Food Chem.* 26:561-563.

Brown, D., and R. F. Keeler. 1978b. Structure-activity relation of steroid teratogens. 2. N-substituted jervines. *J. Agric. Food Chem.* 26:564-566.

Brown, D., and R. F. Keeler. 1978c. Structure-activity relation of steroid teratogens. 3. Solanidan epimers. *J. Agric. Food Chem.* 26:566-569.

Brown, N., and A. Scialli, eds. 1986. *Reproductive toxicology: a medical letter on environmental hazards to reproduction.* Washington, DC: Reproductive Toxicology Center 5:17-22.

Brown, K. S., M. C. Johnston, and J. D. Niswander. 1972. Isolated cleft palate in mice after transportation during gestation. *Teratology* 5:119-124.

Brown, L. P., O. P. Flint, T. C. Orton, and G. G. Gibson. 1986. Chemical teratogenesis: Testing methods and the role of metabolism. *Drug Metab. Rev.* 17:221-260.

Buelke-Sam, J., C. A. Kimmel and J. Adams. 1985a. Design considerations in screening for behavioral teratogens: Results of the collaborative behavioral teratology study. *Neurobehav. Toxicol. Teratol.* 7:537-792.

Buelke-Sam, J., C. A. Kimmel, J. Adams, C. J. Nelson, C. V. Vorhees, D. C. Wright, V. St. Omer, B. A. Korol, R. E. Butcher, M. A. Geyer, J. F. Holson, C. L. Kutscher, and M. J. Wayner. 1985b. Collaborative behavioral teratology study: Results. *Neurobehav. Toxicol. Teratol.* 7:591-624.

Burton, D. S., R. R. Maronpot, and F. L. Howard, III. 1979. Frequency of hydronephrosis in Wistar rats. *Lab. Anim. Sci.* 29:642-644.

Butcher, R. E., C. V. Vorhees, and C. A. Kimmel. 1972. Learning impairment from maternal salicylate treatment in rats. *Nature New Biol.* 236:211-212.

Buzin, C. H., and N. Bournias-Vardiabasis. 1984. Teratogens induce a subset of small heat shock proteins in Drosophila primary embryonic cell cultures. *Proc. Natl. Acad. Sci.* 81:4075-4079.

Cameron, I. L., W. C. Lawrence, and J. B. Lum. 1985. Medaka eggs as a model system for screening potential teratogens. In: M. Marois, ed. *Prevention of Physical and Mental Congenital Defects, Part C: Basic and Medical Science Education and Future Strategies.* New York: Alan R. Liss, Inc., 239-243.

Chahoud, I., G. Bochert, and L. Dietzel-Roehl. 1984. Relation of fetal body weight (mouse) on day 18 of gestation to dam, litter size, number of fetuses per horn and intrauterine position. *Teratology* 30:21A.

Chang, L. W., and J. A. Sprecher. 1976. Degenerative changes in the neonatal kidney following in utero exposure to methylmercury. *Environ. Res.* 11:392-406.

Chao, S. T., and M. R. Juchau. 1983. Placental drug metabolism. In: E. M. Johnson and D. M. Kochhar, eds. *Teratogenesis and Reproductive Toxicology.* East Berlin: Springer-Verlag, 31-48.

Chatot, C. L., N. W. Klein, and N. J. Pierro. 1980. Successful culture of rat embryos on human serum: Use in the detection of teratogens. *Science* 207:471-473.

Chernoff, N., and R. J. Kavlock. 1982. An in vivo teratology screen utilizing pregnant mice. *J. Toxicol. Environ. Health* 10:541-550.

Chernoff, N., and R. J. Kavlock. 1983. A teratology test system which utilizes postnatal growth and viability in the mouse. In: M. Waters, S. Sandhu, J. Lewtas, L. Claxton, N. Chernoff, and S. Nesnow, eds. *Short-Term Bioassays in the Analysis of Complex Environmental Mixtures.* New York: Plenum Press, 417-427.

Chernoff, N., R. J. Kavlock, P. E. Beyer, and D. Miller. 1987. The potential relationship of maternal toxicity, general stress, and fetal outcome. *Teratogenesis Carcinog. Mutagen.* 7:241-253.

Chez, R. A., D. Haire, E. J. Quilligan, and M. B. Wingate. 1976. High-risk Pregnancies: Maternal medical disorders. In: R. L. Brent and M. I. Harris, eds. *Prevention of Embryonic, Fetal and Perinatal Disease.* Washington, DC: U.S. Government Printing Office, 67-95.

Chitlik, L. D., Q. Q. Bui, G. J. Burin, and S. C. Dapson. 1985. *Hazard Evaluation Division Standard Evaluation Procedure.* Teratology Studies. Washing-ton, DC: U.S. Environmental Protection Agency, Office of Pesticide Programs.

Christian, M. S. 1983. Postnatal alterations of gastrointestinal physiology, hematology, clinical chemistry, and other non-CNS parameters. In: E. M. Johnson and D. M. Kochhar, eds. *Teratogenesis and Reproductive Toxicology.* East Berlin: Springer-Verlag, 263-286.

Christian, M. S., and E. M. Johnson. 1979. Postnatal alteration of non-CNS physiology evaluated in rats treated with teratogens during the fetal period. *Teratology* 19:23A.

Christian, M. S., and P. E. Voytek. 1983. In vivo reproductive and mutagenicity tests. In: F. Homburger, J. A. Hayes, and E. W. Pelikan, eds. *A Guide to General Toxicology.* Basel, Switzerland: S. Karger, 294-325.

Christian, M. S., A. M. Hoberman, and E. A. Lochry. 1987. Currently used alternatives to the Chernoff-Kavlock short-term in vivo reproductive toxicity assay. *Teratogenesis Carcinog. Mutagen.* 7:65-71.

Clark, J. H., and S. McCormack. 1977. Clomid or nafoxidine administered to neonatal rats causes reproductive tract abnormalities. *Science* 197:164-165.

Clark, R. L., R. T. Robertson, D. H. Minsker, S. M. Cohen, D. J. Tocco, H. L. Allen, M. L. James, and D. L. Bokelman. 1984. Diflunisal-induced maternal anemia as a cause of teratogenicity in rabbits. *Teratology* 30:319-332.

Clark, R. L., R. T. Robertson, C. P. Peter, J. A. Bland, T. E. Nolan, L. Oppenheimer, and D. L. Bokelman. 1986. Association between adverse maternal and embryo-fetal effects in norfloxacin-treated and food-deprived rabbits. *Fundam. Appl. Toxicol.* 7:272-286.

Clarkson, T. W., G. F. Nordberg, and P. R. Sager. 1983. *Reproductive and developmental toxicity of metals.* New York: Plenum Press.

Clayton, R. M., and A. Zehir. 1982. The use of cell culture methods for exploring teratogenic susceptibility. In: K. Snell, ed. *Developmental Toxicology.* New York: Praeger, 59-92.

Clegg, E. D., C. S. Sakai, and P. E. Voytek. 1986. Assessment of reproductive risks. *Biol. Reprod.* 34:5-16.

Cole, L. J., and Bachuber, L. J. 1914. Effects of lead on the germ cells of the male rabbit and fowl as indicated by their progeny. *Proc. Soc. Exp. Biol. Med.* 12:24-29.

Collins, T. F. X. 1987. Teratological research using in vitro systems. V. Nonmammalian model systems. *Environ. Health Perspect.* 72:237-249.

Collins, T. F. X., J. J. Welsh, T. N. Black, K. E. Whitby, and M. W. O'-Donnell, Jr. 1987. Potential reversibility of skeletal effects in rats exposed *in utero* to caffeine. *Food Chem. Toxicol.* 25:647-662.

Committee for the Working Conference on Principles of Protocols for Evaluating Chemicals in the Environment. 1975. Environmental chemicals as potential hazards to reproduction. In: *Principles for Evaluating Chemicals in the Environment.* Washington, DC: National Academy of Sciences.

Copeland, M. F., R. J. Kavlock, L. A. Oglesby, L. L. Hall, M. T. Ebron-McCoy, and P. E. Beyer. 1988. Evaluation of an approach to embryonic dosimetry: An analysis of the in vivo and in vitro effects of p-iodophenol (p-IP). *Teratology* 37:451.

Copp, A. J. 1983. Teratology and experimental embryology: The pathogenesis of neural tube defects. In: J. B. Warshaw, ed. *The biological basis of reproductive and developmental medicine.* New York: Elsevier Biomedical, 155-178.

Cordero, J. F., and P. M. Layde. 1983. Vaginal spermicides, chromosomal abnormalities and limb reduction defects. *Fam. Plann. Perspect.* 15:1618.

Cox, D. R. 1966. Some procedures connected with the logistic qualitative response curve. In: F. N. David, ed. *Research Papers in Statistics: Festschrift for J. Neyman.* New York: John Wiley and Sons, 55-71.

Cozens, D. O. 1965. Abnormalities of the external form and of the skeleton of the New Zealand white rabbit. *Food Cosmet. Toxicol.* 3:695-700.

Crary, D. E., and R. R. Fox. 1980. Frequency of congenital abnormalities and of anatomical variations among JAX rabbits. *Teratology* 21:113-121.

Cresteil, T., E. LeProvost, J.-P. Flinois, and J.-P. Leroux. 1982. Enzymatic and immunological evidences that phenobarbital induces cytochrome P-450 in fetal and neonatal rat liver. *Biochem. Biophys. Res. Commun.* 106:823-830.

Crocker, J. F. S., S. R. Blecher, and S. H. Safe. 1983. Chemically induced polycystic kidney disease. In: R. J. Kavlock and C. T. Grabowski, eds. *Abnormal Functional Development of the Heart, Lungs and Kidneys: Approaches to Functional Teratology.* New York: Alan R. Liss, Inc., 281-296.

Cummings, A. J. 1983. A survey of pharmacokinetic data from pregnant women. *Clin. Pharmacokinet.* 8:344-345.

D'Ambrosio, S. M., M. J. Samuel, T. A. Dutta-Choudhury, and A. A. Wani. 1987. O^6-methylguanine-DNA methyltransferase in human fetal tissue. *Cancer Res.* 47:51-55.

Danes, B. S., ed. 1980. *In Vitro Epithelia and Birth Defects.* New York: Alan R. Liss, Inc.

Daston, G. P. 1983. Effects of maternal cadmium exposure in the rat on prenatal maturation of the pulmonary surfactant system. In: R. J. Kavlock and C. T. Grabowski, eds. *Abnormal Functional Development of the Heart, Lungs and Kidneys: Approaches to Functional Teratology.* New York: Alan R. Liss, Inc., 143-156.

Daston, G. P., J. M. Rogers, and T.D. Sabourin. 1989. Interspecies comparison of A/D ratios. *Toxicologist* 9:32.

Davidson, J. M. 1980. The urinary system. In: F. E. Hutten and G. Chamberlain, eds. *Clinical Physiology in Obstetrics.* Oxford, England: Blackwell, 289-327.

Dawson, D. A., C. A. McCormick, and J. A. Bantle. 1985. Detection of teratogenic substances in acidic mine water samples using the frog embryo teratogenesis assay—Xenopus (FETAX). *J. Appl. Toxicol.* 5:234-244.

Dean, J. 1983. Preimplantation development: Biology, genetics and mutagenesis. In: D. R. Mattison, ed. Reproductive Toxicology. *Progress in Clinical and Biological Research, Vol. 117.* New York: Alan R. Liss, Inc., 31-49.

Dean, B. J., and G. Hodson-Walker. 1979. Organ-specific mutations in Chinese hamsters induced by chemical carcinogens. *Mutat. Res.* 64:407-413.

Dean, B. J., and K. R. Senner. 1977. Detection of chemically induced somatic mutation in Chinese hamsters. *Mutat. Res.* 46:403-407.

Dedrick, R. L. 1973. Physiological pharmacokinetics. *J. Dyn. Syst. Meas. Cont. Trans.* ASME Sept.:255-257.

Dencker, L. and B. R. G. Danielsson. 1987. Transfer of drugs to the embryo and fetus after placentation. In: H. Nau and W. J. Scott, Jr., eds. *Pharmacokinetics in Teratogenesis, Vol. 1.* Boca Raton: CRC Press, Inc., 55-69.

Dencker, L., and R. M. Pratt. 1981. Association between the presence of the Ah receptor in embryonic murine tissues and sensitivity to TCDD-induced cleft palate. *Teratogenesis Carcinog. Mutagen.* 1:399-406.

DeSesso, J. M. 1987. Maternal factors in developmental toxicity. *Teratogenesis Carcinog. Mutagen* 7:225-240.

deSwiet, M. 1980a. The cardiovascular system. In: F. E. Hytten and G. Chamberlain, eds. *Clinical Physiology in Obstetrics.* Oxford, England: Blackwell, 3-42.

deSwiet, M. 1980b. The respiratory system. In: F. E. Hytten and G. Chamberlain, eds. *Clinical Physiology in Obstetrics*. Oxford, England: Blackwell, 79-100.

Devereux, T. R., and J. R. Fouts. 1975. Effect of pregnancy or treatment with certain steroids on N,N'-dimethylaniline demethylation and N-oxidation by rabbit liver or lung microsomes. *Drug Metab. Dispos.* 3:254-258.

Dimant, I. N., and D. S. Beniashvili. 1978. The significance of some modifying factors during transplacental blastomogenesis by ethylnitrosourea in rabbits. *Neoplasma* 25:453-460.

Dixon, R. L., and J. L. Hall. 1982. Reproductive toxicology. In: A. W. Hayes ed. *Principles and Methods of Toxicology*. New York: Raven Press, 107-140.

Dixon, R. L., and I. P. Lee. 1980. Pharmacokinetic and adaptation factors involved in testicular toxicity. *Fed. Proc.* 39:66-72.

Dixon, R. L., N. Chernoff, E. M. Eddy, S. R. Glasser, J. C. Lamb, IV, G. W. Lucier, D. R. Mattison, M. L. Meistrich, R. A. Pederson, and P. E. Voytek. 1986. Reproductive and developmental effects of 139 environmental agents. In: NIEHS. *Human Health and the Environment—Some Research Needs. Report of the Third Task Force for Research Planning in Environmental Health Science. NIH Publ. No. 86-1277.* Washington, DC: U.S. Government Printing Office, 47-88.

Dobson, R. L., and J. S. Felton. 1983. Female germ cell loss from radiation and chemical exposures. *Am. J. Ind. Med.* 4:175-190.

Domarus, H. V., T. Louton, and F. Lange-Wuhlisch. 1986. The position effect in mice on day 14. *Teratology* 34:73-80.

Dorner, G., F. Gotz, and W.-D. Docke. 1983. Prevention of demasculinization and feminization of the brain in prenatally stressed male rats by perinatal androgen treatment. *Exper. Clin. Endocrinol.* 81:88-90.

Dostal, M. 1977. The technique of intraamniotic drug application in mice. In: D. Neubert, H.-J. Merker, and T. E. Kwosigroch, eds. *Methods in Prenatal Toxicology*. Stuttgart: George Thieme Publishers, 281-288.

Dostal, M., and R. Jelinek. 1979. Embryotoxicity of transplacentally and intraamniotically administered 6-azauridine in mice. *Teratology* 19:143-148.

Draper, N. R., and H. Smith. 1981. *Applied Regression Analysis, 2nd ed.* New York: John Wiley and Sons.

Druckrey, H. 1973. Chemical structure and action in transplacental carcinogenesis and teratogenesis. *Int. Agency Res. Cancer Sci. Pub.* 4:45-58.

Dubowitz, V. 1974. The infant of inappropriate size. In: K. Elliott and J. Knight, eds. *Size at Birth*. New York: Associated Scientific Publishers, 47-64.

Dumpert, K., and E. Zietz. 1984. Platanna (Xenopus laevis) as a test organism for determining the embryotoxic effects of environmental chemicals. *Ecotoxicol. Environ. Safety* 8:55-74.

Dunlop, W. 1981. Serial changes in renal haemodynamics during normal human pregnancy. *Br. J. Obset. Gynecol.* 88:1-9.

Dunnett, C. W. 1955. A multiple comparisons procedure for comparing several treatments with a control. *J. Am. Stat. Assoc.* 50:1096-1121.

Durham, F. M., and H. M. Woods. 1932. Alcohol and inheritance: An experimental study. *Med. Res. Council. Spec. Rep. Series.* London: H.M.S.O. No. 168.

Dutton, G. J. 1978. Developmental aspects of drug conjugation with special reference to glucuronidation. *Ann. Rev. Pharmacol. Toxicol.* 18:17-36.

Edmonds, L. D., P. M. Layde, L. M. James, J. W. Flynt, J. D. Erickson, and G. P. Oakley, Jr. 1981. Congential malformations surveillance: Two American systems. *Int. J. Epidemiol.* 10:247-252.

Edwards, M. J., D. A. Walsh, W. S. Webster, and A. H. Lipson. 1986. Hyperthermia: Is it a "direct" embryonic teratogen? *Teratology* 33:375-376.

Efron, B. 1982. *The jackknife, the bootstrap and other resampling plans.* Philadelphia: Society for Industrial and Applied Mathematics.

Ehling, V. H., and H. V. Malling. 1968. 1,4-Di(methane-sulfonoxy)butane (myleran) as a mutagenic agent in mice. *Genetics* 60:174-175.

Eibs, H.-G., and H. Spielman. 1977. Differential sensitivity of preimplantation mouse embryos to UV irradiation and evidence for past replication repair. *Radiat. Res.* 71:367-376.

El Batawi, M. A., V. Fomenko, K. Hemminki, M. Sorsa and T. Vergieva, eds. 1987. *Effects of Occupational Health Hazards on Reproductive Functions.* Geneva: World Health Organization, Office of Occupational Health.

Elkind, M. E., and G. F. Whitmore. 1967. *The radiobiology of cultured mammalian cells.* New York: Gordon and Breach.

Enders, A. C. 1982. Whither studies of comparative placental morphology? *J. Reprod. Fertil.* 31:9-15.

Endo, A., and T. Watanabe. 1988. Interlitter variability in fetal body weight in mouse offspring from continuous, overnight, and short-period matings. *Teratology* 37:63-67.

Enslein, K. 1984. Estimation of toxicological endpoints by structure-activity relationships. *Pharmacol. Rev.* 36:131S-135S.

Enslein, K., T. R. Lander, and J. R. Strange. 1983. Teratogenesis: A statistical structure-activity model. *Teratogenesis Carcinog. Mutagen.* 3:289-309.

Environmental Health Criteria 30. 1984. Principles for evaluating health risks to progeny associated with exposure to chemicals during pregnancy. Geneva: World Health Organization.

Erickson, J. D., J. Mulinare, P. W. McClain, T. G. Fitch, I. M. James, A. B. McClearn, and M. J. Adams. 1984. Vietnam veterans risks for fathering babies with birth defects. *JAMA* 252:903-912.

Ewing, L. L., and D. R. Mattison. 1987. Introduction: Biological markers of male reproductive toxicology. *Environ. Health Perspect.* 74:11-13.

Fabro, S. 1985. On predicting environmentally induced human reproductive hazards: An overview and historical perspectives. *Fundam. Appl. Toxicol.* 5:609-614.

Fabro, S., G. Shull, and N. A. Brown. 1982. The relative teratogenic index and teratogenic potency: Proposed components of developmental toxicity risk assessment. *Teratogenesis Carcinog. Mutagen.* 2:61-76.

Fantel, A. G. 1982. Culture of whole rodent embryos in teratogen screening. *Teratogenesis Carcinog. Mutagen.* 2:231-242.

Fantel, A. G., J. C. Greenaway, M. R. Juchau, and T.H. Shepard. 1979. Teratogenic bioactivation of cyclophosphamide in vitro. *Life Sci.* 25:67-72.

FASEB. 1986. Predicting neurotoxicity and behavioral dysfunction from preclinical toxicologic data. *Report to the Center for Food Safety and Applied Nutrition, U. S. Food and Drug Administration.* Bethesda: Federation of American Societies for Experimental Biology.

Fasel, N., and J. Schowing. 1980. Embryonic development of NMRI mice: Relationship between the weight, age and ossification of embryos. *Lab. Anim.* 14:243-246.

Faustman, E. M. 1988. Short-term tests for teratogens. *Mutat. Res.* 205:355-384.

Faustman, E. M., P. L. Stapleton, and D. L. Eaton. 1988. Characterization of rodent embryonic glutathione S-transferase activity toward various substrates. *Toxicologist* 8:186.

Faustman-Watts, E., J. C. Greenaway, M. J. Namkung, A. G. Fantel, and M. R. Juchau. 1983. Teraogenicity in vitro of 2-acetylaminofluorene: Role of biotransformation in the rat. *Teratology* 27:19-28.

Faustman-Watts, E. M., C. M. Giachelli, and M. R. Juchau. 1986. Carbon monoxide inhibits monooxygenation by the conceptus and embryotoxic effects of proteratogens in vitro. *Toxicol. Appl. Pharmacol.* 83:590-595.

Fein, G. F., J. L. Jacobson, S. W. Jacobson, P. M. Schwartz, and J. K. Dowler. 1984. Prenatal exposure to polychlorinated biphenyls: Effects on birth size and gestational age. *J. Pediatr.* 105:315-320.

Felton, J. S., and R. L. Dobson. 1982. The mouse oocyte toxicity assay. In: M. D. Waters, S. S. Sandhu, J. Lewtas, L. Claxton, N. Chernoff, and S. Nesnow. *Short-term Bioassays in the Analysis of Complex Environmental Mixtures.* New York: Plenum Press, 245-255.

Filler, R., and K. J. Lew. 1981. Developmental onset of mixed-function oxidase activity in preimplantation mouse embryos. *Proc. Natl. Acad. Sci. USA* 78:6991-6995.

Finster, M., H. Pedersen, and H. O. Morishima. 1984a. Differences in drug kinetics between the adult and the newborn and their relation to drug toxicity in man. In: B. Krauer, F. Kraure, F. E. Hytten, and E. del Pozo, eds. *Drugs and Pregnancy. Maternal Drug Handling—Fetal Drug Exposure.* Orlando: Academic Press, 95-99.

Finster, M., H. Pedersen, and H. O. Morishima. 1984b. Principles of fetal exposure to drugs used in obstetric anesthesia. In: B. Krauer, F. Kraure, F. E. Hytten, and E. del Pozo, eds. *Drugs and Pregnancy. Maternal Drug Handling—Fetal Drug Exposure.* Orlando: Academic Press, 100-113.

Firestone, P., and A. Prabhu. 1983. Minor physical anomalies and obstetrical complications: Their relationship to hyperactive, psychoneurotic and normal children and their families. *J. Abnorm. Child Psychol.* 11:207-216.

Fisher, R. A., A. S. Corbet, and C. B. Williams. 1943. The relation between the number of species and the number of individuals in a random sample from an animal population. *J. Anim. Ecol.* 12:42-58.

Flint, O. P. 1981. An assessment of the available in vitro techniques for detecting teratogens. In: D. Neubert and H.-J. Merker, eds. *Culture Techniques. Applicability for Studies on Prenatal Differentiation and Toxicity.* East Berlin: Walter deGruyter, 561-565.

Flynn, T. J. 1987. Teratological research using in vitro systems. I. Mammalian whole embryo culture. *Environ. Health Perspect.* 72:203-210.

Food and Drug Administration. 1982. *Toxicological Principles for Safety Assessment of Direct Food Additives and Color Additives Used in Foods.* Washington, D.C.: Bureau of Foods, Food and Drug Administration.

Francis, E. Z., and W. H. Farland. 1987. Application of the preliminary developmental toxicity screen for chemical hazard identification under the Toxic Substances Control Act. *Teratogenesis Carcinog. Mutagen.* 7:107-117.

Fraser, F. C. 1977. Interactions and multiple causes. In: J. G. Wilson and F. C. Fraser, eds. *Handbook of Teratology, Vol. 1. General Principles and Etiology.* New York: Plenum Press, 445-463.

Fraser, F. C. 1980. Animal models for craniofacial disorders. In: M. Melnick, D. Bixler, and E. D. Shields, eds. *Etiology of Cleft Lip and Cleft Palate.* New York: Alan R. Liss, Inc., 1-23.

Fraser, B. A., and A. A. Travill. 1978. The relation of aberrant vasculogenesis to skeletal malformation in the hamster fetus. *Anat. Embryol.* 154:111-120.

Freedman, M. A., G. A. Gay, J. E. Brockert, P. W. Potrzebowski, and C. J. Rothwell. 1988. The 1989 revisions of the U.S. standard certificates of live births and deaths and the U.S. standard report of fetal death. *Am. J. Public Health* 78:168-172.

Freeman, S. J., and J. B. Lloyd. 1983. Inhibition of proteolysis in rat yolk sac as a cause of teratogenesis. Effects of leupeptin in vitro and in vivo. *J. Embryol. Exp. Morph.* 78:183-193.

Freeman, S. J., R. L. Brent, and J. B. Lloyd. 1982. The effect of teratogenic antiserum on yolk-sac function in rat embryos cultured in vitro. *J. Embryol. Exp. Morph.* 71:63-74.

Freese, E. 1982. Use of cultured cells in the identification of potential teratogens. *Teratogenesis Carcinog. Mutagen.* 2:355-360.

Friedberg, E. C. 1985. *DNA repair.* New York: W. H. Freeman and Co.

Friedler, G. 1985. Effects of limited paternal exposure to xenobiotic agents on the development of progeny. *Neurobehav. Toxicol. Teratol.* 7:739-743.

Friedman, L. 1987. Teratological research using in vitro systems. II. Rodent limb bud culture system. *Environ. Health Perspect.* 72:211-219.

Fritz, H. 1975. Prenatal ossification in rabbits as indicative of fetal maturity. *Teratology* 11:313-320.

Fujii, T. 1976. Mitigation of caffeine-induced fetopathy in mice by pretreatment with beta-adrenergic blocking agents. *Jpn. J. Pharmacol.* 26:751-756.

Fujii, T., and H. Nishimura. 1974. Reduction in frequency of fetapathic effects of caffeine in mice by pretreatment with propranolol. *Teratology* 10:149-152.

Fulton, M. H., and J. E. Chambers. 1985. The toxic and teratogenic effects of selected organophosphorous compounds on the embryos of three species of amphibians. *Toxicol. Lett.* 26:175-180.

Fulton, M., G. Raab, G. Thomson, D. Laxen, R. Hunter, and W. Hepburn. 1987. Influence of blood lead on the ability and attainment of children in Edinburgh. *Lancet* 1:1221-1226.

Gaffield, W., and R. F. Keeler. 1984. Structure and stereochemistry of steroidal amine teratogens. *Adv. Exp. Med. Biol.* 177:241-251.

Gale, T. F. 1984. The amelioration of mercury-induced embryotoxic effects by simultaneous treatment with zinc. *Environ. Res.* 35:405-412.

Galloway, S. M., P. E. Perry, J. Meneses, D. W. Nebert, and R. A. Pedersen. 1980. Cultured mouse embryos metabolize benzo[a]pyrene during early gestation: Genetic differences detectable by sister chromatid exchange. *Proc. Natl. Acad. Sci. USA* 77:3524-3528.

Garbis-Berkvens, J. M., and P. W. J. Peters. 1987. Comparative morphology and physiology of embryonic and fetal membranes. In: H. Nau and W. J. Scott, Jr., eds. *Pharmacokinetics in Teratogenesis, Vol. 1.* Boca Raton: CRC Press, Inc., 13-44.

Garrett, E. R. 1987. Toxicokinetics. In: R. G. Tardiff and J. V. Rodricks, eds. *Toxic Substances and Human Risk, Principles of Data Interpretation.* New York: Plenum Press, 153-235.

Gaulier, M., and C. Roux. 1970. Effect of busulfan on the germinal line of the rat embryo. *C. R. Soc. Biol.* (Paris) 164:2165-2170.

Gaylor, D. W. 1978. Methods and concepts of biometrics applied to teratology. In: J. G. Wilson and F. C. Fraser, eds. *Handbook of Teratology, Vol. 4. Research Procedures and Data Analysis.* New York: Plenum Press, 429-444.

Geber, W. F. 1966. Developmental effects of chronic maternal audiovisual stress on the rat fetus. *J. Embryol. Exp. Morph.* 16:1-16.

Gellert, R. J., J. L. Bakker, and N. L. Lawrence. 1971. Persistent estrus and altered estrogen sensitivity in rats treated neonatally with clomiphene citrate. *Fertil. Steril.* 22:244-250.

Generoso, W. M., K. T. Cain, M. Krishna, and S. W. Huff. 1979. Genetic lesions induced by chemicals in spermatozoa and spermatids of mice are repaired in the egg. *Proc. Natl. Acad. Sci. USA* 76:435-437.

Generoso, W. M., J. C. Rutledge, K. T. Cain, L. A. Hughes, and P. W. Braden. 1987. Exposure of female mice to ethylene oxide within hours after mating leads to fetal malformation and death. *Mutat. Res.* 176:269-274.

Generoso, W. M., J. C. Rutledge, K. T. Cain, L. A. Hughes, and D. J. Downing. 1988. Mutagen-induced fetal anomalies and death following treatment of females within hours after mating. *Mutat. Res.* 99:175-181.

Generoso, W. M., M. Katoh, K. T. Cain, L. A. Hughes, L. B. Foxworth, T. J. Mitchell, and J. B. Bishop. 1989. Chromosome malsegregation and embryonic lethality induced by treatment of normally ovulated mouse oocytes with nocodazole. *Mutat. Res.* 210:313-322.

Gerhardsson L., and A. Ahlmark. 1985. Silicosis in women. Experience from the Swedish Pneumoconiosis Register. *J. Occup. Med.* 27:347-350.

Geyer, M. A., and L. W. Reiter. 1985. Strategies for the selection of test methods. *Neurobehav. Toxicol. Teratol.* 7:661-662.

Giachelli, C. M., and C. J. Omiecinski. 1986. Regulation of cytochrome P-450b and P-450e mRNA expression in the developing rat: Hybridization to synthetic oligodeoxyribo-nucleotide probes. *J. Biol. Chem.* 261:1359-1363.

Giachelli, C. M., and C. J. Omiecinski. 1987. Developmental regulation of cytrochrome P-450 genes in the rat. *Mol. Pharmacol.* 31:477-484.

Gibaldi, M., and D. Perrier. 1982. *Pharmacokinetics, 2nd ed.* New York: Marcel Dekker.

Gibbons, A. F. E., and M. C. Chang. 1973. Indirect effects of x-irradiation on embryonic development: Irradiation of the exteriorized rat uterus. *Biol. Reprod.* 9:133-141.

Gibson, J. E. 1976. Perinatal nephropathies. *Environ. Health Perspect.* 15:121-130.

Gillert, R. J., J. L. Bakker, and N. L. Lawrence. 1971. Persistent estrus and altered estrogen sensitivity in rats treated neonatally with clomiphene citrate. *Fertil. Steril.* 22:244-250.

Gillette, J. R. 1977. Factors that affect drug concentrations in maternal plasma. In: J. G. Wilson and F. C. Fraser, eds. *Handbook of Teratology, Vol. 3. Comparative, Maternal and Epidemiologic Aspects.* New York: Plenum Press, 35-77.

Gillette, J. R. 1987. Dose, species, and route extrapolation: General aspects. In: *Pharmacokinetics in Risk Assessment, Drinking Water and Health, Vol. 8.* Washington, DC: National Academy Press, 96-158.

Gladen, B. 1979. The use of the jackknife to estimate proportions from toxicological data in the presence of litter effects. *J. Am. Stat. Assoc.* 74:278-283.

Goerttler, K., and H. Loehrke. 1976. Diaplacental carcinogenesis: Initiation with the carcinogens dimethylbenzanthracene (DMBA) and urethane during fetal life and postnatal promotion with the phorbol ester TPA in a modified 2-stage Berenblum/Mottram Experiment. *Virchows Arch. A. Path. Anat. Histol.* 372:29-38.

Goldman, A. S. 1977. Abnormal organogenesis in the reproductive system. In: J. G. Wilson and F. C. Fraser, eds. *Handbook of Teratology, Vol. 2. Mechanisms of Pathogenesis.* New York: Plenum Press, 391-419.

Goldman, A. S., and W. C. Yakovac. 1963. The enhancement of salicylate teratogenicity by maternal immobilization in the rat. *J. Pharmacol. Exp. Ther.* 142:351-357.

Goldman, A. S., L. Baker, R. Piddington, B. Marx, R. Herold, and J. Egler. 1985. Hyperglycemia induced teratogenesis is mediated by a functional deficiency of arachidonic acid. *Proc. Natl. Acad. Sci.* 82:8227-8231.

Goodman, D. R., R. C. James, and R. D. Harbison. 1982. Placental toxicology. *Food Chem. Toxicol.* 20:123-128.

Goss, L. B., and T. D. Sabourin. 1985. Utilization of alternative species for toxicity testing: An overview. *J. Appl. Toxicol.* 5:193-219.

Goto, N., Y. Nakajima, K. Imamura, and T. Yoshida. 1985. Influence of testosterone on hydronephrosis in the inbred mouse strain DDD. *Lab. Anim.* 19:85-88.

Gottschewski, G. M. H. 1964. Mammalian blastopathies due to drugs. *Nature* 201:1232-1233.

Grabowski, C. T. 1983. The electrocardiogram of fetal and newborn rats and dysrhythmias induced by toxic exposure. In: R. J. Kavlock and C. T. Grabowski, eds. *Abnormal Functional Development of the Heart, Lungs and Kidneys: Approaches to Functional Teratology.* New York: Alan R. Liss, Inc., 185-206.

Grabowski, C. T., and G. P. Daston. 1983. Functional teratology of the cardiovascular and other organ systems. In: H. Kalter, ed. *Issues and Reviews in Teratology, Vol. 1.* New York: Plenum Press, 285-308.

Grabowski, C. T., and D. B. Payne. 1980. An electrocardiographic study of cardiovascular problems in Mirex-fed rat fetuses. *Teratology* 22:167-177.

Grabowski, C. T., and D. B. Payne. 1983a. The causes of perinatal death induced by prenatal exposure of rats to the pesticide, mirex. Part I: Preparturition observations of the cardiovascular system. *Teratology* 27:7-11.

Grabowski, C. T., and D. B. Payne. 1983b. The causes of perinatal death induced by prenatal exposure of rats to the pesticide, mirex. Part II: Postnatal observations. *J. Toxicol. Environ. Health* 11:301-315.

Grabowski, C. T., and A. C. Tunstall. 1977. An electrocardiographic study of rat fetuses treated with Trypan blue. *Teratology* 15:32A.

Graham, J. M. 1983. Limb anomalies as a consequence of spatially-restricting uterine environments. In: J. R. Fallon and A. I. Caplan, eds. *Limb development and Regeneration, Part A.* New York: Alan R. Liss, Inc., 413-422.

Gray, L. E., and R. J. Kavlock. 1984. An extended evaluation of an in vivo teratology screen utilizing postnatal growth and viability in the mouse. *Teratogenesis Carcinog. Mutagen.* 4:403-426.

Gray, L. E., R. J. Kavlock, and J. Ostby. 1983. Assessment of the utility of postnatal testing following prenatal exposure to forty chemicals. In: R. J. Kavlock and C. T. Grabowski, eds. *Abnormal Functional Development of the Heart, Lungs and Kidneys: Approaches to Functional Teratology.* New York: Alan R. Liss, Inc., 39-62.

Greenaway, J. C., A. G. Fantel, and M. R. Juchau. 1986. On the capacity of nitroheterocyclic compounds to elicit an unusual axial asymmetry in cultured rat embryos. *Toxicol. Appl. Pharmacol.* 82:307-315.

Greenberg, J. H. 1983. Detection of teratogens using cells in culture. In: E. M. Johnson and D. M. Kochhar, eds. *Teratogenesis and Reproductive Toxicology.* East Berlin: Springer-Verlag, 289-299.

Grice, H. C., I. C. Munroe, D. R. Krewski, and H. Blumenthal. 1981. In utero exposure in chronic toxicity/carcinogenicity studies. *Food Cosmet. Toxicol.* 19:373-379.

Gulamhusein, A. P., W. J. Moore, M. Gupta, and F. Beck. 1982. Trypan blue teratogenesis in the rat: Further observations in vitro. *Teratology* 26:289-297.

Gupta, C., M. Katsumata, A. S. Goldman, R. Herold, and R. Piddington. 1984. Glucocorticoid-induced phospholipase A2-inhibitory proteins mediate glucocorticoid teratogenicity in vitro. *Proc. Natl. Acad. Sci.* 81:1140-1143.

Hales, B. F. and A. H. Neims. 1976. A sex difference in hepatic glutathione S-transferase B and the effect of hypophysectomy. *Biochem. J.* 160:223-229.

Hales, B. F., S. Smith, and B. Robaire. 1986a. Cyclophosphamide in the seminal fluid of treated males: Transmission to females by mating and effect on pregnancy outcome. *Toxicol. Appl. Pharmacol.* 84:423-430.

Hales, B. F., S. Smith, and B. Robaire. 1986b. Reversibility of the effects of chronic paternal exposure to cyclophosphamide (CPA) on pregnancy outcome in rats. *Teratology* 33:82C.

Hall, S. M., and F. J. Zeman. 1968. Kidney function of the progeny of rats fed a low protein diet. *J. Nutr.* 95:49-54.

Hanawalt, P. C., P. K. Cooper, A. K. Ganesan, and C. A. Smith. 1979. DNA repair in bacteria and mammalian cells. *Annu. Rev. Biochem.* 48:783-836.

Hardin, B. D. 1987. A recommended protocol for the Chernoff-Kavlock preliminary developmental toxicity test and a proposed method for assigning priority scores based on results of that test. *Teratogenesis Carcinog. Mutagen.* 7:85-94.

Hardin, B. D., R. A. Becker, R. J. Kavlock, J. M. Seidenberg, and N. Chernoff. 1987a. Overview and summary: Workshop on the Chernoff/Kavlock preliminary developmental toxicity test. *Teratogenesis Carcinog. Mutagen.* 7:119-127.

Hardin, B. D., R. L. Schuler, J. R. Burg, G. M. Booth, H. P. Hazelden, K. M. MacKenzie, V. J. Piccirillo, and K. N. Smith. 1987b. Evaluation of 60 chemicals in a preliminary developmental toxicity test. *Teratogenesis Carcinog. Mutagen.* 7:29-48.

Hart, W. L., R. C. Reynolds, W. J. Krasavage, T. S. Ely, R. H. Bell, and R. L. Raleigh. 1988. Evaluation of developmental toxicity data: A discussion of some pertinent factors and a proposal. *Risk Anal.* 8:59-69.

Hartel, A., and G. Hartel. 1960. Experimental study of teratogenic effect of emotional stress in rats. *Science* 132:1483-1484.

Haseman, J. K. 1983. A reexamination of false-positive rates for carcinogenesis studies. *Fundam. Appl. Toxicol.* 3:334-339.

Haseman, J. K., and M. D. Hogan. 1975. Selection of the experimental unit in teratology studies. *Teratology* 12:165-172.

Haseman, J. K., and L. L. Kupper. 1979. Analysis of dichotomous response data from certain toxicological experiments. *Biometrics* 35:281-293.

Hassell, J. R., and E. A. Horigan. 1982. Chondrogenesis: A model developmental system for measuring teratogenic potential of compounds. *Terato-genesis Carcinog. Mutagen.* 2:325-331.

Hassoun, E., R. d'Argy, L. Dencker, and G. Sundstrom. 1984. Teratological studies on the TCDD congener 3,3',4,4'-tetrachloroazoxybenzene in sensitive and nonsensitive mouse strains: Evidence for direct effect on embryonic tissues. *Arch. Toxicol.* 5:20-26.

Hayasaka, I., and T. Fujii. 1977. Potentiation of the fetopathic effects of caffeine in mice by pargyline or cocaine. *Cong. Anom.* 17:487-492.

Healey, G. F. 1987. Power calculations in toxicology. *ATLA* 15:132-139.

Hemm, R. D., L. Arslanoglau, and J. J. Pollock. 1977. Cleft palate following prenatal food restriction in mice: Association with elevated maternal corticosteroids. *Teratology* 15:243-248.

Hemminki, K., and P. Vineis. 1985. Extrapolation of the evidence on teratogenicity of chemicals between humans and experimental animals: Chemicals other than drugs. *Teratogenesis Carcinog. Mutagen.* 5:251-318.

Hemsworth, B. N. 1968. Embryopathies in the rat due to alkane sulfonates. *J. Reprod. Fertil.* 17:325-334.

Hendrickx, A. G. 1984. Disorders of fertilization, transport, and implantation. In: J. E. Lockey, G. K. Lemasters, and W. R. Keye, Jr., eds. *Reproduction: The New Frontier in Occupational and Environmental Health Research.* New York: Alan R. Liss, Inc., 211-227.

Hendrickx, A. G., P. E. Binkerd, and J. M. Rowland. 1983. Developmental toxicity and nonhuman primates: Interspecies comparisons. In: H. Kalter, ed. *Issues and Reviews in Teratology, Vol. 1.* New York: Plenum Press, 149-180.

Herbst, A. L., R. E. Seully, and S. J. Robboy. 1979. Prenatal diethylstilbestrol exposure and human genital tract abnormalities. *Natl. Cancer Inst. Mono.* 51:25-35.

Herring, S. W., and T. C. Lakars. 1981. Craniofacial development in the absence of muscle contraction. *J. Craniofac. Genet. Devel. Biol.* 1:341-357.

Hettmansperger, T. P. 1984. *Statistical inference based on ranks.* New York: John Wiley and Sons.

Highman, B., R. J. Wordinger, and H. J. Schumacher. 1979. Use of the periodic acid schiff stain to grade retarded fetal renal development in mice. *Toxicol. Lett.* 4:61-69.

Hill, R. 1983. Model systems and their predictive value in assessing teratogens. *Fundam. Appl. Toxicol.* 3:229-232.

Hinkley, D. V., and G. Runger. 1984. The analysis of transformed data. *J. Am. Stat. Assoc.* 79:302-309.

Hirshfield, A. N. 1987. Histological assessment of follicular development and its applicability to risk assessment. *Reprod. Toxicol.* 1:71-79.

Hogan, M. D., and D. G. Hoel. 1982. Extrapolation to man. In: A. W. Hayes, ed. *Principles and Methods of Toxicology.* New York: Raven Press, 711-731.

Holmes, L. B., C. Cann, and C. Cook. 1985. Examination of infants for both minor and major malformations to evaluate for possible teratogenic exposures. In: M. Marois, ed. *Prevention of Physical and Mental Congenital Defects, Part B: Epidemiology, Early Detection and Therapy, and Environmental Factors.* New York: Alan R. Liss Inc., 59-63.

Holy, A. 1982. Novel adenosine analogues with broad-spectrum biological activity: Structure and mechanism of action. *Nucleic Acid Res., Symp. Ser.* 11:199-202.

Hood, R. D. 1985. *Cacodylic Acid: Agricultural Uses, Biologic Effects and Environmental Fate*. Washington, DC: U.S. Government Printing Office.

Hood, R. D., and D. G. Davis. 1984. A Drosophila screen for teratogens. *J. Am. Coll. Toxicol*. 3:164.

Hood, R. D., and C. T. Pike. 1972. BAL alleviation of arsenate induced teratogenesis in mice. *Teratology* 6:235-237.

Hood, R. D., and G. C. Vedel-Macrander. 1984. Evaluation of the effect of BAL (2,3-dimercaptopropanol) on arsenite induced teratogenesis in mice. *Toxicol. Appl. Pharmacol*. 73:1-7.

Hose, J. E. 1985. Potential uses of sea urchin embryos for identifying toxic chemicals: Description of a bioassay incorporating cytologic, cytogenetic and embryologic endpoints. *J. Appl. Toxicol*. 5:245-254.

Hoyme, H. E. 1987. Minor Malformations. Significant or insignificant? *Am. J. Dis. Child*. 141:947.

Hudson, R., and H. Distal. 1986. The potential of the newborn rabbit for behavioral teratological research. *Neurobehav. Teratol*. 8:209-212.

Husain, S. M., M. Belanger-Barbeau, and M. Pellerin. 1970. Malformation in the progeny of thalidomide-treated male rats. *Can. Med. Assoc. J*. 103:163-164.

Hutchings, D. E. 1983. Behavioral teratology: A new frontier in behavioral research. In: E. M. Johnson and D. M. Kochhar, eds. *Teratogenesis and Reproductive Toxicology*. New York: Springer-Verlag.

Hutchings, D. E. 1985. Prenatal opioid exposure and the problem of causal inference. In: T. M. Pinkert, ed. *Current Research on the Consequences of Maternal Drug Use*. Natl. Inst. on Drug Abuse Res. Series. DHHS Pub. No. (ADM)85-1400. Washington, DC: U.S. Government Printing Office, 6-19.

Hutchings, D. E. 1987. Drug abuse during pregnancy: Embryopathic and neurobehavioral effects. In: M. C. Braude and A. M. Zimmerman, eds. *Genetic and Perinatal Effects of Abused Substances*. New York: Academic Press, 131-151.

Hutchings, D. E., and W. P. Fifer. 1986. Neurobehavioral effects in human and animal offspring following prenatal exposure to methadone. In: E. Riley and C. Vorhees, eds. *Handbook of Behavioral Teratology*. New York: Plenum Press, 141-161.

Hytten, F. E. 1980a. The alimentary system. In: F. E. Hytten and G. Chamberlain, eds. *Clinical Physiology in Obstetrics*. Oxford, England: Blackwell Scientific Publications Ltd., 147-162.

Hytten, F. E. 1980b. Weight gain in pregnancy. In: F. E. Hytten and G. Chamberlain, eds. *Clinical Physiology in Obstetrics*. Oxford, England: Blackwell Scientific Publications Ltd., 193-233.

Hytten, F. E. 1984. Physiological changes in the mother related to drug handling. In: B. Krauer, F. Krauer, F. E. Hytten, and E. del Pozo, eds.

Drugs and Pregnancy, Maternal Drug Handling-Fetal Drug Exposure. London: Academic Press, 7-15.

Hytten, F. E., and G. Chamberlain. 1980. *Clinical Physiology in Obstetrics.* Oxford, England: Blackwell Scientific Publications Ltd.

Hytten, F. E., and I. Leitch. 1971. *The Physiology of Human Pregnancy.* 2nd ed. Oxford, England: Blackwell Scientific Publications Ltd.

Iannaccone, P. M., N. L. Bossert, and C. S. Connelly. 1987. Disruption of embryonic and fetal development due to preimplantation chemical insults: A critical review. *Am. J. Obstet. Gynecol.* 157:476-484.

Inman, O., and C. R. Markivee. 1963. Gross effects on rabbit embryos and membranes of x-irradiation on the blastocyst stage. *Anat. Rec.* 147: 139-147.

Interagency Regulatory Liaison Group (IRLG). 1981. Recommended Guideline for Teratogenicity Studies in the Rat, Mouse, Hamster, or Rabbit.

Irikura, T., H. Suzuki, and T. Sugimato. 1981. Reproduction studies of AM-715 in mice II. Teratological study. *Chemotherapy* (Tokyo) 29:895-915.

Ivankovic, S. 1969. Erzeugung von genitalkrebs bei trachtigen ratten. *Arzneimittel Forsch.* 19:1040.

Jelinek, R. 1977. The chick embryotoxicity screening test (CHEST). In: D. Neubert, H.-J. Merker, and T. E. Kwasigroch, eds. *Methods in Prenatal Toxicology.* Stuttgart: George Thieme Publishers, 381-386.

Jelinek, R. 1982. Use of chick embryo in screening for embryotoxicity. *Teratogenesis Carcinog. Mutagen.* 2:255-261.

Jelinek, R., M. Peterka, and Z. Rychter. 1985. Chick embryotoxicity screening test — 130 substances tested. *Ind. J. Exp. Biol.* 23:588-595.

Joffe, J. M., and L. F. Soyka. 1981. Effects of drug exposure on male reproductive processes and progeny. *Period. Biol.* 83:351-362.

Johnson, E. M. 1980a. A subvertebrate system for rapid determination of potential teratogenic hazards. *J. Environ. Pathol. Toxicol.* 4:153-156.

Johnson, E. M. 1980b. Screening for teratogenic potential: Are we asking the proper question? *Teratology* 21:259.

Johnson, E. M. 1981. Screening for teratogenic hazards: Nature of the problems. *Annu. Rev. Pharmacol. Toxicol.* 21:417-429.

Johnson, E. M. 1983a. Current status of, and considerations for, estimation of risk to the human conceptus from environmental chemicals. In: W. M. Galbraith, P. Voytek, and M. G. Ryon, eds. *Assessment of Risks to Human Reproduction and to Development of the Human Conceptus from Exposure to Environmental Substances.* Oak Ridge, TN: U.S. EPA, 99-115.

Johnson, E. M. 1983b. *Quantitative assessments of reproductive outcomes.* Discussion paper. Prepared by ICAIR Systems, Division Life Systems, Inc., Cleveland, OH, for U.S. EPA, Washington, DC.

Johnson, E. M. 1984. A prioritization and biological decision tree for developmental toxicity safety evaluations. *J. Am. Coll. Toxicol.* 3:141-147.

Johnson, D. R., and L. Kleinman. 1979. Effects of lead exposure on renal function in young rats. *Toxicol. Appl. Pharmacol.* 48:361-367.

Johnson, E. M., and M. S. Christian. 1984. When is a teratology study not an evaluation of teratogenicity? *J. Am. Coll. Toxicol.* 3:431-434.

Johnson, E. M., and B. E. G. Gabel. 1982. Application of the hydra assay for rapid detection of developmental hazards. *J. Am. Coll. Toxicol.* 1:57-71.

Johnson, E. M., and B. E. G. Gabel. 1983. An artificial "embryo" for detection of abnormal developmental biology. *Fundam. Appl. Toxicol.* 3:243-249.

Johnson, N. L., and S. Kotz. 1969. *Discrete Distributions.* New York: John Wiley and Sons.

Johnson, E. M., R. M. Gorman, B. E. G. Gabel, and M. E. George. 1982. The Hydra attenuata system for detection of teratogenic hazards. *Teratogenesis Carcinog. Mutagen.* 2:263-276.

Johnson, E. M., B. E. G. Gabel, and J. Larson. 1984. Developmental toxicity and structure/activity correlates of glycols and glycol ethers. *Environ. Health Perspect.* 57:135-139.

Johnson, E. M., M. S. Christian, L. Dansky, and B. E. G. Gabel. 1987. Use of the adult developmental relationship in prescreening for developmental hazards. *Teratogenesis Carcinog. Mutagen.* 7:273-285.

Johnston, M. C., and K. K. Sulik. 1979. Some abnormal patterns of development in the craniofacial region. In: M. Melnick and R. Jorgenson, eds. *Developmental Aspects of Craniofacial Dysmorphology.* New York: Alan R. Liss, Inc., 23-42.

Jollie, W. P. 1986. Review article: Ultra-structural studies of protein transfer across rodent yolk sac. *Placenta* 7:263-281.

Jonsson, N. A. 1972a. Chemical structure and teratogenic properties. III. A review of available data on structure-activity relationships and mechanism of action of thalidomide analogues. *Acta Pharm. Suec.* 9:521-542.

Jonsson, N. A. 1972b. Chemical structure and teratogenic properties. IV. An outline of a chemical hypothesis for the teratogenic action of thalidomide. *Acta Pharm. Suec.* 9:543-562.

Jonsson, N. A., L. Mikiver, and U. Selberg. 1972. Chemical structure and teratogenic properties. II. Synthesis and teratogenic activity in rabbits of some derivatives of phthalimide, isoindoline-1-one,1,2- benzisothiazoline-3-one-1,1-dioxide and 4(3H)-quinazolinone. *Acta Pharm. Suec.* 9:431-446.

Juchau, M. R. 1976. Drug biotransformation reactions in the placenta. In: B.L. Mirkin, ed. *Perinatal Pharmacology and Therapeutics*. New York: Academic Press, 71-118.

Juchau, M. R. 1980. Drug biotransformation in the placenta. *Pharmacol. Ther.* 8:501-524.

Juchau, M. R. 1981. Enzymatic bioactivation and inactivation of chemical teratogens and transplacental carcinogens/mutagens. In: M. R. Juchau, ed. *The Biochemical Basis of Chemical Teratogenesis*. New York: Elsevier/North-Holland, Inc., 63-94.

Juchau, M. R. 1982. The role of the placenta in developmental toxicology. In: K. Snell, ed. *Developmental Toxicology*. New York: Praeger, 189-209.

Juchau, M. R., and E. Faustman-Watts. 1983. Pharmacokinetic considerations in the maternal-placental fetal unit. *Clin. Obstet. Gynecol.* 26:379-390.

Juchau, M. R., S. T. Chao, and C. J. Omiecinski. 1980. Drug metabolism by the human fetus. *Clin. Pharmacokin.* 5:320-339.

Juchau, M. R., C. M. Giachelli, A. G. Fantel, J. C. Greenaway, T. H. Shepard, and E. M. Faustman-Watts. 1985. Effects of 3-methylcholanthrene and phenobarbital on the capacity of embryos to bioactivate teratogens during organogenesis. *Toxicol. Appl. Pharmacol.* 80:137-146.

Jurand, A. 1985. The interference of naloxone hydrochloride in the teratogenic activity of opiates. *Teratology* 31:235-240.

Jusko, W. J. 1972. Pharmacodynamic principles in chemical teratology: Dose-effect relationships. *J. Pharmacol. Exp. Ther.* 183:469-480.

Kalland, T. 1980a. Alterations of antibody response in female mice after neonatal exposure to diethylstilbestrol. *J. Immunol.* 124:194-198.

Kalland, T. 1980b. Reduced natural killer activity in female mice after neonatal exposure to diethylstilbestrol. *J. Immunol.* 124:1297-1300.

Kallen, B. 1979. Errors in differentiation of the central nervous system. In: N. C. Myrianthopoulas and D. Bergsma, eds. *Recent Advances in the Developmental Biology of Central Nervous System Malformations*. New York: Alan R. Liss, Inc., 43-53.

Kalter, H. 1978. The structure and uses of genetically homogeneous lines of animals. In: J. G. Wilson and F. C. Fraser, eds. *Handbook of Teratology, Vol. 4. Research Procedures and Data Analysis*. New York: Plenum Press, 155-190.

Kalter, H. 1980. The relation between congenital malformations and prenatal mortality in experimental animals. In: I. H. Porter and E. B. Hook, eds. *Human Embryonic and Fetal Death*. New York: Academic Press, 29-44.

Kalter, H. 1981. Dose-response studies with genetically homogeneous lines of mice as a teratology testing and risk-assessment procedure. *Teratology* 24:79-86.

Kameyama, Y. 1985. Comparative developmental pathology of malformations of the central nervous system. In: M. Marios, ed. *Prevention of Physical and Mental Congenital Defects, Part A: The Scope of the Problem.* New York: Alan R. Liss, Inc., 143-156.

Kaplan, L. C., R. Matsuoka, E. F. Gilbert, J. M. Opitz, and D. M. Kurnit. 1985. Ectopia cardis and cleft sternum: Evidence for mechanical teratogenesis following rupture of the charion or yolk sac. *Am. J. Med. Genet.* 21:187-199.

Karkinen-Jaaskelainen, M. 1985. Early fetal development-sensitive periods. In: K. Hemminki, M. Sorsa, and H. Vainio, eds. *Occupational Hazards and Reproduction.* New York: Hemisphere Publ. Corp., 17-29.

Karnofsky, D. A. 1965. Mechanisms of action of certain growth inhibiting drugs. In: J. G. Wilson and J. Warkany, eds. *Teratology: Principles and Techniques.* Chicago: University of Chicago Press, 185-213.

Karotkin, E. H., M. Kido, R. A. Redding, W. J. Cashore, W. Douglas, L. Stern, and W. Oh. 1976. The inhibition of pulmonary maturation in the fetal rabbit by maternal treatment with phenobarbital. *Am. J. Obstet. Gynecol.* 124:529-531.

Karp, W. B., T. F. Gale, S. B. Subramanyam, and R. H. DuRant. 1985. The effect of mercuric acetate on selected enzymes of maternal and fetal hamsters at different gestational ages. *Environ. Res.* 36:351-358.

Katayama, S., and N. Matsumoto. 1985. Toxic effects of chemicals on mouse postblastocyst development — A trial to establish a testing system for embryotoxicity. *Acta Obstet. Gynecol.* Japan 37:421-430.

Katoh, M., N. L. A. Cacheiro, C. V. Cornett, K. T. Cain, J. C. Rutledge, and W. M. Generoso. 1989. Fetal anomalies produced subsequent to treatment of zygotes with ethylene oxide or ethyl methanesulfonate are not likely due to the usual genetic causes. *Mutat. Res.* 210:337-344.

Kavlock, R. J., and G. P. Daston. 1983. Detection of renal dysfunction in neonatal rats: Methodologies and applications. In: R. J. Kavlock and C. T. Grabowski, eds. *Abnormal Functional Development of the Heart, Lungs and Kidneys: Approaches to Functional Teratology.* New York: Alan R. Liss, Inc., 339-356.

Kavlock, R. J., and J. A. Gray. 1983. Morphometric, biochemical, and physiological assessment of perinatally induced renal dysfunction. *J. Toxicol. Environ. Health* 11:1-13.

Kavlock, R. J., N. Chernoff, and E. H. Rogers. 1985. The effect of acute maternal toxicity on fetal development in the mouse. Teratogenesis Carcinog. Mutagen. 5:3-13.

Kavlock, R. J., E. H. Rogers, and B. F. Rehnberg. 1986. Renal functional teratogenesis resulting from adriamycin exposure. *Teratology* 33:213-220.

Kavlock, R. J., R. D. Short, Jr., and N. Chernoff. 1987. Further evaluation of an in vivo teratology screen. *Teratogenesis Carcinog. Mutagen.* 7:7-16.

Keller, W. C., C. T. Olson, K. C. Back, and C. L. Gaworski. 1984. Teratogenic assessment of three methylated hydrazine derivatives in the rat. *J. Toxicol. Environ. Health* 13:125-131.

Keller, S. J., and M. K. Smith. 1982. Animal virus screens for potential teratogens. 1. Poxvirus morphogenesis. *Teratogenesis Carcinog. Mutagen.* 2:361-374.

Kennedy, L. A., and T. V. N. Persaud. 1977. Pathogenesis of developmental defects induced in the rat by amniotic sac puncture. *Acta Anat.* 97:23-35.

Kerster, H. W., and D. J. Schaeffer. 1983. Brine shrimp (Artemia salina) nauplii as a teratogen test system. *Ecotoxicol. Environ. Safety* 7:342-349.

Khera, K. S. 1981. Common fetal aberrations and their teratologic significance: A review. *Fundam. Appl. Toxicol.* 1:13-18.

Khera, K. S. 1984a. Adverse effects in humans and animals of prenatal exposure to selected therapeutic drugs and estimation of embryo-fetal sensitivity of animals for human risk assessment. In: H. Kalter, ed. *Issues and Reviews in Teratology, Vol. 2.* New York: Plenum Press, 399-507.

Khera, K. S. 1984b. Maternal toxicity—A possible factor in fetal malformations in mice. *Teratology* 29:411-416.

Khera, K. S. 1985. Maternal toxicity: A possible etiological factor in embryo-fetal deaths and fetal malformations of rodent-rabbit species. *Teratology* 31:129-153.

Khera, K. S. 1986. Reply to Hyperthermia: Is it a "direct" embryonic teratogen? *Teratology* 33:377-378.

Khera, K. S. 1987a. Maternal toxicity of drugs and metabolic disorders—a possible etiologic factor in the intrauterine death and congenital malformation: A critique on human data. *CRC Crit. Rev. Toxicol.* 17:345-375.

Khera, K. S. 1987b. Maternal toxicity in humans and animals: Effects on fetal development and criteria for detection. *Teratogenesis Carcinog. Mutagen.* 7:287-295.

Kimmel, C. A. 1981a. A profile of developmental toxicity. In: C. A. Kimmel and J. Buelke-Sam, eds. *Developmental Toxicology.* New York: Raven Press, 321-331.

Kimmel, G. L. 1981b. Developmental aspects of chemical interaction with cellular receptors. In: Kimmel, C. A. and J. Buelke-Sam, eds. *Developmental Toxicology.* New York: Raven Press, 115-130.

Kimmel, G. L. 1985. In vitro tests in screening teratogens: Considerations to aid the validation process. In: M. Marios, ed. *Prevention of Physical and Mental Congenital Defects, Part C: Basic and Medical Science, Education, and Future Strategies.* New York: Alan R. Liss, Inc., 259-263.

Kimmel, G. L. 1987. Short-term developmental toxicity testing: Considerations in the validation process. *Teratogenesis Carcinog. Mutagen.* 7:1-6.

Kimmel, C. A., and J. Buelke-Sam. 1985. Collaborative behavioral teratology study. Background and overview. *Neurobehav. Toxicol. Teratol.* 7:541-546.

Kimmel, C. A., and J. F. Young. 1983. Correlating pharmacokinetics and teratogenic endpoints. *Fundam. Appl. Toxicol.* 3:250-255.

Kimmel, C. A., R. O. Cook, and R. E. Staples. 1976. Teratogenic potential of noise in mice and rats. *Toxicol. Appl. Pharmacol.* 36:239-245.

Kimmel, G. L., K. Smith, D. M. Kochhar, and R. M. Pratt. 1982. Overview of in vitro teratogenicity testing: Aspects of validation and application to screening. *Teratogenesis Carcinog. Mutagen.* 2:221-229.

Kimmel, C. A., J. F. Holson, C. J. Hogue, and G. L. Carlo. 1984. *Reliability of Experimental Studies for Predicting Hazards to Human Development.* Final Report for Experiment 6015. Jefferson, AR: National Center for Toxicological Research.

Kimmel, C. A., J. Buelke-Sam, and J. Adams. 1985. Collaborative behavioral teratology study: Implications, current applications and future directions. *Neurobehav. Toxicol. Teratol.* 7:669-773.

Kimmel, C. A., G. L. Kimmel, and V. Frankos. 1986. Interagency Regulatory Liaison Group workshop on reproductive toxicity risk assessment. *Environ. Health Perspect.* 66:193-221.

Kimmel, G. L., C. A. Kimmel, and E. Z. Francis. 1987. Implications of the consensus workshop on the evaluation of maternal and developmental toxicity. *Teratogenesis Carcinog. Mutagen.* 7:329-338.

King, B. F. 1982. Comparative anatomy of the placental barrier. *Bibl. Anat.* 22:13-28.

Kirk, K. M., and M. F. Lyon. 1984. Induction of congenital malformations in the offspring of male mice treated with x-rays at pre-meiotic and post-meiotic stages. *Mutat. Res.* 125:75-85.

Kistler, A. 1985. Inhibition of chondrogenesis by retinoids: Limb bud cell cultures as a test system to measure the teratogenic potential of compounds? In: F. Homburger, ed. *Organs, Cells, Primitive Organisms.* Basel, Switzerland: S. Karger, 86-100.

Kitchin, K. T., and M. T. Ebron. 1984. Combined use of a water-insoluble chemical delivery system and a metabolic activation system in whole embryo culture. *J. Toxicol. Environ. Health* 13:499-509.

Kitchin, K. T., M. K. Sanyal, and B. P. Schmid. 1981. A coupled microsomal-activating/embryo culture system: Toxicity of reduced b-nicotinamide adenine dinucleotide phosphate (NADPH). *Biochem. Pharmacol.* 30(9):985-992.

Kitchin, K. T., B. P. Schmid, and M. K. Sanyal. 1986. Rodent whole embryo culture as a teratogen screening method. *Meth. Find. Exp. Clin. Pharmacol.* 8:291-301.

Klassen, R. W., and T. V. N. Persaud. 1979. Experimental studies on the influence of male alcoholism on testicular function, pregnancy and progeny. In: T. V. N. Persaud, ed. *Teratological Testing*. Lancaster, England: MTP Press Ltd., 239-256.

Kleihues, P. 1982. Developmental carcinogenicity. In: K. Snell, ed. *Developmental Toxicology*. New York: Praeger, 211-246.

Klein, N. W., and L. J. Pierro. 1983. Whole embryos in culture. In: E. M. Johnson and D. M. Kochhar, eds. *Teratogenesis and Reproductive Toxicology*. East Berlin: Springer-Verlag, 315-333.

Kline, J., Z. Stein, B. Strobino, M. Susser, and D. Warburton. 1977. Surveillance of spontaneous abortions. Power in environmental monitoring. *Am. J. Epidemiol*. 106:345-350.

Klose, J., J. Blohm, and I. Gerner. 1977. The use of isoelectric focusing and electrophoresis to obtain highly complex protein patterns of mouse embryos. In: D. Neubert, H.-J. Merker, and T. E. Kwasigroch, eds. *Methods in Prenatal Toxicology*. Stuttgart: George Thieme Publishers, 303-313.

Klug, S., C. Lewandowski, and D. Neubert. 1985. Modification and standardization of the culture of early postimplantation embryos for toxicological studies. *Arch. Toxicol*. 58:84-88.

Koch, H. P., and M. J. Czejka. 1986. Evidence for the intercalation of thalidomide into DNA: Clue to the molecular mechanism of thalidomide teratogenicity? *Z. Naturforsch*. 41c:1057-1061.

Kocher, W. 1977a. Action and interaction of chemical and genetic factors in teratogenesis of the limb. In: D. Bergsma and W. Lenz, eds. *Morphogenesis and Malformation of the Limbs*. New York: Alan R. Liss, Inc., 1-18.

Kocher, W. 1977b. Special strains of mice (breeding systems, mutants) in teratological evaluation and planning. In: D. Neubert, H.-J. Merker, and T. E. Kwasigroch, eds. *Methods in Prenatal Toxicology*. Stuttgart: George Thieme Publishers, 72-76.

Kochhar, D. M. 1975. The use of in vitro procedures in teratology. *Teratology* 11:273-288.

Kochhar, D. M. 1981. Embryo explants and organ cultures in screening of chemicals for teratogenic effects. In: C. A. Kimmel and J. Buelke-Sam, eds. *Developmental Toxicology*. New York: Raven Press, 303-319.

Kochhar, D. M. 1983. Embryonic organs in culture. In: E. M. Johnson and D. M. Kochhar, eds. *Teratogenesis and Reproductive Toxicology*. East Berlin: Springer-Verlag, 301-314.

Kochhar, D. M., J. Kraft, and H. Nau. 1987. Teratogenicity and disposition of various retinoids in vivo and in vitro. In: H. Nau and W. J. Scott, Jr., eds. *Pharmacokinetics in Teratogenesis, Vol. II*. Boca Raton: CRC Press, Inc., 173-186.

REFERENCES 243

Koeter, H. B. W. M. 1983. Relevance of parameters related to fertility and reproduction in toxicity testing. *Am. J. Ind. Med.* 4:81-86.

Kollar, E. J. 1985. Embryonic induction and teratology of the developing skin and oral mucosa. In: H. Kalter, ed. *Issues and Reviews in Teratology, Vol. 3.* New York: Plenum Press, 219-237.

Korhonen, A., K. Hemminki, and H. Vainio. 1982. Embryotoxicity of industrial chemicals on the chicken embryo: Thiourea derivatives. *Acta Pharmacol. Toxicol.* 51:38-44.

Korte, R., F. Vogel, and I. Osterburg. 1987. The primate as a model for hazard assessment of teratogens in humans. Mechanisms and models in toxicology. *Arch. Toxicol., Suppl.* 11:115-121.

Krasner, J. 1972. Drug-protein interaction. *Pediatr. Clin. North Am.* 19:51-63.

Krauer, B. 1987. Physiological changes and drug disposition during pregnancy. In: H. Nau and W. J. Scott, Jr., eds. *Pharmacokinetics in Teratogenesis, Vol. 1.* Boca Raton: CRC Press, Inc., 3-12.

Krauer, B., and F. Krauer. 1977. Drug kinetics in pregnancy. *Clin. Pharmacokinet.* 2:167-181.

Krokan, H., A. Haugen, B. Myrnes, and P. H. Guddal. 1983. Repair of premutagenic DNA lesions in human fetal tissues: Evidence for low levels of O^6-methylguanine-DNA methyltransfrase and uracil-DNA glycosylase activity in some tissues. *Carcinogenesis* 4:1559-1564.

Kulkarni, A.P., and M. F. Kenel. 1987. Human placental lipid peroxidation. Some characteristics of the NADPH-supported microsomal reaction. *Gen. Pharmacol.* 18:491-496.

Kulkarni, A.P., B. Strohm, and W. H. Houser. 1985. Human placental indanol dehydrogenase: Some properties of the microsomal enzyme. *Xenobiotica* 15:513-519.

Kundomal, Y. R., and J. M. Baden. 1985. Toxicity and teratogenicity of inhaled anesthetics in Drosophila melanogaster. *Toxicol. Lett.* 25:287-291.

Kupper, L. L., and J. K. Haseman. 1978. The use of a correlated binomial model for the analysis of certain toxicological experiments. *Biometrics* 34:69-76.

Kupper, L. L., C. Portier, M. D. Hogan, and E. Yamamoto. 1986. The impact of litter effects on dose-response modeling in teratology. *Biometrics* 42:85-98.

Kurppa, K., P. C. Holmberg, K. Rantala, T. Nurminen and L. Saxen. 1985. Birth defects and exposure to video display terminals during pregnancy. *Scand. J. Work Environ. Health* 11:353-356.

Kwasigroch, T. E., and R. G. Skalko. 1983. Development of mouse limbs in organ culture: Dose dependent retinoic acid-induced defects evaluated using image analysis. *Prog. Clin. Biol. Res. 110* (pt. A):335-344.

244REFERENCES

Kwasigroch, T. E., and R. G. Skalko. 1985. The teratogenic interaction of hydroxyurea and 5-bromodeoxyuridine examined with the aid of limb culture and image analysis. *Fundam. Appl. Toxicol.* 5:1161-1173.

Laale, H. W. 1981. Teratology and early fish development. *Am. Zool.* 21:517-533.

Lamb, J. C., T. A. Marks, and J. K. Haseman. 1981. Development and viability of offspring of male mice treated with chlorinated phenoxy acids and 2,3,7,8-tetrachlorodibenzo-p-dioxin. *J. Toxicol. Environ. Health* 8:835-844.

Lamb, J. C., IV, M. D. Ross, and R. E. Chapin. 1986. Experimental methods for studying male reproductive function in standard toxicology studies. *J. Am. Coll. Toxicol.* 5:225-234.

Lammer, E. J., D. T. Chen, R. M. Hoar, N. D. Agnish,, P. J. Benke, J. T. Braun, C. J. Curry, P. M. Fernhoff, A. W. Grix, and I. T. Lott. 1984. Retinoic acid embryopathy. *New Eng. J. Med.* 313:837-841.

Langman, J., W. Webster, and P. Rodier. 1975. Morphological and behavioral abnormalities caused by insults to the CNS in the perinatal period. In: C. L. Berry and D. E. Poswillo, eds. *Teratology: Trends and Applications.* New York: Springer-Verlag, 182-200.

Lary, J. M., R. D. Hood, and R. Lindahl. 1982. Interactions between cycloheximide and T-locus alleles during mouse embryogenesis. *Teratology* 25:345-349.

Leavitt, W. W., and D. N. Meisner. 1967. Persistent anovulatory estrus (PAE) caused by clomiphene or coumestrol. *Fed. Proc.* 26:426.

Lee, M. 1985. Potentiation of chemically induced cleft palate by ethanol ingestion during gestation in the mouse. *Teratogenesis Carcinog. Mutagen.* 5:433-440.

Legraverend, C., T. M. Guenther, and D. W. Nebert. 1984. Importance of the route of administration for genetic differences in benzo[a]pyrene-induced in utero toxicity and teratogenicity. *Teratology* 29:35-48.

Lehmann, E. L. 1975. *Nonparametrics: Statistical methods based on ranks.* San Francisco: Holden-Day.

Leonard, A., G. Linden, and G. B. Gerber. 1973. Etude, chez la souris, des effets genetiques et cytogenetique d'une contamination par le plomb. *Proceedings International Symposium Environmental Health Aspects of Lead.* Luxembourg, Belgium: CID, 303-309.

Levin, A. A., and R. K. Miller. 1981. Fetal toxicity of cadmium in the rat: Decreased utero-placental blood flow. *Toxicol. Appl. Pharmacol.* 58:297-306.

Levy, G. 1984. Protein binding of drugs in the maternal-fetal unit and its potential clinical signficance. In: B. Krauer and F. Krauer, eds. *Drugs and Pregnancy Maternal Drug Handling—Fetal Drug Exposure.* London: Academic Press, 29-42.

Lewis, P. J. 1980. Drug metabolism. In: F. E. Hytten and G. Chamberlain, eds. *Clinical Physiology in Obstetrics.* Oxford, England: Blackwell, 270-286.

Lewis, P. J. 1983. *Clinical Pharmacology in Obstetrics.* Boston: Wright PSG.

Lin, F. O., and J. K. Haseman. 1976. A modified Jonckheere test against ordered alternatives when ties are present at a single extreme value. *Biometr. Zeitschr.* 18:623-631.

Lindbohm, M-L., and K. Hemminki. 1988. Use of registered data in studies of occupational exposure and pregnancy outcome. In: V. K. Meyers, ed. *Teratogens: Chemicals Which Cause Birth Defects.* New York: Elsevier, 260-270.

Lindstedt, S. L. 1987. Allometry: Body size constraints in animal design. In: *Pharmacokinetics in Risk Assessment, Drinking Water and Health, Vol. 8.* Washington, DC: National Academy Press, 65-79.

Lloyd, J. B., F. Beck, and A. Griffiths. 1965. Structure-activity studies for the teratogenic effects of disazo dyes. *J. Pharm. Pharmacol.* 17:126S-128S.

Loch-Caruso, R., and J. E. Trosko. 1985. Inhibited intercellular communication as a mechanistic link between teratogenesis and carcinogenesis. *CRC Crit. Rev. Toxicol.* 16:157-183.

Lochry, E. A., A. M. Hoberman, and M. S. Christian. 1985. Comparative sensitivity of pup body weight and commonly used developmental landmarks. *Teratology* 32:28A.

Longo, L. D., and H. Bartels. 1973. *Respiratory Gas Exchange and Blood Flow in the Placenta.* U. S. Department of Health, Education and Welfare. DHEW Publication (NIH) 73-361.

Lovecchio, J. L., J. Krasner, and S. J. Yaffe. 1981. Serum protein binding of salicylate during pregnancy and the puerperium. *Dev. Pharmacol. Ther.* 2:172-179.

Lucier, G. W., and O. S. McDaniel. 1979. Developmental toxicology of the halogenated aromatics: Effects on enzyme development. *Ann. N. Y. Acad. Sci.* 320:449-457.

Lui, E. M. K., and G. P. Wysocki. 1987. Reproductive tract defects induced in adult male rats by postnatal 1,2-dibromo-3-chloropropane exposure. *Toxicol. Appl. Pharmacol.* 90:299-314.

Lum, J. T., and P. G. Wells. 1986. Pharmacological studies on the potentiation of phenytoin teratogenicity by acetaminophen. *Teratology* 33:53-72.

Luster, M. I., R. E. Faith, and J. A. McLachlan. 1978. Alterations of the antibody response following in utero exposure to diethylstilbestrol. *Bull. Environ. Contam. Toxicol.* 20:433-437.

Luster, M. I., R. E. Faith, J. A. McLachlin, and G. C. Clark. 1979. Effect of in utero exposure to diethylstilbestrol on the immune response in mice. *Toxicol. Appl. Pharmacol.* 47:279-285.

Luster, M. I., G. A. Boorman, J. H. Dean, M. W. Harris, R. W. Luebke, M. L. Padarathsingh, and J. A. Moore. 1980. Examination of bone marrow, immunologic parameters and host susceptibility following pre- and postnatal exposure to 2,3,7,8-tetrachlorodibenzo-p-dioxin (TCDD). *Int. J. Immunopharmacol.* 2:301-310.

Lutwak-Mann, C. 1964. Observations on progeny of thalidomide-treated male rabbits. *Br. Med. J.* 1:1090-1091.

Lutz, R. J., and R. L. Dedrick. 1987. Implications of pharmacokinetic modeling in risk assessment analysis. *Environ. Health Perspect.* 76:97-106.

MacDowell, E. C., and E. M. Lord. 1927. Reproduction in alcoholic mice: Treated males. Study of prenatal mortality and sex ratios. *Arch. Entwicklungsmech. Org.* 110:427-449.

MacDowell, E. C., E. M. Lord, and C. G. MacDowell. 1926a. Heavy alcoholization and prenatal mortality in mice. *Proc. Soc. Exp. Med.* 23:652-654.

MacDowell, E. C., E. M. Lord, and C. G. MacDowell. 1926b. Sex ratio of mice from alcoholized fathers. *Proc. Soc. Exp. Med.* 23:517-519.

Mactutus, C. F., and H. A. Tilson. 1986. Psychogenic and neurogenic abnormalities after perinatal insecticide exposure: A critical review. In: E. P. Riley and C. V. Vorhees, eds. *Handbook of Behavioral Teratology.* New York: Plenum Press, 335-390.

Manchester, D., and E. Jacoby. 1984. Decreased placental monooxygenase activities associated with birth defects. *Teratology* 30:31-37.

Mankes, R. F., R. LeFevre, K. F. Benitz, I. Rosenblum, H. Bates, A. I. T. Walker, R. Abraham, and W. Rockwood. 1982. Paternal effects of ethanol in the Long-Evans rat. *J. Toxicol. Environ. Health* 10:871-878.

Mann, T., and C. Lutwak-Mann. 1982. Passage of chemicals into human and animal semen: Mechanisms and significance. *CRC Crit. Rev. Toxicol.* 2:1-14.

Manson, J. M. 1981. Developmental toxicity of alkylating agents: Mechanism of action. In: M. R. Juchau, ed. *The Biochemical Basis of Chemical Teratogenesis.* North Holland, NY: Elsevier, 95-136.

Manson, J. M., and R. Simons. 1979. In vitro metabolism of cyclophosphamide in limb bud culture. *Teratology* 19:149-158.

Marhan, O., and R. Jelinek. 1979. Efficiency of embryotoxicity testing procedures. II. Comparison between the official, MEST and CHEST methods. *Toxicol. Lett.* 4:389-392.

Marks, T. A., T. A. Ledoux, and J. A. Moore. 1982. Teratogenicity of a commercial xylene mixture in the mouse. *J. Toxicol. Environ. Health* 9:97-105.

Mast, T. J., H. Nau, W. Wittfoht and A. G. Hendrickx. 1987. Tertogenicity and pharmacokinetics of valproic acid in the rhesus monkey. In: H. Nau and W. J. Scott, Jr., eds. *Pharmacokinetics in Teratogenesis, Vol. 1.* Boca Raton: CRC Press, Inc., 131-147.

Masui, Y., and R. A. Pedersen. 1975. Ultraviolet light-induced unscheduled DNA synthesis in mouse oocytes during meiotic maturation. *Nature* 257:705-706.

Mattison, D. R. 1983. The mechanisms of action of reproductive toxins. *Am. J. Ind. Med.* 4:65-79.

Mattison, D. R. 1986. Physiological variations in pharmacokinetics during pregnancy. In: S. Fabro and A. R. Scialli, eds. *Drug and Chemical Action in Pregnancy.* New York: Marcel Dekker Inc., 37-102.

Mattison, D. R., and F. R. Jelovsek. 1987. Pharmacokinetics and expert systems as aids for risk assessment in reproductive toxicology. *Environ. Health Perspect.* 76:107-119.

Mattison, D. R., M. S. Nightingale, and K. Shiromizu. 1983. Effects of toxic substances on female reproduction. *Environ. Health Perspect.* 48:43-52.

Mattison, D. R., K. Shiromizu, and M. S. Nightingale. 1985. The role of metabolic activation in gonadal and gamete toxicity. In: K. Hemminki, M. Sorsa, and H. Vainio, eds. *Occupational Hazards and Reproduction.* Washington, DC: Hemisphere Publishing Corp., 87-111.

McCormack, S., and J. H. Clark. 1979. Clomid administration to pregnant rats causes abnormalities of the reproductive tract in offspring and mothers. *Science* 204:629-631.

McCormack, K. M., A. Abuelgasim, V. L. Sanger, and J. B. Hook. 1980. Postnatal morphology and functional capacity of the kidney following prenatal treatment with dinoseb in rats. *J. Toxicol. Environ. Health* 6:633-643.

McLachlan, J. A., R. R. Newbold, K. S. Korach, J. C. Lamb IV, and Y. Suzuki. 1981. Transplacental toxicology: Prenatal factors influencing postnatal fertility. In: C. A. Kimmel and J. Buelke-Sam, eds. *Developmental Toxicology.* New York: Raven Press, 213-232.

McLaren, A., and D. Michie. 1959. The spacing of implantations in the mouse uterus. *Mem. Soc. Endocrinol.* 6:65-74.

McLaren, A., and D. Michie. 1960. Congenital runts. In: G. E. Wolstenholme and G. M. O'Connor, eds. *Ciba Foundation Symposium on Congenital Malformations.* London: Churchill, 178-193.

McMichael, A. J., P. A. Baghurst, N. R. Wigg, G. V. Vimpani, E. F. Robertson, and R. J. Roberts. 1988. Port Pirie cohort study: Environmental exposure to lead and children's abilities at the age of four years. *N. Engl. J. Med.* 319:468-475.

Mehes, K. 1985. Minor malformations in the neonate: Utility in screening infants at risk of hidden major defects. In: M. Marois, ed. *Prevention of Physical and Mental Congenital Defects, Part C: Basic and Medical*

Science, Education, and Future Strategies. New York: Alan R. Liss, Inc., 45-49.

Meistrich, M. 1983. *Quantitative assessments of reproductive outcomes.* Discussion paper: Work assignment for ICAIR Systems Division, Life Systems, Inc., Cleveland, OH.

Melnick, M. 1979. The genesis of craniofacial malformations: A four-dimensional perspective. In: M. Melnick and R. Jorgensen, eds. *Developmental Aspects of Craniofacial Dysmorphology.* New York: Alan R. Liss, Inc., 3-9.

Menkes, B., S. Sander, and A. Ilies. 1970. Cell death in teratogenesis. In: D. H. M. Woolam, ed. *Advances in Teratology.* New York: Academic Press, 169-215.

Meyer, S. L., and E. P. Riley. 1986. Behavioral teratology of alcohol. In: E. Riley and C. Vorhees, eds. *Handbook of Behavioral Teratology.* New York: Plenum Press.

Miller, R. W. 1966. Relation between cancer and congenital defects in man. *N. Engl. J. Med.* 275:87-93

Miller, R. W. 1977. Relationship between human teratogens and carcinogens. *JNCI* 58:471-474.

Miller, R. G., Jr. 1981. *Simultaneous Statistical Inference, 2nd ed.* New York: Springer-Verlag.

Miller, R. K. 1983. Perinatal toxicology: Its recognition and fundamentals. *Am. J. Ind. Med.* 4:205-244.

Miller, R. K., and W. O. Berndt. 1975. Mechanisms of transport across the placenta: An in vitro approach. *Life Sci.* 16:7-30.

Miller, R. W., and W. J. Blot. 1972. Small head size after in utero exposure to atomic radiation. *Lancet* 2:784-787.

Miller, R. K., T. R. Koszalka, and R. L. Brent. 1976. Transport mechanisms for molecules across placental membranes. In: G. Poste and G. Nicolson, eds. *The Cell Surface in Animal Embryogenesis and Development.* Amsterdam: Elsevier/North-Holland, 145-232.

Miller, R. K., W. W. Ng, and A. A. Levin. 1983. The placenta: Relevance to toxicology. In: T.W. Clarkson, G.F. Nordberg, and P.R. Sager, eds. *Reproductive and Developmental Toxicity of Metals.* New York: Plenum Press, 569-607.

Mirkes, P. E. 1985. Cyclophosphamide teratogenesis: A review. *Teratogenesis Carcinog. Mutagen.* 5:75-88.

Mirkes, P. E., J. C. Greenaway, and T. H. Shepard. 1983. A kinetic analysis of rat embryo response to cyclophosphamide exposure in vitro. *Teratology* 28:249-256.

Mohr, U., M. Emura, and H.-B. Richter-Reichhelm. 1980. Transplacental carcinogenesis. *Invest. Cell Pathol.* 3:209-229.

Morgan, H. B., G. S. Danford, F. M. Holland, K. C. Miller, E. T. Owens, B. E. Ricci, S. Y. Uppulari, and J. S. Wassom. 1988. How to obtain information about the teratogenic potential of chemicals. In: V. K. Myers, ed. *Teratogens: Chemicals Which Cause Birth Defects*. New York: Elsevier, 6-41.

Moriguchi, M., and W. J. Scott, Jr. 1986. Prevention of caffeine-induced limb malformations by maternal adrenalectomy. *Teratology* 33:319-322.

Morishita, H., K. Nakago, K. Ki, T. Hashimoto, M. Kawamoto, T. Tanaka, K. Higuchi, Y. Miyauchi, and T. Ozasa. 1979. Anovulation and oviductal hyperplasia in rats treated with clomiphene citrate 5 days after birth. *Acta Endocrinol.* (Copenh.) 92:577-584.

Mosier, H. D., L. C. Dearden, R. A. Jansons, R. C. Roberts, and C. S. Biggs. 1982. Disproportionate growth of organs and body weight following glucocorticoid treatment of the rat fetus. *Dev. Pharmacol. Ther.* 4:89-105.

Moskowitz, S. B., S. M. Bloch, and W. L. Lappenbusch. 1983. Issues Paper: *Multiple Chemicals in Drinking Water*. Washington, DC: U.S. Environmental Protection Agency.

Mossman, H. W. 1987. *Vertebrate Fetal Membranes: Comparative Ontogeny and Morphology, Evolution, Phylogenetic Significance, Basic Functions, Research Opportunities*. New Brunswick, NJ: Rutgers University Press.

Muller, R., and M. F. Rajewsky. 1983. Elimination of O^6-ethylguanine from the DNA of brain, liver, and other rat tissues exposed to ethylnitrosourea at different stages of prenatal development. *Cancer Res.* 43:2897-2904.

Murphy, S. 1981. *General Principles in the Assessment of Toxicity of Chemical Mixtures*. Paper presented at NIEHS Conference, Fall Inc., Research Triangle Park, NC.

National Academy of Sciences. 1984. *Toxicity Testing: Strategies to Determine Needs and Priorities*. Washington, DC: National Research Council, National Academy of Sciences.

National Academy of Sciences. 1985. *Models for Biomedical Research, A New Perspective*. Washington, DC: National Academy Press.

National Center for Health Statistics. 1981. *Data Systems of the National Center for Health Statistics*. Vital In-Health Statistics, Series No. 1, 16 DHAF (No. PHF 82-1318) Public Health Service. Washington, DC: U.S. Government Printing Office.

Nakatsuka, T., and T. Fujii. 1979. Comparative teratogenicity study of diflunisal (MK-647) and aspirin in the rat. *Oyo Yakuri* 17:551-557.

Nau, H. 1986a. Species differences in pharmacokinetics and drug teratogenesis. *Environ. Health Perspect.* 70:113-129.

Nau, H. 1986b. Valproic acid teratogenicity in mice after various administration and phenobarbital-pretreatment regimens: The parent drug and not one of the metabolites assayed is implicated as teratogen. *Fundam. Appl. Toxicol.* 6:662-668.

Nau, N. 1987. Species differences in pharmacokinetics, drug metabolism, and teratogenesis. In: H. Nau and W. J. Scott, Jr., eds. *Pharmacokinetics in Teratogenesis, Vol. 1.* Boca Raton: CRC Press, Inc., 81-106.

Nau, H., and W. J. Scott, Jr., eds. 1987. *Pharmacokinetics in Teratogenesis, Vol. 1 and 2.* Boco Raton: CRC Press, Inc.

Nau, H., and W. J. Scott. 1987. Teratogenicity of valproic acid and related substances in the mouse: Drug accumulation and pH$_i$ in the embryo during organogenesis and structure-activity considerations. Mechanisms and models in toxicology. *Arch. Toxicol., Suppl.* 11:128-139.

Nau, H., H. Spielmann, C. M. Lo Turco Mortler, K. Winckler, L. Riedel, and G. Obe. 1982. Mutagenic, teratogenic and pharmacokinetic properties of cyclophosphamide and some of its deuterated derivatives. *Mutat. Res.* 95:105-118.

Nebert, D. W. 1983. Genetic differences in drug metabolism: Proposed relationship to human birth defects. In: E. M. Johnson and D. M. Kochhar, eds. *Teratogenesis and Reproductive Toxicology.* East Berlin: Springer-Verlag, 49-62.

Nebert, D. W., and S. Shum. 1980. Reply to the letter of Doctors Shepard and Fantel. *Teratology* 22:349-350.

Neims, A. H., M. Warner, P. M. Loughnan, and J. V. Aranda. 1976. Developmental aspects of the hepatic cytochrome P-450 monooxygenase system. *Ann. Rev. Pharmacol. Toxicol.* 16:427-446.

Nelson, V. A. 1972. The use of Grassostrea gigas larva to access the hazard associated with zinc-65 and elevated rearing water temperatures. Ph.D. Thesis, University of Washington School of Fisheries, Seattle, WA.

Nelson, B. K. 1981. Dose/effect relationships in developmental neurotoxicology. *Neurobehav. Toxicol. Teratol.* 3:255.

Nelson, C. J., and J. F. Holson. 1978. Statistical analysis of teratologic data: Problems and advancements. *J. Environ. Pathol. Toxicol.* 2:187-199.

Nelson, J. L., and A. P. Kulkarni. 1986. Peroxidase activity in the mouse uterus, placenta and fetus during pregnancy. *Biochem. Int.* 13:131-138.

Nelson, C. J., R. P. Felton, C. A. Kimmel, J. Buelke-Sam, and J. Adams. 1985. Collaborative behavioral teratology study: Statistical approach. *Neuro-behav. Toxicol. Teratol.* 7:587-590.

Nelson, B. K., W. S. Brightwell, D. R. Mackenzie-Taylor, J. R. Burg, and V. J. Massari. 1988. Neurochemical, but not behavioral, deviations in the offspring of rats following prenatal or paternal inhalation exposure to ethanol. *Neurotoxicol. Teratol.* 10:15-22.

Netzloff, M. L., K. P. Chepenik, E. M. Johnson, and S. Kaplan. 1968. Respiration of rat embryos in culture. *Life Sci.* 7:401-405.

Neubert, D. 1981. On the predictability of developmental toxicity—especially prenatal toxicity—on the basis of culture experiments. In: D. Neubert and H.-J. Merker, eds. *Culture Techniques.* Berlin: Walter de Gruyter, 567-583.

Neubert, D. 1985. Benefits and limits of model systems in developmental biology and toxicology (in vitro techniques). In: M. Marois, ed. *Prevention of Physical and Mental Congenital Defects, Part A: The scope of the problem.* New York: Alan R. Liss, Inc., 91-96.

Neubert, D., and H.-J. Barrach. 1977a. Significance of in vitro techniques for the evaluation of embryotoxic effects. In: D. Neubert, H.-J. Merker, and T. E. Kwasigroch, eds. *Methods in Prenatal Toxicology.* Stuttgart: George Thieme Publishers, 202-209.

Neubert, D., and H.-J. Barrach. 1977b. Techniques applicable to study morphogenetic differentiation of limb buds in organ culture. In: D. Neubert, H.-J. Merker, and T. E. Kwasigroch, eds. *Methods in Prenatal Toxicology.* Stuttgart: George Thieme Publishers, 241-251.

Neubert, D., and H.-J. Barrach. 1979. Effect of environmental agents on embryonic development and the applicability of in vitro techniques for teratological testing. In: A. R. Kolber, T. K. Wong, L. D. Grant, R. S. DeWoskin, and T. J. Hughes, eds. *In Vitro Toxicity Testing of Environmental Agents.* New York: Plenum Press, 147-172.

Neubert, D., and R. Krowke. 1983. Effect of thalidomide-derivatives on limb development in culture. *Prog. Clin. Biol. Res.* 110(A):387-397.

Neubert, D., H.-J. Barrach, and H.-J. Merker. 1980. Drug-induced damage to the embryo or fetus. In: E. Grundmann, ed. *Current Topics in Pathology.* 69:242-331.

Neubert, D., G. Blankenburg, C. Kwandawski, and S. Klug. 1985. Misinterpre-tations of results and creation of "artifacts" in studies on developmental toxicity using systems simpler than in vitro systems. In: J. W. Lash and L Saxen, eds. *Developmental Mechanisms: Normal and Abnormal.* New York: Alan R. Liss, Inc., 241-266.

Neubert, D., I. Chahoud, T. Platzek, and R. Meister, 1987. Principles and problems in assessing prenatal toxicity. *Arch. Toxicol.* 60:238-245.

New, D. A. T. 1970. Culture of fetuses in vitro. In: G. Raspe, ed. *Advances in Biosciences.* New York: Pergamon, 367-378.

Newman, L. M., and E. M. Johnson. 1983. Abnormal lung function induced by prenatal insult. In: E. M. Johnson and D. M. Kochhar, eds. *Teratogenesis and Reproductive Toxicology, Vol. 65. Handbook of Experimental Pharmacology.* Berlin: Springer-Verlag, 237-261.

Nieuwkoop, P. D. 1985. Inductive interaction and determination: A new approach to an old problem. In: G. M. Edelman, ed. *Molecular Determinants of Animal Form.* New York: Alan R. Liss, Inc., 59-71.

Nisbet, I. C. T., and N. J. Karch. 1983. Chemical hazards to human reproduction. Park Ridge, NJ: Noyes Data Corp.

Nishimura, M., M. Iizuka, S. Iwaki, and A. Kast. 1982. Repairability of drug-induced "wavy ribs" in rat offspring. *Drug Res.* 32:1518-1522.

Nomura, T. 1982. Parental exposure to x-rays and chemicals induces heritable tumors and anomalies in mice. *Nature* 296: 575-577.

Norman, N. A., and N. W. Bruce. 1979. Fetal and placental weight relationships in the albino rat near term. *Teratology* 19:245-250.

Oakley, G. P. 1985. Population and case-controlled surveillance with search for environmental causes of birth defects. In: M. Marois, ed. *Prevention of Physical and Mental Congenital Defects, Part B: Epidemiology, Early Detection and Therapy, and Environmental Factors*. New York: Alan R. Liss, Inc., 27-32.

Ogawa, K., K. Yokokawa, T. Tomoyori, and T. Onoe. 1982. Induction of 8-glutamyltranspeptidase-positive altered hepatocyte lesions by combination of transplacental initiation and postnatal selection. *Int. J. Cancer* 29:333-336.

Oglesby, L. A., M. T. Ebron, P. E. Beyer, B. D. Carver, and R. J. Kavlock. 1986. Co-culture of rat embryos and hepatocytes: In vitro detection of a proteratogen. *Teratogenesis Carcinog. Mutagen.* 6:129-138.

Oglesby, L. A., M. T. Ebron, P. E. Beyer, L. Hall, and R. J. Kavlock. 1987. The embryotoxicity of a series of para substituted phenols: An in vitro structure-activity study. *Teratology* 35:75A.

Opitz, J. M. 1979. The developmental field concept in clinical genetics. In: M. Melnick and R. Jorgensen, eds. *Developmental Aspects of Craniofacial Dysmorphology*. New York: Alan R. Liss, Inc., 107-112.

Organization for Economic Cooperation and Development (OECD). 1981. Guidelines for testing of chemicals – Teratogenicity.

Ornoy, A. 1984. Experimental animal models to test teratogenicity of drugs in man. In: J. G. Schenker, E. T. Rippmann, and D. Weinstein, eds. *Recent Advances in Pathophysiological Conditions in Pregnancy*. New York: Elsevier Science Publishers, 318-322.

Osimitz, T. G., and A. P. Kulkarni. 1982. Oxidative metabolism of xenobiotics during pregnancy: Significance of microsomal flavin containing mono-oxygenase. *Biochem. Biophys. Res. Commun.* 109:1164-1171.

Otake, M., and W. J. Schull. 1984. In utero exposure to A-bomb radiation and mental retardation, a reassessment. *Br. J. Radiol.* 57:409-414.

Overstreet, J. W. 1984. Assessment of disorders of spermatogenesis. In: J. E. Lockey, G. K. Lemasters, and W. R. Keye, Jr., eds. *Reproduction: The New Frontier in Occupational and Environmental Health Research*. New York: Alan R. Liss, Inc., 275-292.

Palmer, A. K. 1968. Spontaneous malformations of the New Zealand white rabbit: The background to safety evaluation tests. *Lab. Anim.* 2:195-206.

Palmer, A. K. 1969. The concept of the uniform animal relative to teratogenicity. *Carworth Eur. Collect. Pap.* 3:101-113.

Palmer, A. K. 1974. Statistical analysis and choice of sampling units. *Teratology* 10:301-302.

Palmer, A. K. 1976. Assessment of current test procedures. *Environ. Health Perspect.* 18:97-104.

Palmer, A. K. 1977. Incidence of sporadic malformations, anomalies and variations in random bred laboratory animals. In: D. Neubert, H.-J. Merker, and T. E, Kwasigroch, eds. *Methods in Prenatal Toxicology.* Stutt-gart: George Thieme Publishers, 52-70.

Palmer, A. K. 1978. The design of subprimate animal studies. In: J. G. Wilson and F. C. Fraser, eds. *Handbook of Teratology, Vol. 4. Research Procedures and Data Analysis.* New York: Plenum Press, 215-253.

Palmer, A. K. 1980. Teratology and safety evaluation. In: C. L. Galli, S. D. Murphy, and R. Paoletti, eds. *The Principles and Methods in Modern Toxicology.* New York: Elsevier/North Holland Biomedical Press, 139-157.

Palmer, A. K. 1981. Regulatory requirements for reproductive toxicology: Theory and practice. In: C. A. Kimmel and J. Buelke-Sam, eds. *Developmental Toxicology.* New York: Raven Press, 259-288.

Palmer, A. K. 1985. Use of mammalian models in teratology. In: M. Marois, ed. *Prevention of Physical and Mental Congenital Defects, Part A: The Scope of the Problem.* New York: Alan R. Liss, Inc., 97-106.

Palmer, A. K. 1987. An indirect assessment of the Chernoff/Kavlock assay. *Teratogenesis Carcinog. Mutagen.* 7:95-106.

Palmer, A. K. 1988. The relevance of minor structural differences. *Teratology* 38:6A.

Palmer, A. K., R. J. Kavlock, et al. 1987. Consensus workshop on the evaluation of maternal and developmental toxicity. Work Group II Report. Study design considerations. *Teratogenesis Carcinog. Mutagen.* 7:311-319.

Parra, A., D. Santos, C. Cervantes, I. Sojo, A. Carranco, and V. Cortes-Gallegos. 1978. Plasma gonadotropins and gonadal steroids in children treated with cyclophosphamide. *J. Pediatr.* 92:117-124.

Paul, S. R. 1982. Analysis of proportions of affected fetuses in teratological experiments. *Biometrics* 38:361-370.

Pearn, J. H. 1983. Teratogens and the male: An analysis with special reference to herbicide exposure. *Med. J. Australia* 2:16-20.

Pedersen, R. A. 1987. Analysis of cell lineage during early mouse embryogenesis. *Banbury Report* 26:57-72.

Pedersen, R. A., and J. E. Cleaver. 1975. Repair of UV damage to DNA of implantation-stage mouse embryos in vitro. *Exp. Cell. Res.* 95:247-253.

Pedersen, R. A., and F. Mangia. 1978. Ultraviolet-light-induced unscheduled DNA synthesis by resting and growing mouse oocytes. *Mutat. Res.* 49:425-429.

Pelkonen, O. 1980. Developmental drug metabolism. In: P. Jenner and B. Teshs, eds. *Concepts of Drug Metabolism.* New York: Marcel Dekker Inc., 285-309.

Pelkonen, O., and N. T. Karki. 1973. Drug metabolism in human fetal tissues. *Life Sci.* 12:1163-1180.

Pelkonen, O., P. Korhonen, P. Jouppila, and N. T. Karki. 1975. Placental transfer and fetal metabolism of drugs. In: P. L. Morselli, S. Garattini, and F. Sereni, eds. *Basic and Therapeutic Aspects of Perinatal Pharmacology.* New York: Raven Press, 65-74.

Pelkonen, O., N. T. Karki, P. Korhonen, M. Koivisto, R. Tuimala, and A. Kauppila. 1979. Human placental and hydrocarbon hydroxylase: Genetics and environmental influences. In: P. W. Jones and P. Leber, eds. *Polynuclear Aromatic Hydrocarbons.* Ann Arbor: Ann Arbor Science Publishers, 765-778.

Pelkonen, O., N. T. Karki, and R. Tuimala. 1981. A relationship between cord blood and maternal blood lymphocytes and term placentas in the induction of arylhydrocarbon hydroxylase activity. *Cancer Lett.* 13:103-110.

Pennisi, A., C. N. Grushkin, and E. Lieberman. 1975. Gonadal function in children with nephrosis treated with cyclophosphamide. *Am. J. Dis. Child.* 129:315-318.

Perin-Roussel, O., N. Barat, and F. Zajdela. 1985. Formation and removal of dibenzo[a,e]fluoranthene-DNA adducts in mouse embryo fibroblasts. *Carcinogenesis* 6:1791-1796.

Perraud, J. 1976. Levels of spontaneous malformations in the CD rat and the CD-1 mouse. *Lab. Anim. Sci.* 26:293-300.

Perraud, J., J. Stadler, M. J. Kessedjian, and A. M. Munro. 1984. Reproductive studies with the anti-inflammatory agent, piroxicam: Modification of classical protocols. *Toxicology* 30:59-63.

Persaud, T. V. N. 1985. Critical phases of intrauterine development. In: T. V. N. Persaud, A. E. Chudley, and R. G. Skalko, eds. *Basic Concepts in Teratology.* New York: Alan R. Liss, Inc., 23-29.

Pfeifer, W. D., J. R. MacKinnon, and R. L. Seiser. 1977. Adverse effects of paternal alcohol consumption on offspring in rat. *Bull. Psychonom. Sco.* 10:246.

Philipson, A. 1979. Pharmacokinetics of antibiotics in pregnancy and labor. *Clin. Pharmacokinet.* 4:297-309.

Pillans, P. I., P. I. Folb, and S. F. Ponzi. 1988. The effects of in vivo administration of teratogenic doses of vitamin A during the preimplantation period in the mouse. *Teratology* 37:7-11.

Pinto-Machado, J. 1970. Influence of prenatal administration of busulfan on the postnatal development of mice: Production of a syndrome including hypoplasia of the thymus. *Teratology* 3:363-370.

Pinto-Machado, J. 1985. External examination of limb positions in near-term mouse fetuses: An experimental study and review of the literature published in teratology. *Teratology* 31:413-423.

Plasterer, M. R., W. S. Bradshaw, G. M. Booth, M. W. Carter, R. L. Schuler, and B. D. Hardin. 1985. Developmental toxicity of nine selected compounds following prenatal exposure in the mouse: Naphthalene, p-nitrophenol, sodium selenite, dimethyl phthalate, ethylenethiourea, and four glycol ether derivatives. *J. Toxicol. Environ. Health* 15:25-38.

Poland, A., and E. Glover. 1973. Chlorinated dibenzo-p-dioxins: Potent inducers of aminolevulinic acid synthetase and aryl hydrocarbon hydroxylase. *Mol. Pharmacol.* 9:736-747.

Poland, A., and E. Glover. 1980. 2,3,7,8-Tetrachlorodibenzo-p-dioxin: Segregation of toxicity with the Ah locus. *Mol. Pharmacol.* 17:86-94.

Politch, J. A., and L. R. Herrenkohl. 1984. Effects of prenatal stress on reproduction in male and female mice. *Physiol. Behav.* 32:95-99.

Prasad, M. R. N. 1984. The in vitro sperm penetration test: A review. *Int. J. Androl.* 7:5-22.

Pratt, R. M. 1984. Hormones, growth factors, and their receptors in normal and abnormal prenatal development. In: H. Kalter, ed. *Issues and Reviews in Teratology, Vol. 2.* New York: Plenum Press, 189-217.

Pratt, R. M. 1985. Receptor dependent mechanisms of glucocorticoid and dioxin-induced cleft palate. *Environ. Health Perspect.* 61:35-40.

Pratt, R. M., and R. L. Christiansen, eds. 1980. *Current Research Trends in Prenatal Craniofacial Development.* New York: Elsevier/North Holland Biomedical Press.

Pratt, R. M., and W. D. Willis. 1985. In vitro screening assay for teratogens using growth inhibition of human embryonic cells. *Proc. Natl. Acad. Sci.* 82:5791-5794.

Pratt, R. M., A. L. Wilk, E. A. Horigan, J. H. Greenberg, and G. R. Martin. 1980. Screening for teratogens in vitro. In: M. Melnick, D. Bixler, and E. D. Shields, eds. *Etiology of Cleft Lip and Cleft Palate.* New York: Alan R. Liss, Inc., 169-172.

Pratt, R. M., R. I. Grove, and W. D. Willis. 1982. Prescreening for environmental teratogens using cultured mesenchymal cells from the human embryonic palate. *Teratogenesis Carcinog. Mutagen.* 2:313-318.

Pratt, R. M., E. H. Goulding, and B. D. Abbott. 1987. Retinoic acid inhibits migration of cranial neural crest cells in the cultured mouse embryo. *J. Craniofacial Genet. Devel. Biol.* 7:205-217.

Prentice, R. L. 1986. Binary regression using an extended beta-binomial distribution, with discussion of correlation induced by co-variate measurement errors. *J. Am. Stat. Assoc.* 81:321-327.

Radulovic, L. L., J. J. LaFcrla, and A. P. Kulkarni. 1986. Human placental glutathione S-transferase mediated metabolism of methyl parathion. *Biochem. Pharmacol.* 35:3473-3480.

Radulovic, L. L., W. C. Dauterman, and A. P. Kulkarni. 1987. Biotransformation of methyl parathion by human fetal liver glutathione S-transferases: An in vitro study. *Xenobiotica* 17:105-114.

Rai, K., and J. Van Ryzin. 1985. A dose response for teratological experiments involving quantal responses. *Biometrics* 41:1-10.

Ramsey, E. M. 1982. *The placenta human and animal.* New York: Praeger Publishers, 7-56.

Randall, C. L., T. A. Burling, E. A. Lochry, and P. B. Sutker. 1982. The effect of paternal alcohol consumption on fetal development in mice. *Drug Alcohol Depend.* 9:89-95.

Rands, D. L., C. L. Newhouse, J. L. Stewart, and W. S. Bradshaw. 1982a. Indicators of developmental toxicity following prenatal administration of hormonally active compounds in the rat. II. Pattern of maternal weight gain. *Teratology* 25:45-51.

Rands, D. L., R. D. White, M. W. Carter, J. D. Allen, and W. S. Bradshaw. 1982b. Indicators of developmental toxicity following prenatal administration of hormonally active compounds in the rat. I. Gestational length. *Teratology* 25:37-43.

Ranganathan, S., D. G. Davis, and R. D. Hood. 1987. Developmental toxicity of ethanol in Drosophila melanogaster. *Teratology* 36:45-49.

Rao, M. C., and G. Gibori. 1987. Corpus luteum: Animal models of possible relevance to reproductive toxicology. *Reprod. Toxicol.* 1:61-69.

Rao, R. S., B. A. Schwetz, and C. N. Park. 1981. Reproductive toxicity risk assessment of chemicals. *Vet. Hum. Toxicol.* 23:167-175.

Raub, J. A., R. R. Mercer, and R. J. Kavlock. 1983. Effects of prenatal nitrogen exposure on postnatal lung function in the rat. In: R. J. Kavlock and C. T. Grabowski, eds. *Abnormal Functional Development of the Heart Lungs, and Kidneys: Approaches to Functional Teratology.* New York: Alan R. Liss, Inc., 119-134.

Rawlings, S. J., D. E. G. Shuker, M. Webb, and N. A. Brown. 1985. The teratogenic potential of alkoxy acids in post implantation rat embryo culture: Structure-activity relationships. *Toxicol. Lett.* 128:49-58.

Reiners, J., W. Wittfoht, H. Nau, R. Vogel, B. Tenschert, and H. Spielmann. 1987. Teratogenesis and pharmacokinetics of cyclophosphamide after drug infusion as compared to injection in the mouse during day 10 of gestation. In: H. Nau and W. J. Scott, Jr., eds. *Pharmacokinetics in Teratogenesis, Vol. 2.* Boca Raton: CRC Press, Inc., 41-48.

Rice, J. M. 1973. An overview of transplacental chemical carcinogenesis. *Teratology* 8:113-125.

Rice, J. M. 1976. Carcinogenesis: A late effect of irreversible toxic damage during development. *Environ. Health Perspect.* 18:133-139.

Rice, J. M. 1979. Perinatal period and pregnancy: Intervals of high risks for chemical carcinogens. *Environ. Health Perspect.* 29:23-27.

Rice, J. M. 1981. Prenatal susceptibility to carcinogenesis by xenobiotic substances including vinyl chloride. *Environ. Health Perspect.* 41:179-188.

Ritter, E. J. 1977. Altered biosynthesis. In: J. G. Wilson and F. C. Fraser, eds. *Handbook of Teratology, Vol. 2. Mechanisms of Pathogenesis.* New York: Plenum Press, 89-116.

Ritter, E. J. 1984. Potentiation of teratogenesis. *Fundam. Appl. Toxicol.* 4:352-359.

Robertson, D., J. Frohlich, K. Carr, T. Watson, J. Hollifield, D. Shand, and J. Oates. 1978. Effects of caffeine on plasma renin activity, catecholamines and blood pressure. *N. Engl. J. Med.* 298:181-186.

Rogan, W. J., B. C. Gladen, K.-L. Hung, S.-L. Koong, L.-Y. Shih, J. S. Taylor, Y.-C. Wu, D. Yang, N. B. Ragan, and C.-C. Hsu. 1988. Congenital poisoning by polychlorinated biphenyls and their contaminants in Taiwan. *Science* 241:334-336.

Roger, J. C., D. G. Upshall, and J. E. Casida. 1969. Structure-activity and metabolism studies on organophosphate teratogens and their alleviating agents in developing hen eggs with special emphasis on bidrin. *Biochem. Pharmacol.* 18:373-392.

Rogers, J. M. 1987. Comparison of maternal and fetal toxic dose responses in mammals. *Teratogenesis Carcinog. Mutagen.* 7:297-306.

Rosenkrantz, J. G., F. P. Lynch, and W. W. Frost. 1970. Congenital anomalies in the pig: Teratogenic effects of trypan blue. *J. Ped. Surg.* 5:232-237.

Rosenzweig, S., and F. M. Blaustein. 1970. Cleft palate in A/J mice resulting from restraint and deprivation of food and water. *Teratology* 3:47-52.

Ross, R. H. 1985. Teratogenicity. In: M. G. Ryon and D. S. Sawhney, eds. *Scientific Rationale for the Selection of Toxicity Testing Methods. II. Teratology, Immunotoxicology, and Inhalation Toxicology.* Washington, DC: Office of Toxic Substances, U.S. Environmental Protection Agency, 9-67.

Rossi, L., O. Barbieri, M. Sanguinetti, A. Staccione, L. F. Santi, and L. Santi. 1983. Carcinogenic activity of benzo[a]pyrene and some of its synthetic derivatives by direct injection into the mouse fetus. *Carcinogenesis* 4:153-156.

Rugh, R., and E. Grupp. 1959. Exencephalia following x-irradiation of the pre-implantation mammalian embryo. *J. Neuropath. Exp. Neurol.* 18:468-481.

Russell, L. B. 1950. X-ray induced developmental abnormalities in the mouse and their use in the analysis of embryological patterns. I. External and gross visceral changes. *J. Exp. Zool.* 114:545-602.

Russell, L. B. 1956. X-ray induced developmental abnormalities in the mouse and their use in the analysis of embryological patterns. II. Abnormalities of the vertebral column and thorax. *J. Exp. Zool.* 131:329-390.

Russell, L. B., and C. S. Montgomery. 1966. Radiation-sensitivity differences within cell-division cycles during mouse cleavage. *Int. J. Radiat. Biol.* 10:151-164.

Russell, L. B., and K. F. Stelzner. 1988. High frequency of mosaic mutants from ENU treatment of mouse zygotes. *Environ. Mol. Mutagen.* 11:90.

Rustia, M., and P. Shubik. 1979. Effects of transplacental exposure to diethylstilbestrol on carcinogenic susceptibility during postnatal life in hamster progeny. *Cancer Res.* 39:4636-4644.

Rutledge, J. C., and W. M. Generoso. 1989. The fetal pathology produced by ethylene oxide treatment of the murine zygote. *Teratology* 39:563-572.

Sabourin, T. D., R. T. Faulk, and L. B. Goss. 1985. The efficacy of three non-mammalian test systems in the identification of chemical teratogens. *J. Appl. Toxicol.* 5:227-233.

Sadler, T. W. 1985. The role of mammalian embryo culture in developmental biology and teratology. In: H. Kalter, ed. *Issues and Reviews in Teratology, Vol. 3*. New York: Plenum Press, 273-294.

Sadler, T. W., and C. W. Warner. 1984. Use of whole embryo culture for evaluating toxicity and teratogenicity. *Pharmacol. Rev.* 36:1455-1505.

Sadler, T. W., W. E. Horton, and C. W. Warner. 1982. Whole embryo culture: A screening technique for teratogens? *Teratogenesis Carcinog. Mutagen.* 2:243-253.

Sadler, T. W., L. Shum, C. W. Warner, and M. Kate Smith. 1988. The role of pharmacokinetics in determining the response of rodent embryos to teratogens in whole-embryo culture. *Toxic. in Vitro* 2:175-180.

Salomon, D. S. 1983. Hormone receptors and malformations. In: E. M. Johnson, and D. M. Kochhar, eds. *Teratogenesis and Reproductive Toxicology*. East Berlin: Springer-Verlag, 113-134.

Saxen, L. 1977. Abnormal cellular and tissue interactions. In: J. G. Wilson and F. C. Fraser, eds. *Handbook of Teratology, Vol. 2. Mechanisms and Pathogenesis*. New York: Plenum Press, 171-197.

Saxen, L. 1979. In vitro model systems for chemical teratogenesis. In: A. Kolber, T. K. Wang, L. D. Grant, R. S. DeWoskin, and T. J. Hughes, eds. *In Vitro Toxicity Testing of Environmental Agents, Part B*. New York: Plenum Publishing Co., 173-190.

Saxen, L. 1983. Twenty years of study of the etiology of congenital malformations in Finland. In: H. Kalter, ed. *Issues and Reviews in Teratology, Vol. 1*. New York: Plenum Publishing Co., 73-110.

Saxen L. 1985. Prediction and detection of teratogenicity. In: K. Hemminki, M. Sorsa, and H. Vainio, eds. *Occupational Hazards and Reproduction*. New York: Hemisphere Publishing Corp., 189-199.

Schardein, J. L. 1976a. Evaluation of teratogenicity and other effects. In: J. L. Schardein, ed. *Drugs as Teratogens*. Cleveland: CRC Press, Inc., 35-48.

Schardein, J. L. 1976b. Principles for testing teratogenic effects in animals. In: J. L. Schardein, ed. *Drugs as Teratogens*. Cleveland: CRC Press, Inc., 9-33.

Schardein, J. L. 1983. Teratogenic risk assessment: Past, present, and future. In: H. Kalter, ed. *Issues and Reviews in Teratology, Vol. 1*. New York: Plenum Press, 181-214.

Schardein, J. L. 1985. *Chemically Induced Birth Defects*. New York: Marcel Dekker.

Schardein, J. L. 1987. Approaches to defining the relationship of maternal and developmental toxicity. *Teratogenesis Carcinog. Mutagen.* 7:255-271.

Schardein, J. L., B. A. Schwetz, and M. F. Kenel. 1985. Species sensitivities and prediction of teratogenic potential. *Environ. Health Perspect.* 61:55-67.

Schmid, B. 1987. Old and new concepts in teratogenicity testing. *Trends Pharmacol. Sci.* 8:133-137.

Schmidt, R. R. 1984. Altered development of immunocompetence following prenatal or combined prenatal-postnatal insult: A timely review. *J. Am. Coll. Toxicol.* 3:57-72.

Schmidt, R. R., and P. K. Abbott. 1983. Altered postnatal mitogenic responsiveness of adult rat splenic lymphocytes following in utero exposure to corn oil. *Teratology* 27:411-416.

Schneider, H., M. Panigel, and J. Dancis. 1972. Transfer across the perfused human placenta of antipyrine, sodium, and leucine. *Am. J. Obstet. Gynecol.* 114:822-828.

Schuler, R. L., B. D. Hardin, and R. W. Niemeier. 1982. Drosophila as a tool for the rapid assessment of chemicals for teratogenicity. *Teratogenesis Carcinog. Mutagen.* 2:293-301.

Schuler, R. L., B. D. Hardin, R. W. Niemeier, G. Booth, K. Hazelden, V. Piccirillo, and K. Smith. 1984. Results of testing fifteen glycol ethers in a short-term in vivo reproductive toxicity assay. *Environ. Health Perspect.* 57:141-146.

Schuler, R. L., M. A. Radike, B. D. Hardin, and R. W. Niemeier. 1985. Pattern of response of intact Drosophila to known teratogens. *J. Am. Coll. Toxicol.* 4:291-303.

Schumacher, H. J., J. G. Wilson, and R. L. Jordan. 1969. Potentiation of the teratogenic effects of 5-fluorouracil by natural pyrimidines. II. Biochemical aspects. *Teratology* 1:99-105.

Schwetz, B. A., and M. P. Moorman. 1987. Assessment of adult toxicity in developmental versus prechronic toxicology studies. *Teratogenesis Carcinog. Mutagen.* 7:211-223.

Schwetz, B. A., R. W. Tyl, et al. 1987. Consensus workshop on the evaluation of maternal and developmental toxicity. Work Group III report: Low dose extrapolation and other considerations for risk assessment-models and applications. *Teratogenesis Carcinog. Mutagen.* 7:321-327.

Scott, Jr., W. J. 1977. Cell death and reduced proliferative rate. In: J. G. Wilson and F. C. Fraser, eds. *Handbook of Teratology, Vol. 2. Mechanisms and Pathogenesis.* New York: Plenum Press, 81-98.

Scott, Jr., W. J., and H. Nau. 1987. Accumulation of weak acids in the young mammalian embryo. In: H. Nau and W. J. Scott, Jr., eds. *Pharmacokinetics in Teratogenesis, Vol. 1.* Boca Raton: CRC Press, Inc., 71-77.

Searle, S. R. 1971. Linear Models. New York: John Wiley and Sons.

Second Task Force for Research Training in Environmental Health Science. 1977. *Human Health and the Environment — Some Research Needs.* DHEW Publication No. NIH 77-1277. Washington, DC: U.S. Government Printing Office, 319, 322.

Seidenberg, J. M., and R. A. Becker. 1987. A summary of the results of 55 chemicals screened for developmental toxicity in mice. *Teratogenesis Carcinog. Mutagen.* 7:17-28.

Seidenberg, J. M., D. G. Anderson, and R. A. Becker. 1986. Validation of an in vivo developmental toxicity screen in the mouse. *Teratogenesis Carcinog. Mutagen.* 6:361-374.

Selevan, S. G., K. Hemminki, and M. L. Lindbohm. 1986. Linking data to study reproductive effects of occupational exposures. In: Z. A. Stein and M. C. Hatch, eds. *Reproductive Problems in the Workplace.* Philadelphia: Hanley and Belfus, 445-455.

Seller, M. J., K. J. Perkins, and M. Adinolfi. 1983. Differential response of heterozygous curly-tail mouse embryos to vitamin A teratogenesis depending on maternal genotype. *Teratology* 28:123-129.

Sharma, R. K., D. Jacobson-Kram, M. Lemmon, J. Bakke, I. Galperin, and W. F. Blazak. 1985. Sister-chromatid exchange and cell replication kinetics in fetal and maternal cells after treatment with chemical teratogens. *Mutat. Res.* 158:217-231.

Shepard, T. H., A. G. Fantel, P. E. Mirkes, J. C. Greenaway, E. Faustman-Watts, M. Campbell, and M. R. Juchau. 1983. Teratology testing: I. Development and status of short term prescreens. II. Biotransformation of teratogens as studied in whole embryo culture. In: S. M. MacLeod, A. B. Okey, and S. P. Spielberg, eds. *Developmental Pharmacology.* New York: Alan R. Liss, Inc., 147-164.

Shirley, E. A. C., and R. Hickling. 1981. An evaluation of some statistical methods for analysing numbers of abnomalities found amongst litters in teratology studies. *Biometrics* 37:819-829.

Shull, G. E. 1984. Differential inhibition of protein synthesis: A possible biochemical mechanism of thalidomide teratogenesis. *J. Theor. Biol.* 110:461-486.

Shum, S., N. M. Jensen, and D. W. Nebert. 1979. The murine Ah locus: In vitro toxicity and teratogenesis associated with genetic differences in benzo[a]pyrene metabolism. *Teratology* 20:365-376.

Simmons, D. L., D. M. Valentine, and W. S. Bradshaw. 1984. Different patterns of developmental toxicity in the rat following prenatal administration of structurally diverse chemicals. *J. Toxicol. Environ. Health* 14:121-136.

Singh, J., and R. D. Hood. 1985. Maternal protein deprivation enhances the teratogenicity of ochratoxin A in mice. *Teratology* 32:381-388.

Singh, J., and R. D. Hood. 1986. Effects of protein deficiency on the teratogenicity of cytochalasins in mice. *Teratology* 35:87-93.

Skalko, R. G. 1981. Biochemical mechanisms in developmental toxicology. In: C. A. Kimmel and J. Buelke-Sam, eds. *Developmental Toxicology.* New York: Raven Press, 1-11.

Skalko, R. G. 1985a. Cellular mechanisms in teratogenesis. In: T. V. N. Persaud, A. E. Chudley, and R. G. Skalko, eds. *Basic Concepts in Teratology.* New York: Alan R. Liss, Inc., 103-118.

Skalko, R. G. 1985b. Chemical interactions in teratogenesis. In: T. V. N. Persaud, A. E. Chudley, and R. G. Skalko, eds. *Basic Concepts in Teratology.* New York: Alan R. Liss, Inc., 119-129.

Skalko, R. G., and T. E. Kwasigroch. 1983. The interaction of chemicals during pregnancy: An update. *Biol. Res. Preg. Perinatal.* 4:26-35.

Skalko, R. G., S. M. Tucci, P. A. Eretto, and F. Schoen. 1978. 5-Bromodeoxyuridine teratogenesis in the mouse: Modulation by hydroxyurea. In: D. Neubert, H.-J. Merker, H. Nau, and J. Langman, eds. *Role of Pharmaco-kinetics in Prenatal and Perinatal Toxicology.* Stuttgart: George Thieme Publishers, 549-573.

Skalko, R. G., E. M. Johnson, et al. 1987. Consensus workshop on the evaluation of maternal and developmental toxicity. Work Group I report: End points of maternal and developmental toxicity. *Teratogenesis Carcinog. Mutagen.* 7:307-310.

Sleet, R. B., and K. Brendel. 1983. Brine shrimp, Artemia salina: A potential screening organism for initial teratology screening. *Proc. West. Pharmacol. Soc.* 26:169-170.

Sleet, R. B., and K. Brendel. 1985. Homogeneous populations of Artemia nauplii and their potential use for in vitro testing in developmental toxicology. *Teratogenesis Carcinog. Mutagen.* 5:41-54.

Slikker, Jr., W. 1987. Disposition of selected naturally occurring and synthetic steroids in the pregnant rhesus monkey. In: H. Nau and W. J. Scott, Jr., eds. *Pharmacokinetics in Teratogenesis, Vol. 1.* Boca Raton: CRC Press, Inc., 149-176.

Slikker, Jr., W., J. R. Bailey, G. D. Newport, G. W. Lipe, and D. E. Hill. 1982. Placental transfer and metabolism of 17a-Ethynylestradiol-17b and Estradiol-17b in the Rhesus monkey. *J. Pharm. Exper. Thera.* 223:483-489.

Slotkin, T. A. 1983. The cardiac-sympathetic axis as a teratological model. In: R. J. Kavlock and C. T. Grabowski, eds. *Abnormal Functional Development of the Heart, Lungs, and Kidneys: Approaches to Functional Teratology.* New York: Alan R. Liss, Inc., 237-248.

Smith, C. G. 1983. Reproductive toxicity: Hypothalamic-pituitary mechanisms. *Am. J. Ind. Med.* 4:107-112.

Smith, M. K., G. L. Kimmel, D. M. Kochhar, T. H. Shepard, S. D. Spielberg, and J. G. Wilson. 1983. A selection of candidate compounds for in vitro teratogenesis test validation. *Teratogenesis Carcinog. Mutagen.* 3:461-480.

Snell, K. 1983. In vitro reproductive toxicity studies. In: M. Balls, R. J. Riddell, and A. N. Worden, eds. *Animals and Alternatives in Toxicity Testing.* London: Academic Press, 207-213.

Snow, M. H. L. 1987. Uncoordinated development of embryonic tissue following cytoxic damage. In: F. Welsch, ed. *Approaches to Elucidate Mechanisms in Teratogenesis.* Washington, DC: Hemisphere Publishing Corp., 83-98.

Snow, M. H. L., and P. P. L. Tam. 1979. Is compensatory growth a complicating factor in mouse teratology? *Nature* 279:555-557.

Solt, D., and E. Farber. 1976. New principle for the analysis of chemical carcinogenesis. *Nature* 263:701-703.

Soyka, L. F., and J. M. Joffe. 1980. Male mediated drug effects on offspring. In: R. H. Schwarz and S. J. Yaffe, eds. *Drug and Chemical Risks to the Fetus and Newborn.* New York: Alan R. Liss, Inc., 49-66.

Soyka, L. F., J. M. Joffe, and S. M. Smith. 1980. Influence of concurrent testosterone on the effects of methadone on male rats and their progeny. *Devel. Pharmacol. Ther.* 1:182-188.

Spielberg, S. S. 1984. Pharmacogenetics and teratology. In: B. Krauer, ed. *Drugs and Pregnancy.* London: Academic Press, 85-93.

Spielberg, S.P. 1987. Phenytoin-induced birth defects: The role of pharmacogenetic differences in areneoxide detoxification. In: H. Nau and J. Scott, Jr., eds. *Pharmacokinetics in Teratogenesis, Vol. 1.* Boca Raton: CRC Press, Inc., 225-232.

Spielhoff, R., H. Breasch, M. Honig, and U. Mohr. 1974. Milk as transport agent for dimethylnitrosamine in Syrian golden hamsters. *J. Natl. Cancer Inst.* 53:281-282.

Spielmann, H. 1976. Embryo transfer technique and action of drugs on the preimplantation embryo. *Curr. Top. Pathol.* 62:87-103.

Spielmann, H., and R. Vogel. 1987. Transfer of drugs into the embryo before and during implantation. In: H. Nau and W. J. Scott, Jr., eds. *Pharmacokinetics in Teratogenesis, Vol. 1.* Boca Raton: CRC Press, Inc., 45-53.

Spielmann, H., H.-G. Eibs, and H.-J. Merker. 1977. Effects of cyclophosphamide treatment before implantation on the development of rat embryos after implantation. *J. Embryol. Exp. Morph.* 41:65-78.

Spielmann, H., H.-G. Eibs, and U. Jacob-Muller. 1979. Cyclophosphamide treatment prior to implantation: The effects on embryonic development. In: T. V. N. Persaud, ed. *Teratological Testing.* Lancaster, England: MTP Press, Ltd., 95-112.

Stadler, J., M.-J. Kessedjian, and J. Perraud. 1983. Use of the New Zealand white rabbit in teratology: Incidence of spontaneous and drug induced malformations. *Food Chem. Toxicol.* 21:631-636.

Staples, R. E. 1975. Potential of direct application techniques for detection of teratogens. In: D. Neubert and H. J. Merker, eds. *New Approaches to the Evaluation of Abnormal Embryonic Development.* Stuttgart: George Thieme Publishers, 71-81.

Staples, R. E. 1979. Teratology. *J. Assoc. Off. Anal. Chem.* 62:833-839.

Steele, C. E. 1985. The role of postimplantation mammalian embryo culture in the study of teratogenic mechanisms. In: M. Marois, ed. *Prevention of Physical and Mental Congenital Defects, Part C: Basic and Medical Science, Education and Future Strategies.* New York: Alan R. Liss, Inc., 271-276.

Steinberger, E., and J. A. Lloyd. 1985. Chemicals affecting the development of reproductive capacity. In: R. L. Dixon, ed. *Reproductive Toxicology.* New York: Raven Press, 1-20.

Stephens, T. D. 1988. Proposed mechanisms of action in thalidomide embryopathy. *Teratology* 38:229-239.

Stern, L. 1982. In vivo assessment of the teratogenic potential of drugs in man. *Devel. Pharmacol. Ther.* 4(Suppl. 1):10-18.

Sterz, H., G. Hebold, and G. Sponer. 1982. The induction of wavy ribs in fetuses by xenobiotics and its prevention. *Pharmacol. Toxicol. Veterin.* 8:273-276.

Sterz, H., G. Sponer, P. Neubert, and G. Hebold. 1985. A postulated mechanism of beta-sympathomimetic induction of rib and limb anomalies in rat fetuses. *Teratology* 31:401-412.

Stjernfeldt, M., J. Lindsten, K. Berglund, and J. Ludvigsson. 1986. Maternal smoking during pregnancy and risk of childhood cancer. *Lancet*, June 14: 1350-1352.

Stockard, C. R. 1913. The effect on the offspring of intoxicating the male parent and the transmission of the defects to subsequent generations. *Am. Nat.* 47:641-682.

Stowe, H. D., and R. A. Goyer. 1971. The reproductive ability and progeny of F_1 lead-toxic rats. *Fertil. Steril.* 22:755-760.

Stuckhardt, J. L., M. N. Brunden, and S. B. Harris. 1981. Influence of intrauterine position on fetal weight in Dutch belted rabbits. *J. Toxicol. Environ. Health* 8:777-786.

Swinyard, C. A. 1982. Concepts of multiple congenital contractures (arthro-gryposis) in man and animals. *Teratology* 25:247-258.

Tabacova, S., B. Nikiforov, and L. Balabaeva. 1983. Carbon disulphide intrauterine sensitization. *J. Appl. Toxicol.* 3:223-229.

Takeuchi, I. K. 1984. Teratogenic effects of methylnitrosourea on pregnant mice before implantation. *Experientia* 40:879-881.

Tanaka, H., N. Suzuki, and M. Arima. 1982. Experimental studies on the influence of male alcoholism on fetal development. *Brain Devel.* 4:1-6.

Teorell, T. 1937. Kinetics distribution of substances administered to the body. *Arch. Int. Pharmacodyn. Therap.* 57:205-240.

Teramoto, S., M. Kaneda, H. Aoyama, and Y. Shirasu. 1981. Correlation between the molecular structure of N-alkylureas and N-alkylthioureas and their teratogenic properties. *Teratology* 23:335-342.

Tesh, J. M., J. W. Ross, A. L. Pritchard, M. McIntyre, S. A. Tesh, and O. K. Wilby. 1982. MK-366: *Effects of oral administration upon pregnancy in the rat.* Life Science Research Report No. 82/MED009/253, Occold, Suffolk, England.

Tomatis, L., and U. Mohr, eds. 1973. *Transplacental Carcinogenesis. IARC Scientific Publications No. 4.* Lyon, France: International Agency for Research on Cancer.

Tomatis, L., J. R. P. Cabral, A. J. Likhachev, and V. Ponomarkov. 1981. Increased cancer incidence in the progeny of male rats exposed to ethylnitrosourea before mating. *Int. J. Cancer* 28:475-478.

Townsend, J. C., K. M. Bodner, P. F. D. VanPeenen, R. D. Olson, and R. R. Cook. 1982. Survey of reproductive events of wives of employees exposed to chlorinated dioxins. *Am. J. Epidemiol.* 115:695-713.

Trasler, D. G., D. Kemp, and T. A. Trasler. 1984. Increased susceptibility to 6-aminonicotinamide-induced cleft lip of heterozygote dancer mice. *Teratology* 29:101-104.

Trasler, J. M., B. F. Hales, and B. Robaire. 1985. Paternal cyclophosphamide treatment of rats causes fetal loss and malformations without affecting male fertility. *Nature* 316:144-146.

Trasler, J. M., B. F. Hales, and B. Robaire. 1986. Chronic low dose cyclophosphamide treatment of adult male rats: Effect on fertility, pregnancy outcome and progeny. *Biol. Reprod.* 34:275-283.

Trosko, J. E., C.-C. Chang, and M. Netzloff. 1982. The role of inhibited cell-cell communication in teratogenesis. *Teratogenesis Carcinog. Mutagen.* 2:31-45.

Tuchmann-Duplessis, H. 1972. Teratogenic drug screening. Present procedures and requirements. *Teratology* 5:271-285.

Tuchmann-Duplessis, H. 1977. Selection of animal species for teratological drug testing. In: D. Neubert, H.-J. Merker, and T. E. Kwasigroch, eds. *Methods in Prenatal Toxicology.* Stuttgart: George Thieme Publishers, 25-34.

Tuchmann-Duplessis, H. 1979. *Drug Effects on the Fetus. Monographs on Drugs, Vol. 2.* Sidney, Australia: ADIS Press.

Ugen, K. E., and W. J. Scott, Jr. 1986. Acetazolamide teratogenesis in Wistar rats: Potentiation and antagonism by adrenergic agents. *Teratology* 34:195-200.

Ullberg, S., L. Dencker, and B. Danielsson. 1982. The distribution of drugs and other agents in the fetus. In: K. Snell, ed. *Developmental Toxicology.* London: Croom-Helm, 123-163.

U.S. Congress, Office of Technology Assessment. 1985. *Reproductive Health Hazards in the Workplace.* Washington, DC: U.S. Government Printing Office.

U.S. Department of Health, Education and Welfare. 1966. *Guidelines for Reproduction Studies for Safety Evaluation of Drugs for Human Use.* Washington, DC: Food and Drug Administration.

U.S. Environmental Protection Agency. 1978. Proposed guidelines for registering pesticides in the United States; hazard evaluation: Humans and domestic animals. *Federal Register* 40:37336-37385.

U.S. Environmental Protection Agency. 1984. *Health Effects Test Guidelines.* Developmental Toxicity Study. Washington, DC: Office of Toxic Substances, Office of Pesticides and Toxic Substances.

U.S. Environmental Protection Agency. 1985. *Hazard Evaluation Division Standard Evaluation Procedure.* Teratology Studies. Washington, DC: Office of Pesticide Programs.

U.S. Environmental Protection Agency. 1986a. *Consensus Workshop on the Evaluation of Maternal and Developmental Toxicity.* Rockville, MD, May 12-14.

U.S. Environmental Protection Agency. 1986b. Guidelines for the health assessment of suspect developmental toxicants. *Federal Register* 51:34028-34040.

Urso, P., and N. Gengozian. 1980. Depressed humoral immunity and increased tumor incidence in mice following in utero exposure to benzo[a]pyrene. *J. Toxicol. Environ. Health* 6:569-576.

Uyeki, E. M., J. Doull, C. C. Cheng, and M. Misawa. 1982. Teratogenic and antiteratogenic effects of nicotinamide derivatives in chick embryos. *J. Toxicol. Environ. Health* 9:963-973.

Van Ryzin, J. 1975. Estimating the mean of a random binomial parameter with trial size random. *Sankhya, Series B* 37:10-27.

Van Ryzin, J. 1985. Risk assessment for fetal toxicity. *Toxicol. Indust. Health* 1:299-310.

Vianna, N., and A. Polan. 1984. Incidence of low birth weight among Love Canal residents. *Science* 226:1217-1219.

Vincres, S. A., and A. Koestner. 1982. Reduction of ethylnitrosurea-induced neoplastic proliferation in rat trigeminal nerves by nerve growth factor. *Cancer Res.* 42:1038-1040.

Vojnik, C., and L. S. Hurley. 1977. Abnormal prenatal lung development resulting from maternal zinc deficiency in rats. *J. Nutr.* 107:862-872.

Vogel, R., and H. Spielmann. 1986. Effects of methyl-nitroso-urea (MNU) after treatment during preimplantation period in the mouse. *Teratology* 34:422.

Vorhees, C. V. 1985a. Comparison of the collaborative behavioral teratology study and Cincinnati behavioral teratology test batteries. *Neurobehav. Toxicol. Teratol.* 7:624-625.

Vorhees, C. V. 1985b. Behavioral effects of prenatal d-amphetamine in rats: A parallel trial to the collaborative behavioral teratology study. *Neurobehav. Toxicol. Teratol.* 7:709-716.

Vorhees, C. V. 1985c. Behavioral effects of prenatal methylmercury in rats: A parallel trial to the collaborative behavioral teratology study. *Neurobehav. Toxicol. Teratol.* 7: 717-726.

Vorhees, C. V. 1986. Principles of behavioral teratology. In: E. P. Riley and C. V. Vorhees, eds. *Handbook of Behavioral Teratology*. New York: Plenum Press, 23-48.

Vorhees, C. V. 1987. Fetal hydantoin syndrome in rats: Dose-effect relationships of prenatal phenytoin on postnatal development and behavior. *Teratology* 35:287-303.

Vorhees, C. V., and R. E. Butcher. 1982. Behavioral teratogenicity. In: K. Snell, ed. *Developmental Toxicology*. New York: Praeger, 249-297.

Waddell, W. J., and G. C. Marlowe. 1976. Disposition of drugs in the fetus. In: B. L. Mirkin, ed. *Perinatal Pharmacology and Therapeutics*. New York: Academic Press, 119-268.

Waddell, W. J., and G. C. Marlowe. 1981. Biochemical regulation of the accessibility of teratogens to the developing embryo. In: M. R. Juchau, ed. *The Biochemical Basis of Chemical Teratogenesis*. North Holland: Elsevier, 1-62.

Wagner, J. G. 1979. *Fundamentals of Clinical Pharmacokinetics*. Hamilton, IL: Drug Intelligence Publications.

Walker, A. P. 1984. The work of OECD in the harmonization of the testing and control of chemicals. *Food Chem. Toxicol.* 22:905-908.

Walton, B. T. 1981. Chemical impurity produces extra compound eyes and heads in crickets. *Science* 3:51-53.

Walton, B. T. 1983. Use of the cricket embryo (Acheta domesticus) as an invertebrate teratology model. *Fundam. Appl. Toxicol.* 3:233-236.

Ward, I. L. 1984. The prenatal stress syndrome: Current status. *Psychoneuro-endocrinology* 9:3-11.

Ward, I. L., and J. Weisz. 1984. Differential effects of maternal stress on circulating levels of corticosterone, progesterone, and testosterone in male and female rate fetuses and their mothers. *Endocrinology* 114:1635-1644.

Ward, C. O., M. A. Barletta, and T. Kaye. 1970. Teratogenic effects of audiogenic stress in albino mice. *J. Pharmaceut. Sci.* 59:1661-1662.

Warner, C. W., T. W. Sadler, J. Shockey, and M. K. Smith. 1983. A comparison of the in vivo and in vitro response of mammalian embryos to a teratogenic insult. *Toxicology* 28:271-282.

Wassom, J. S. 1985. Use of selected toxicology information resources in assessing relationships between chemical structure and biological activity. *Environ. Health Perspect.* 61:287-294.

Watkinson, W. P., E. H. Hoke, D. A. Whitehouse, and E. H. Rogers. 1983. Electrocardiographic studies of developing rodents exposed in utero to trypan blue. In: R. J. Kavlock and C. T. Grabowski, eds. *Abnormal Functional Development of the Heart, Lungs, and Kidneys: Approaches to Functional Teratology.* New York: Alan R. Liss, Inc., 207-222.

Ways, S. C., P. B. Blair, H. A. Bern, and M. O. Staskawicz. 1980. Immune responsiveness of adult mice exposed neonatally to diethylstilbestrol, steroid hormones or vitamin A. *J. Environ. Pathol. Toxicol.* 3:207-220.

Weatherall, J. A. C., P. De Wals, and M. F. Lechat. 1984. Evaluation of information systems for the surveillance of congenital malformations. *Int. J. Epidemiol.* 13:193-196.

Weber, H., M. W. Harris, J. K. Haseman, and L. S. Birnbaum. 1985. Teratogenic potency of TCDD, TCDF and TCDD-TCDF combinations in C57BL/6N mice. *Toxicol. Lett.* 26:159-167.

Wechman, R., M. Braun, and F. Hilton. 1985. Intrauterine position affects sex-accessory biochemistry in adult female mice. *Biol. Reprod.* 33:803-807.

Weller, C. V. 1915. The blastophthoric effect of chronic lead poisoning. *J. Med. Res.* 33:271-293.

Welsch, F. 1988. Status and critical evaluation of short term in vivo and in vitro methods to assess developmental toxicity hazard. In: H. Kalter, ed. *Issues and Reviews in Teratology.* New York: Plenum Press.

Welsch, F., and D. B. Stedman. 1984. Inhibition of metabolic cooperation between Chinese hamster V79 cells by structurally diverse teratogens. *Teratogenesis Carcinog. Mutagen.* 4:285-301.

Welsh, J. J. 1987. Teratological research using in vitro systems. IV. Cells in culture. *Environ. Health Perspect.* 72:225-235.

Wendler, D. 1980. The state and future requirements of teratogenic testing. *Arch. Toxicol. Suppl.* 4:274-283.

Whitby, K. E. 1987. Teratological research using in vitro systems. III. Embryonic organs in culture. *Environ. Health Perspect.* 72:221-223.

White, C. G., J. F. Holson, and J. F. Young. 1981. *Extrapolation models in teratogenesis.* Final Report for Experiment #281. Jefferson, AR: National Center for Toxicological Research.

Wickramaratne, G. A. de S. 1987. The Chernoff-Kavlock assay: Its validation and application in rats. *Teratogenesis Carcinog. Mutagen.* 7:73-83.

Wickramaratne, G. A. de S. 1988. The post-natal fate of supernumerary ribs in rat teratogenicity studies. *J. Appl. Toxicol.* 8:91-94.

Wide, M. 1985. Lead exposure on critical days of fetal life affects fertility in the female mouse. *Teratology* 32:375-380.

Wiebe, J. P., K. T. Barr, and K. D. Buckingham. 1982. Lead administration during pregnancy and lactation affects steroidogenesis and hormone receptors in testes of offspring. *J. Toxicol. Environ. Health* 10:653-666.

Wier, P. J., S. C. Lewis, and K. A. Traul. 1987. A comparison of developmental toxicity evident at term to postnatal growth and survival using ethylene glycol monoethyl ether, ethylene glycol monobutyl ether and ethanol. *Teratogenesis Carcinog. Mutagen.* 7:55-64.

Willhite, C. C. 1986. Structure-activity relationships of retinoids in developmental toxicology. II. Influence of the polyene chain of the vitamin A molecule. *Toxicol. Appl. Pharmacol.* 83:563-575.

Willhite, C. C., M. I. Dawson, and K. J. Williams. 1984. Structure-activity relationships of retinoids in developmental toxicology. I. Studies on the nature of the polar terminus of the vitamin A molecule. *Toxicol. Appl. Pharmacol.* 74:397-410.

Williams, D. A. 1975. The analysis of binary responses from toxicological experiments involving reproduction and teratogenicity. *Biometrics* 31:949-952.

Williams, K. E. 1982. Biochemical mechanisms of teratogenesis. In: K. Snell, ed. *Developmental Toxicology.* New York: Praeger, 94-121.

Williams, B. J., and M. E. Abreu. 1983. Cardiotoxicity of perinatal lead exposure. In: R. J. Kavlock and C. T. Grabowski, eds. *Abnormal Functional Development of the Heart, Lungs, and Kidneys: Approaches to Functional Teratology.* New York: Alan R. Liss, Inc., 223-235.

Williams, K. E., G. Roberts, M. E. Kidston, F. Beck, and J. B. Lloyd. 1976. Inhibition of pinocytosis in rat yolk sac by trypan blue. *Teratology* 14:343-354.

Wilson, J. G. 1964. Teratogenic interaction of chemical agents in the rat. *J. Pharmacol. Exp. Ther.* 144:429-436.

Wilson, J. G. 1973. *Environment and Birth Defects.* New York: Academic Press.

Wilson, J. G. 1977a. Current status of teratology. In: J. G. Wilson and F. C. Fraser, eds. *Handbook of Teratology, Vol. 1. General Principles and Etiology.* New York: Plenum Press, 47-74.

Wilson, J. G. 1977b. Survey of in vitro systems: Their potential use in teratogenicity screening. In: J. G. Wilson and F. C. Fraser, eds. *Handbook of Teratology, Vol. 4. Research Procedures and Data Analysis.* New York: Plenum Press, 135-153.

Wilson, J. G. 1977c. Feasibility and design of subhuman primate studies. In: J. G. Wilson and F. C. Fraser, eds. *Handbook of Teratology, Vol. 4. Research Procedures and Data Analysis.* New York: Plenum Press, 255-273.

Wilson, J. G. 1978. Review of in vitro systems with potential for use in teratogenicity screening. *J. Environ. Pathol. Toxicol.* 2:149-167.

Wilson, J. G., R. L. Jordan, and H. Schumaker. 1969. Potentiation of the teratogenic effects of 5-fluorouracil by natural pyrimidines. I. Biological aspects. *Teratology* 1:91-97.

Winick, M. 1983. Nutrition, intrauterine growth retardation and the placenta. *Trophoblast. Res.* 1:7-14.

Winter, C., T. Shen, D. Tocco, R. Robertson, and R. Shackleford. 1981. Diflunisal. In: M. Goldberg, ed. *Pharmacological and Biochemical Properties of Drug Substances, Vol. 3.* Washington, DC: American Pharmaceutical Association, 291-323.

Wise, L. D., and W. J. Scott. 1982. Incorporation of 5-bromo-2'-deoxyuridine into mesenchymal limb-bud cells destined to die: Relationship to polydactyly induction in rats. *J. Embryol. Exp. Morph.* 72:125-141.

Witorsch, R. J. 1986. Use of gonadotropic hormones and sex steroids in assessing male reproduction. *J. Am. Coll. Toxicol.* 5:235-247.

Wolkowski-Tyl, R. 1981. Reproductive and teratogenic effects: No more thalidomides? In: S. K. Bandal, G. J. Marco, L. Golberg, and M. L. Leng, eds. *The Pesticide Chemist and Modern Toxicology.* Washington, DC: American Chemical Society, 115-155.

Woo, Y.-T. 1983. Carcinogenicity, mutagenicity and teratogenicity of carbamates, thiocarbamates and related compounds: An overview of structure-activity relationships and environmental concerns. *J. Environ. Sci. Health.* Cl:97-133.

Woo, D. C., and R. M. Hoar. 1972. "Apparent hydronephrosis" as a normal aspect of renal development in late gestation of rats: The effect of methyl salicylate. *Teratology* 6:191-196.

World Health Organization (WHO). 1967. *Scientific Group on Principles for the Testing of Drugs for Teratogenicity. World Health Organization Technical Report Series 364.* Geneva: World Health Organization, 7.

World Health Organization (WHO). 1984. Principles for evaluating health risks to progeny associated with exposure to chemicals during pregnancy. In: *Environmental Health Criteria*. Geneva: World Health Organization.

Wyrobek, A. J., G. Watchmaker, and L. Gordon. 1984. An evaluation of sperm tests as indicators of germ-cell damage in men exposed to chemical or physical agents. In: J. E. Lockey, G. K. Lemasters, and W. R. Keye, Jr., eds. *Reproduction: The New Frontier in Occupational and Environmental Health Research*. New York: Alan R. Liss, Inc., 385-405.

Yamada, K. M. 1977. Cell morphogenetic movements. In: J. G. Wilson and F. C. Fraser, eds. *Handbook of Teratology, Vol. 2. Mechanisms and Pathogenesis*. New York: Plenum Press, 199-230.

Yanagimachi, R. 1984. Zona-free hamster eggs: Their use in assessing fertilizing capacity and examining chromosomes of human spermatozoa. *Gamete Res.* 10:187-232.

Yang, H.-Y. L., M. J. Namkung, and M. R. Juchau. 1988. Cytochrome P-450-dependent biotransformation of a series of phenoxazone ethers in the rat conceptus during early organogenesis: Evidence for multiple P-450 isoenzymes. *Mol. Pharmacol.* 34:67-73.

Yoneda, T., and R. M. Pratt. 1981. Vitamin B6 reduces cortisone-induced cleft palate in the mouse. *Teratology* 26:255-258.

Young, J. F. 1983. Pharmacokinetic modeling and the teratologist. In: E. M. Johnson and D. M. Kochhar, eds. *Teratogenesis and Reproductive Toxicology*. East Berlin: Springer-Verlag. 7-29.

Young, J. F. 1987. Correlations of various pharmacokinetic parameters with endpoints in teratogencity testing. In: H. Nau and W. J. Scott, Jr., eds. *Pharmacokinetics in Teratogenesis, Vol. 2*. Boca Raton: CRC Press, Inc., 49-59.

Zeindl, E., and K. Sperling. 1977. Chromosomal analysis of embryonic tissues. In: D. Neubert, H.-J. Merker, and T. E. Kwasigroch, eds. *Methods in Prenatal Toxicology*. Stuttgart: George Thieme Publishers, 290-302.

Zeman, F. J. 1968. Effects of maternal protein restriction on the kidney of the newborn young of rats. *J. Nutr.* 94:111-116.

Zeman, F. J. 1983. The effect of prenatal protein-calorie malnutrition on kidney development in the rat. In: R. J. Kavlock and C. T. Grabowski, eds. *Abnormal Functional Development of the Heart, Lungs, and Kidneys: Approaches to Functional Teratology*. New York: Alan R. Liss, Inc., 309-338.

Zenick, H., and E. D. Clegg. 1986. Issues in risk assessment in male reproductive toxicology. *J. Am. Coll. Toxicol.* 5:249-259.

Zenick, H., L. Hastings, M. Goldsmith, and R. J. Niewenhuis. 1982. Chronic cadmium exposure: Relation to male reproductive toxicity and subsequent fetal outcome. *J. Toxicol. Environ. Health* 9:377-387.

INDEX